Total Exposure Health

Environmental and Occupational Health Series

Series Editors:
LeeAnn Racz
Bioenvironmental Engineer, US Air Force, Hurlburt Field, Florida
Adedeji B. Badiru
Professor and Dean, Graduate School of Engineering and Management, AFIT, Ohio

Handbook of Respiratory Protection
Safeguarding Against Current and Emerging Hazards
LeeAnn Racz, Robert M. Eninger, and Dirk P. Yamamoto

Perfluoroalkyl Substances in the Environment
Theory, Practice, and Innovation
David M. Kempisty, Yun Xing, and LeeAnn Racz

Total Exposure Health
An Introduction
Kirk A. Phillips, Dirk P. Yamamoto, and LeeAnn Racz

More Books Forthcoming
More about this series can be found at: https://www.crcpress.com/Environmental-and-Occupational-Health-Series/book-series/CRCENVOCCHEASER

Total Exposure Health
An Introduction

Edited by
Kirk A. Phillips, Dirk P. Yamamoto, and
LeeAnn Racz

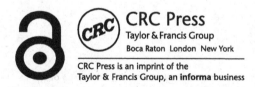

CRC Press
Taylor & Francis Group
Boca Raton London New York

CRC Press is an imprint of the
Taylor & Francis Group, an **informa** business

First edition published 2020
by CRC Press
6000 Broken Sound Parkway NW, Suite 300, Boca Raton, FL 33487-2742

and by CRC Press
2 Park Square, Milton Park, Abingdon, Oxon, OX14 4RN

ISBN: 978-0-367-20139-5 (hbk)
ISBN: 978-0-367-50541-7 (pbk)
ISBN: 978-0-429-26328-6 (ebk)

DOI: 10.1201/9780429263286

Typeset in Times
by codeMantra

The Open Access version of chapter 16 was funded by University of Utah.

Dedicated to the researchers, exposure scientists, environmental health specialists, and industrial hygienists striving to improve exposure assessments and the resulting care.

Contents

SECTION I Overview and Fundamentals

SECTION II Advances in Toxicology and the -Omics

SECTION III Bioethics

Foreword

Over the last several decades, a substantial amount of energy has been directed towards understanding human exposure to chemicals and the risks associated with those exposures. The primary approach to research on this subject has been to study a single chemical or chemical group (e.g., dioxins) at a time. In early risk assessment practices, more than one chemical would also be considered, but there was a relatively poor understanding of how to assess exposures and related potential risks to multiple chemicals. Further, the list of chemicals of concern was often centered on known site-specific chemicals or priority pollutants (126 chemicals out of the many thousands to which people may be exposed) or other similarly limited groups of chemicals. The exposure sciences community's understanding of chemical-outcome associations is often also inhibited by inadequate information on human behaviors that influence exposure over time, including dietary habits, pharmaceutical exposures, personal care product use, and employment and hobbies.

A complete picture of environmental exposures would involve obtaining data for all of one's exposures throughout their lifetimes, as well as the amount and routes of those exposures (chemical concentrations over time via dermal, inhalation, and oral exposures), and the variability in exposures (the exposome approach). However, due to resource, ethical, and technical constraints, we are faced with the fact that obtaining this kind of information completely is difficult at best and ultimately likely impossible.

Fortunately, various visionaries in the field of exposure science have pushed us all to think more comprehensively and creatively about how to do a better job of getting a more complete picture of human exposures and how to link those combined and varying exposures to potential adverse health outcomes. This book is focused on one of these boundary-pushing approaches—*Total Exposure Health*. As described by Kirk A. Phillips in Chapter 1, *Total Exposure Health* "aims to integrate and provide occupational, environmental, lifestyle and clinical exposure-related data from individuals to ensure that controls are established to protect health effectively." This ambitious vision will require interdisciplinary efforts among industrial hygienists, clinicians, computational toxicologists, molecular biologists, and geneticists.

This book describes key aspects of the interdisciplinary activities needed to move us, as the exposure scientists, closer to a more complete understanding of complex human exposures inside and outside of the workplace and to understand how those exposures along with the complexities of the human body relate to human health.

Judy S. LaKind, Ph.D.
President, LaKind Associates, LLC
Adjunct Associate Professor, University of Maryland School of Medicine
Past President, International Society of Exposure Science

Preface

You are about to read about an idea that, I believe, will help you understand that we are on the threshold of advancements in exposure collection which allows us to obtain data for far more people over greater portions of their lives. You will also learn about new discoveries of how exposures that cause disease at the genetic level can be discovered and prevented. As a practicing industrial hygienist and environmental engineer for 30 years, I have watched as advancements in science and the application of prevention strategies have resulted in significant improvement in the lives of workers and communities. Significant gains were achieved, but for many practices, only small incremental changes seem possible now. The great news is that a better understanding of the human body has now carried us as exposure scientists into the advancements of the Fourth Industrial Revolution. The full understanding of the genome and the differences in its expression among people is delivering the possibility of a healthier future as we apply this new information to precision health, ensuring exposures that are "acceptable" for most but harmful to the individual with a genetic proclivity are addressed.

"Was there a way for exposure science to use these knowledge bases to prevent, or at least reduce, disease for everyone, not just a worker in a factory or on a construction project?" I wondered. *Total Exposure Health* (TEH) was the term I coined for a framework that exposure scientists could use to capitalize on the advancements that were rapidly expanding our knowledge base.

Two major areas of improvement stood out as I worked to create this framework to collect information. The first was the development of technologies which promised to multiply our ability to get exposure data beyond the workplace at a lower cost and with less effort than traditional methods. The second was to use the developments in genetics which were identifying how differences in people resulted in different gene expressions to improve health.

The industrial hygienist and the environmental scientist needed to be able to more effectively utilize the rapidly expanding scientific discoveries. My vision was to find a way to deliver a better understanding of how the environment and the human body's reaction to it could be identified and used to give each of us better health. The framework for this information gathering and delivery I named *Total Exposure Health*.

This book allows readers to begin to share my vision of how lifestyle decisions can be made with a clearer understanding of what health issues might be prevented or reduced with more scientific information. Each chapter is designed to cover a discipline necessary to deliver TEH and is written by authors recognized as experts in their fields. We, the editors, are extremely grateful these scientists have chosen to share their expertise. You will receive an overview of how the TEH framework combines the expertise of industrial hygiene and other sciences to deliver true primary prevention.

My co-editors, whom I have worked with for over 20 years, were invaluable in delivering this book. Their encouragement to get TEH codified and their connections to other scientists ensure that this book will give the scientific community a better understanding of how exposures cause diseases at the genetic level and develop interventions to interrupt that process. It is my dream that TEH will allow those alive today to experience true primary prevention.

Acknowledgments

We gratefully acknowledge the many contributors to this book, who dedicated many hours to share their research findings and other ideas on *Total Exposure Health*.

Editors

Kirk A. Phillips is a Managing Principal at LJB, Inc., an engineering firm where he manages a third of the company as the practice leader for the Health, Safety and Environmental which provides risk assessments and engineering solutions externally for a wide range of clients in all markets to include many of the Fortune 100 and Fortune 500 companies. Prior to his current position, Kirk served in the Air Force as a Bioenvironmental Engineer for over 28 years and retired as a Colonel. For the last 8 years of his career, he served as a senior executive where he first developed the overarching environmental, safety and occupational health (ESOH) policy for the Air Force as the senior officer for ESOH in the Air Force Secretariat. He then worked for the Air Force Surgeon General, where he led the Bioenvironmental Engineering career field and directed a worldwide staff of 1,900 Industrial Hygienists, Engineers, Environmental Professionals, Health Physicists, Medical Architects and technicians to deliver the industrial hygiene and occupational and environmental health programs Air Force-wide. While at the Surgeon General's office, Kirk developed the *Total Exposure Health* (TEH) Framework and established it as a strategic objective of the Surgeon General. He was a Certified Industrial Hygienist from 1989 to 2009 when he became a full-time strategic thinker and manager in industrial hygiene. He has a BS in Aerospace Engineering from the University of Missouri (Rolla), an MS in Engineering and Environmental Management from the Air Force Institute of Technology (AFIT) (Ohio), and completed Air War College. Kirk is a member of the American Industrial Hygiene Association (AIHA), where he is the chair of the Total Worker Health Task Force Steering Committee and a member of the Actions Committee. He is also a member of the American Society of Safety Professionals, where he is a member of the Governmental Affairs Committee and the TWH Task Force. Kirk served as the provost for the Industrial Hygiene and Environmental Engineering MS Degrees at AFIT from 2014 to 2017. Kirk has been the keynote speaker at the Toxicology and Risk Assessment Conference, the AIHA Fall Conference on Leadership and Management, and the American Industrial Hygiene Conference and Exposition. Kirk speaks regularly on TEH and is a thought leader in the future of exposure science.

Dirk P. Yamamoto is a US Air Force civil service employee and a Senior Industrial Hygienist at the 711th Human Performance Wing/Airman Readiness Optimization Branch (711th HPW/RHMO) at Wright-Patterson Air Force Base, Dayton, OH. He leads a team of researchers focused on Toxicology and Risk Assessment and is the research lead for *Total Exposure Health*. He retired from military service as a Lieutenant Colonel, having served 23 years as both an Electronics Engineer and Bioenvironmental Engineer with the US Air Force. While on active duty, assignments included serving as an Assistant Professor of Industrial Hygiene and Director of the Graduate Industrial Hygiene Program at the Air Force Institute of Technology (AFIT) in Dayton, OH, along with other positions in Texas, Utah, California, and

North Dakota. He holds a BS in Electrical Engineering from the University of Minnesota, MS in Engineering Systems Management from St. Mary's University (TX), MS Public Health (Industrial Hygiene emphasis) from the University of Utah, and a PhD in Systems Engineering (Industrial Hygiene emphasis) from AFIT. He is a Certified Industrial Hygienist (CIH), Certified Safety Professional (CSP), and is licensed as a Professional Engineer (PE). He also volunteers for various American Industrial Hygiene Association (AIHA) committees and ABET, and served as the Chair for the Board for Global EHS Credentialing (formerly, the American Board of Industrial Hygiene—ABIH).

LeeAnn Racz is a Bioenvironmental Engineer in the US Air Force having served at bases across the globe. Previous assignments have also included Assistant Professor of Environmental Engineering and Director of the Graduate Environmental Engineering and Science Program in the Systems and Engineering Management at the Air Force Institute of Technology. She currently holds the rank of Lieutenant Colonel. She is a licensed professional engineer (PE), Certified Industrial Hygienist (CIH), and Board Certified Environmental Engineer (BCEE). She holds BS in Environmental Engineering from California Polytechnic State University (San Luis Obispo), MS in Biological and Agricultural Engineering from the University of Idaho, and a PhD in Civil and Environmental Engineering from the University of Utah. Her areas of interest include characterizing the fate of chemicals of emerging concern in the natural and engineered environments as well as environmental health issues. She has authored dozens of refereed journal articles, conference proceedings, magazine articles, presentations, and five handbooks. She is a member of several professional associations and honor societies and has received numerous prestigious teaching and research awards.

Contributors

Kim A. Anderson
Food Safety and Environmental
  Stewardship Program
Oregon State University
Corvallis, Oregon

Benjamin E. Berkman
Department of Bioethics
National Human Genome Research
  Institute
National Institutes of Health
Bethesda, Maryland

Christopher E. Bradburne
Asymmetric Operations Sector
Applied Physics Laboratory
and
Department of Genetic Medicine
School of Medicine
Johns Hopkins University
Laurel, Maryland

Sherrod Brown
U.S. Air Force
Airman Readiness Optimization
  Branch
711th Human Performance Wing
Wright-Patterson Air Force Base
Dayton, Ohio

L. Casey Chosewood
Office for Total Worker Health
National Institute for Occupational
  Safety and Health
Centers for Disease Control and
  Prevention
Atlanta, Georgia

Scott Collingwood
Department of Pediatrics
Center of Excellence for Exposure
  Health Informatics
University of Utah
Salt Lake City, Utah

Chia-Chia Chang
Centers for Disease Control and
  Prevention
National Institute for Occupational
  Safety and Health
Washington, District of Columbia

Yaroslav G. Chushak
Henry M. Jackson Foundation for the
  Advancement of Military Medicine
711th Human Performance Wing
Wright-Patterson Air Force Base
Dayton, Ohio

Mollie Cummins
Department of Biomedical Informatics
College of Nursing
Center for Clinical and Translational
  Science
Center of Excellence for Exposure
  Health Informatics
University of Utah
Salt Lake City, Utah

Holly M. Dixon
Food Safety and Environmental
  Stewardship Program
Oregon State University
Corvallis, Oregon

Julio C. Facelli
Department of Biomedical Informatics
Center for Clinical and Translational
  Science
Center of Excellence for Exposure
  Health Informatics
University of Utah
Salt Lake City, Utah

Celia B. Fisher
Department of Psychology
Fordham University
New York

Jeffery M. Gearhart
Henry M. Jackson Foundation for the
  Advancement of Military Medicine
711th Human Performance Wing
Wright-Patterson Air Force Base
Dayton, Ohio

Ashley Golden
Health, Energy and Environment
  Program
Oak Ridge Associated Universities
Oak Ridge, Tennessee

Kenneth W. Goodman
Institute for Bioethics and Health Policy
Miller School of Medicine
University of Miami
Miami, Florida

Ramkiran Gouripeddi
Department of Biomedical Informatics
Center for Clinical and Translational
  Science
Center of Excellence for Exposure
  Health Informatics
University of Utah
Salt Lake City, Utah

Richard Hartman
Independent Consultant
Alexandria, Virginia

Zachariah Hubbell
Health, Energy and Environment
  Program
Oak Ridge Associated Universities
Oak Ridge, Tennessee

Heidi Hudson
U.S. Public Health Service
National Institute for Occupational
  Safety and Health
Centers for Disease Control and
  Prevention
Cincinnati, Ohio

Sneha Kasera
School of Computing
Center of Excellence for Exposure
  Health Informatics
University of Utah
Salt Lake City, Utah

Judy S. LaKind
LaKind Associates, LLC
and
Department of Epidemiology and
  Public Health
University of Maryland School of
  Medicine
Baltimore, Maryland

and

International Society of Exposure
  Science
Herndon, Virginia

Deborah M. Layman
Department of Psychology
Fordham University
New York, New York

Philip Lundrigan
Department of Electrical and Computer
Engineering
Center of Excellence for Exposure
Health Informatics
Brigham Young University
Provo, Utah

Jeffrey R. Miller
Health, Energy and Environment
Program
Oak Ridge Associated Universities
Oak Ridge, Tennessee

Kevin Montgomery
CEO, IoT/AI Inc.
Fremont, California

Mark Oxley
Department of Mathematics and
Statistics
Air Force Institute of Technology
Wright-Patterson Air Force Base
Dayton, Ohio

Heather A. Pangburn
Department of Systems Biology
711th Human Performance Wing
Wright-Patterson Air Force Base
Dayton, Ohio

Kirk A. Phillips
LJB, Inc. Engineering
Washington, District of Columbia

Carolyn M. Poutasse
Food Safety and Environmental
Stewardship Program
Oregon State University
Corvallis, Oregon

LeeAnn Racz
1st Special Operations Operational
Medical Readiness Squadron
U.S. Air Force
Hurlburt Field, Florida

Roland Saldanha
Department of Genomics
711th Human Performance Wing
Wright-Patterson Air Force Base
Dayton, Ohio

N. Cody Schaal
Environmental Health Effects
Laboratory
Naval Medical Research Unit–Dayton
Wright-Patterson Air Force Base
Dayton, Ohio

and

Department of Preventive Medicine and
Biostatistics
F. Edward Hébert School of Medicine
Uniformed Services University
Bethesda, Maryland

Hannah W. Shows
Biological Sciences Department
Wright State University
Dayton, Ohio

Jeremy Slagley
Graduate Industrial Hygiene Program
Department of Systems Engineering
and Management
Air Force Institute of Technology
Wright-Patterson Air Force Base
Dayton, Ohio

Katherine Sward
Department of Biomedical Informatics
College of Nursing
Center for Clinical and Translational
Science
Center of Excellence for Exposure
Health Informatics
University of Utah
Salt Lake City, Utah

Sara L. Tamers
Office for Total Worker Health
National Institute for Occupational
    Safety and Health
Centers for Disease Control and
    Prevention
Atlanta, Georgia

Dirk P. Yamamoto
Airman Readiness Optimization
    Branch
711th Human Performance Wing
Wright-Patterson Air Force Base
Dayton, Ohio

Section I

Overview and Fundamentals

1 Total Exposure Health
An Exposure Science Framework for the Fourth Industrial Age

Kirk A. Phillips
LJB, Inc. Engineering

CONTENTS

DOI: 10.1201/9780429263286-2

1.1   ORIGINS OF TOTAL EXPOSURE HEALTH

Total Exposure Health (TEH) provides today's industrial hygienists (IHs), environmental health specialists (EHS), and safety professionals a framework to more effectively respond to the changing nature of the industrial work environment, the increased availability of technology to obtain exposure monitoring, and the ability of the human body to respond to internal and external exposures at the genetic and molecular biological response levels. TEH can, therefore, be thought of as the way for the exposure scientist to respond in a more effective way to society's desire for healthier life choices.

1.1.2   THE STEADFAST PRACTICE OF INDUSTRIAL HYGIENE

A review of the *Text-Book of Hygiene*, 3rd Ed (Rohé 1898), is an amazing trip through time from an occupational exposure standpoint. It is interesting to note that many of the tables and knowledge in the early edition were pre-American Civil War. So much was learned during the war because Sanitary Engineers, the term for IHs of the day, were embedded with the fighting forces, and revised editions were needed to incorporate significant increases in preventive health knowledge. What makes this textbook amazing today is that much of what is understood about exposures to workers and communities was also understood to some extent back then in each of the primary categories of chemical, physical, and biological agents (Rohé 1898). Chapter 5 of this volume by Yamamoto provides additional historical perspective on the development of the practice of IH.

Due to the limits of science in 1898, Rohé's work was qualitative not quantitative measurements. For example, coal miner's lung was described, and the essential elements of an exposure assessment (anticipation, recognition, evaluation, and control) were used. This early text concluded that the causes of the lung disease were the contaminants in the air along with increased time of exposure. It also carefully tabulated the life expectancy of each job type in the industry. Disease-causing organisms, such as bacteria, were just being understood, and their causes and effects were being debated in scientific communities. Nevertheless, the handbook described the symptoms of cholera, its connection to water, the need to observe spread in a population, and the need to change the water source. Similar descriptions of exposures to arsenic, noise, acids, ammonia, chlorine, mercury, lead, carbon monoxide, carbon disulfide, mineral wools, cotton dust, phosphorous, illness from heat, sedentary lifestyle, mechanical violence, and many more were all covered and applied to populations of people or essentially similar exposure groups (SEGs). Today, the application of IH and environmental health (EH) is significantly enhanced as scientists better understand the functions of organs and systems in the body, develop ways to quantitatively match exposures to observed effect levels, and then establish criteria to reduce or limit the negative effects. What has not changed is the use of population studies to determine the exposure level of concern. This stable application of IH and EH practices through many years led to the realization that TEH could be used to refine the science of IH and EH.

1.1.3 Exposures and Exposed Populations Are Decreasing

The second indicator that a new application of exposure science was needed was the changing nature of exposure from a quantification standpoint both in the levels of exposure and in the number of people being exposed. The nature of work in societies across the industrial world is changing rapidly as the industrial nature of work decreases for many workers (Sterling 2019). The reduction of exposures across the industrial workforce utilizes the full spectrum of the hierarchy of controls. Many manufacturing and heavy industry positions have been modified to decrease exposure to the worker using engineering controls, material substitutions, roboticization, and personal protective equipment (PPE). The result of these efforts is that the occupational and environmental health communities have been successful in identifying, measuring, and reducing exposures for significant portions of the workforce. Although it is true that significant numbers of workers are still being exposed to chemical, physical, and biological agents, the exposures have been reduced. Despite these reductions, IHs still desire to make a difference in the healthfulness of workers and to be able to demonstrate that they are being successful.

The challenge today is that many exposed populations under an IH's or EH's management have few exposures that exceed exposure limits; when exposures do exceed limits, there are controls that place the exposures within acceptable levels. Success, as defined today, is protecting a statistically significant portion of the population by using a standard established to protect the majority of the population. Those individuals who manifest a disease are often thought to be outside of the ability to be protected, or their disease is not considered to have been significantly caused by their exposures.

Over time, the trend will be for exposures of individuals to go lower and for the number of workers in jobs with exposure to continue to decrease (Postelnicu and Câlea 2019). Relevancy of the IH is bound to be questioned by many business owners and workplace supervisors. There will still be disease and the exposures will still have an impact on workers, but the overall cost to the business will decrease and make the job of the IH *seem* irrelevant.

1.1.4 Sensors Are (Almost) Ubiquitous

IHs, by definition, take care of exposures in the workplace, but to effectively protect workers, they must consider the environment outside of the workplace. A worker who plays in a rock band as a hobby or for a secondary income is not likely to have the requisite hours of quiet needed for recovery if he or she is exposed to noise at work, and alternative allowable exposure levels and intervals should be considered in determining his or her overall health. Other examples of outside of the work environment issues would be workers with hobbies like small engine repair or artists who use spray can paints or those whose hobbies use significant amounts of volatile organic chemicals. Such environments must have their exposures considered so that the combination of all exposures does not exceed a unity calculation for chemicals with similar metabolic mechanisms or organ targets. In these situations, IHs should inquire about these outside exposures, but many do not; if they do, they rely on generalized estimations of exposures of concern based on a narrative given by the worker.

A concerned person might ask, "Why not just send a sensor home with the worker to collect data on these exposures?" Often, the answer is that IHs who desire to collect data outside of the workplace have concerns with the legal implications of sampling outside the workplace and/or the instrumentation is too expensive and in limited quantities and there simply are not enough resources to gather data for periods of non-work. However, sensors are becoming smaller and cheaper to the point that individuals are buying them and using them in their everyday lives.

The fact that sensors are becoming cheaper and more available gives the IHs new tools that can be incorporated into their practices and obtained from the EH community to ensure exposures to individuals are accounted for regardless of location and time exposed. For a more in-depth discussion of this new possibility, refer to the chapters in the "Advances in Exposure Sciences" and "Bioethics" sections in this volume. The important aspects that led to the creation of TEH are the availability of the data under the IHs control and the data being collected through sensors owned by others.

1.1.5 EXPANDED KNOWLEDGE OF DISEASE, MECHANISMS OF DISEASE, AND GENETICS

Historically, exposure limits have been derived occasionally from actual human exposures when significant numbers of humans were being exposed to sufficient toxic levels. These exposures were not intentionally given in order to develop an exposure limit; they just occurred, and occupational health benefitted. Disease-producing agents, noise, asbestos, and lead are commonly understood to be in this category. However, it is difficult to get the exact data needed through human exposure due to the ethics of intentionally exposing a human.

The animal study has been the gold standard for exposure-based science, and toxicologists apply the science of exposure to these populations and then apply the observed exposure effects from an animal model to a human model. These studies look for significant changes that can alter cell viability or organ performance. This approach has been effective in the past and is the present source of many exposure limits. However, these studies document numerous limitations and introduce some fairly significant and potentially large safety factors. They all additionally have the limitation of applying to a population which cannot account for outlier members of the populations but instead provides protection for the majority.

Three professions are diligently working on a better understanding of the human body at the cellular level: computational toxicologists, molecular biologists, and geneticists. More will be discussed in this text, but for now, it is sufficient to understand that IHs and EHS have not, as a community, necessarily begun to see these science disciplines as partners in the exposure science community and valuable team members to achieve the goal of disease prevention among workers and non-workers.

1.2 AIMS OF TOTAL EXPOSURE HEALTH

True prevention will be achieved when all relevant exposures are measured and controlled, regardless of where they occur, and sensitive or genetically at-risk sub-populations are provided exposure limits that protect them. TEH provides the new framework to use the technological and medical advancements and apply them to the exposure science that IHs and EHS practice. There are no other professions specifically bringing these formerly disparate science professions together. IHs and EHS are in the ideal professions to bring the data from these disciplines together and apply them in practice. IHs already use the data from all these sciences to apply exposure limits to humans, and they serve a large percentage of the exposed population, the workers, regularly. With the risk to relevancy looming as fewer workers are exposed and fewer are exposed above exposure limits, it becomes increasingly important to provide exposure-based disease prevention to those individuals at risk due to increased sensitivity wherever exposed and whether or not they are workers.

1.3 THE TOTALS EXPLAINED

The terms Total, Worker, Exposure, and Health are often heard in various combinations: Total Worker Health® (TWH), Total Worker Exposure (TWE), and TEH are the three most interrelated and confused in the practice of IH today. Each of these totals has overlapping areas of concern which is the primary reason there is confusion. The key to describing the differences is to think of the population which is covered by the term, the exposures that are covered by the term and, finally, the preventive health practices which are incorporated into the definition.

1.3.1 TOTAL WORKER HEALTH®

Chapter 4 of this volume by Tamers et al. provides a comprehensive review of TWH and contains a figure that lists the issues relevant to TWH from the National Institute for Occupational Safety and Health (NIOSH) of the Centers for Disease Control and Prevention (CDC). NIOSH defines Total Worker Health® (TWH) as policies, programs, and practices that integrate protection from work-related safety and health hazards with promotion of injury and illness prevention efforts to advance worker well-being (NIOSH 2015). The most important consideration from an exposure standpoint is that TWH needs IHs and EHS who are participating in the process to define which exposures are included. The limitations imposed by TWH only

TABLE 1.1

Areas of Concern—TWH

Population	Worker
Health	Occupational and environmental health and primary care
Exposures	Workplace, environmental, and lifestyle (hobbies/home life)

require the exposures to impact workers. This then allows for and expects exposures that occur external to the workplace under the "Built Environmental Supports" and "Community Supports" categories, namely healthy community design, healthy housing, safe and clean environment, and quality healthcare. TWH does not specifically or separately categorize precision medicine, but under the quality healthcare category, the practice of medicine is increasingly adding precision health to medical care. Precision health, which includes genomic health, is also covered later in this volume in the "Advances in Toxicology" section, and the quickly expanding scientific fields identified as "-omics" are becoming increasingly important to the professional community seeking to provide quality healthcare. TWH does not cover non-workers in its definition but does cover psychosocial factors to provide flexible work arrangements such as working from home, work-life programs, housing, green spaces, productive aging, and health information privacy which are all significant parts of the non-work environment and have exposure aspects. See Table 1.1.

1.3.2 Total Worker Exposure (TWE)

Originally coined by the American Industrial Hygiene Association (AIHA; www.aiha.org), TWE was established as a content priority (i.e., focus area) of AIHA. There is not much formally written about TWE, but it is used in both the TWH and IH communities. TWE takes the classic at-work exposure concerns, which IHs have seen as part of the application of industrial hygiene, and adds the exposures to the worker primarily from the environment and from work not associated with the primary employer. See Table 1.2. In a TWE delivery model of IH, the IH professional takes special care to identify and include exposures that occur during the working day but not from the work itself (the at-work environment). Some examples of these types of exposures are personal smoking, chemical exposures from ambient air when there is infiltration from a waste plume under a slab at a workplace, airborne exposures from nearby industrial operations, radiation from natural sources such as the

TABLE 1.2

Areas of Concern—TWE

Population	Worker
Health	Occupational and environmental health applied to population exposure limits
Exposures	Workplace and environmental

sun and radon, ingestion exposures from water sources, and hand-to-mouth environmental contamination transfer. TWE also considers exposures that are received from multiemployer individuals who receive exposures from the multiple jobs they hold. TWE could include exposures in an alternative work environment such as a home office worker or a worker without an office such as a truck driver or a salesperson. For these workers, TWE attempts to capitalize on the increased availability (lower cost, ease of collections, etc.) of sensors to gain exposure data on these alternative work environments. Just as in TWH, it is important to understand what TWE does not specifically include. First, it does not include exposures from locations that are not at a workplace; therefore, it only covers the workforce but not other members of society. TWE gathers exposure data and then applies an exposure profile of all related work exposures to the standard exposure limits established using population-based statistics commonly referred to as occupational exposure limits (OELs).

1.3.3 TOTAL EXPOSURE HEALTH (TEH)

TEH considers exposure from four primary areas: Occupational, Environmental, Lifestyle, and Clinical (Figure 1.1). TEH does not limit its use to workers alone, although workers do comprise a significant portion of the population which benefits. IHs often find themselves applying their exposure collection and knowledge in environmental and community exposure positions and work closely with EHS. This is because the knowledge needed to be a good IH exposure scientist is nearly the

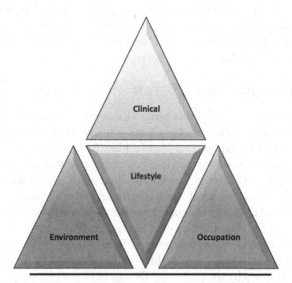

Total Exposure Health (TEH) Incorporates Environmental,
Workplace Lifestyle and Clinical Exposures Improving

"Health and Well Being"

FIGURE 1.1   Exposures relevant to TEH.

TABLE 1.3

Areas of Concern—TEH

Population	Workers and Non-workers
Health	Precision health
Exposures	Workplace, environmental, lifestyle (hobbies/home life), and clinical

same as being an environmental or community exposure scientist, e.g., EHS. The differences are in a few sampling methods and the way the laws treat the exposures from a regulatory standpoint. The TEH framework acknowledges this skill and envisions its use to combine the workplace environmental exposures and work exposures together for the worker (like in TWE). Likewise, IHs have the expertise to collect and assess exposures from the full environment, a person's lifestyles (at home and hobbies), and clinical exposures and adds these when at relevant levels to impact prevention of disease. TEH likewise addresses the need to capture exposures for the non-working population similar to how community health and EH communities apply exposure science to a community, but TEH then adds in exposures from lifestyle (home and hobby) and clinical testing and treatment (Table 1.3). Finally, TEH considers individual proclivity to disease when possible. Genetically, every human is different and has the potential to respond differently to an exposure. Present guidelines do not account for this genetic predisposition but instead use population-based limits to protect the majority population which potentially overprotect one population subset and underprotect another population subset. *TEH, therefore, of the three frameworks includes the greatest population set, the greatest exposure set and acknowledges and uses the latest medical understanding of individuality and precision medicine to deliver true primary prevention.*

1.4 TEH EXPOSURES OF CONCERN

It is a common misunderstanding that under TEH, every exposure *must* be identified. While this would certainly be the optimum, it is not possible. Total exposure, therefore, represents as many exposures as can be identified and have the potential to be relevant. Relevancy, as mentioned earlier, can be because they are additive to other exposures and this total must be considered. Relevancy also considers exposures which may be more concerning at low levels for an individual but not for a population overall. IHs and EHS already consider some of these relative exposures such as exposure concerns for breastfeeding mothers and mothers to be, individuals with compromised or reduced organ function (e.g., liver or lung), and/or individuals with a chemical hypersensitivity (e.g., formaldehyde or isocyanates). Relevant exposures not currently addressed by the practicing IH and EHS are genetic predisposition or proclivity to negative effects from an exposure.

The different exposures which can be part of the total may or may not be easily obtained and readily available. Those easy to obtain can, of course, still be used. For the exposures which are more difficult to obtain, new tools and techniques are being developed, and the IH and EHS communities need to recognize and be ready to use these new sources. Another chapter in this volume discusses silicone wristbands as just one example of a new tool available to gather exposures. These wristbands collect volatile organic chemicals at a low cost and deliver a simplified way to measure exposures at multiple time intervals. One interval can be selected as the workday, and another interval can record non-working hours and easily provide a total exposure for a large number of organic chemicals. The practicing IH and EHS may not readily imagine all the exposures which occur and should be considered in TEH. To begin to appreciate the expanded possibilities that are becoming available, each of the four primary exposure areas is now discussed in detail.

1.4.1 OCCUPATIONAL

TEH as a framework includes all the current IH exposure practices and uses the established exposure limits and associated regulatory standards. For more information, Chapter 5 by Yamamoto provides a comprehensive review of current IH exposure practices. TEH acknowledges and expects the use of regulated standards since there need to be guidelines employers can follow to know that the population of workers under their management are being taken care of to a recognized standard. Using recognized minimum standards for SEGs is still possible. However, with the desire to move toward more personalized medicine and with the increased ability to collect exposure data with smaller, cheaper, and more easily used sensors, the TEH framework that provides individual exposures is preferred. Exposures for at-home workers are not likely to be from their actual work processes, so these exposures would be captured under a different category. Exposures from work at a second employer may be available if the second employer has a quality IH program. Often the secondary forms of employment do not have this type of monitoring, and in these cases, these exposures are best handled as exposures based on lifestyle.

1.4.2 ENVIRONMENT

Environmental exposures occur all the time. An individual experiences environmental exposure simply by being present in a particular environment. Common environmental exposures are chemicals in drinking water, ambient air with the potential to have waste products or naturally occurring chemicals (PM10, PM2.5, ozone, mercury, etc.), solar radiation, and naturally occurring radioactive materials (radon). Less common environmental exposures can be infiltration of a living or working space's air from an underground chemical plume, pesticide, or fungicide overspray from farming operations, naturally occurring hazardous materials like asbestos deposits, heavy metal-laden soils (ingestion or inhalation), noise from nearby aircraft operations, traffic corridor and traffic congestion exposures, and many more. These exposures can be identified in several ways. The EHS in the EH community collects data on many exposures of concern, and these are documented and published. The IH can get this data from the internet easily and apply it to an individual. The specific quantification of exposure is not available through these data sources, but estimates are possible. If the exposure is relevant, then specific testing can be done to measure an individual's exposure.

1.4.3 LIFESTYLE

Lifestyle exposures include exposures that apply to people due to the specific aspects of their living situations and the hobbies or activities they choose. Many lifestyle exposures can approach exposure levels which would be experienced in an occupational setting. For example, some hobbies which have noise exposure in excess of the exposure limits are attending concerts, listening to music with headphones, playing an instrument, volunteering as a firefighter, going to a bar, and flying a private plane. Hobbies involving vehicles and engines such as engine repair, car racing, motorcycle riding, and car restoration can have noise and vibration issues. Artistic hobbies such as spray paint art which uses volatile organic compounds (VOCs), woodworking which generates dust and VOCs, and stained-glass art which can cause ingestion of lead from hand-to-mouth contact all can have exposures of concern.

Secondary jobs can have exposures of concern such as noise for bartenders and musicians, chemicals from farm jobs, and radiation and biological hazards in medical positions. Finally, exposures can be from lifestyle choices. Some examples of these types of exposures are noise and exhaust gases from a long and congested commute, noise from mowing a large yard or caring for a crying baby, gardening which increases exposure to solar radiation, usage of pesticides and herbicides, and maintenance of a household with potentially toxic chemicals. These exposures may or may not exceed an exposure limit on their own, but they definitely add to the overall daily exposure. An IH can be practicing TEH if he or she asks about these types of exposures and considers them when applying the exposure limits. The IH can go beyond present recognized exposure guidelines with more targeted questioning of individual choices, collect some exposure data to quantify the additional exposures, and consider the additional exposures when applying controls. The important thing is not to ignore these exposures as they can be significant.

1.4.4 CLINICAL

Clinical exposures are often completely ignored by practicing IHs. There are a number of reasons why this occurs. The first reason is privacy. Under the Health Insurance Portability and Accountability Act (HIPAA), medical information is private and releasable only when specific permission is given by the individual whom the information is about and there is a medical need. While there can be a medical need from an exposure standpoint, IHs are not connected well to the medical community other than through the occupational health function. While the health community has the needed information, it is reasonable for the IH to feel the wall of privacy prevents him or her from having any information. The second primary reason clinical exposures are ignored is that clinical testing to provide medical care is considered a fact-of-life and of limited duration and not taking place at work anyway. Therefore, under normal IH practice, a worker regularly monitored for ionizing radiation exposure receives a clinically necessary medical X-ray without any concern about the additive exposure.

Pharmaceuticals also represent a clinical exposure, and these are more likely to be longer term or ongoing. Pharmaceuticals, by their very design, are bioactive.

Drugs can impact the organ functions of the kidneys and liver which are key to detoxifying and eliminating chemicals that enter the body. There are hundreds of drugs with ototoxic properties that encompass nearly every drug class (Bisht and Bist 2011) and can be a cause of hearing loss beyond noise-induced hearing loss (NIHL). For these exposures, the IH community needs to work with the medical community to ensure that the standards being developed for innovative medicine, such as electronic health records, can integrate clinical and nonclinical exposures to inform the conversation between patient and provider and provide recommended practices to protect the patient.

The onset of pregnancy is a good example of a present integration where informed dialogue is beneficial; a provider tells a patient there are special actions that should be taken to protect the health of the baby. The patient now in TEH terms is a member of society who chooses to reduce personal exposures, such as limiting her alcohol intake, and has the option to inform her employer and ask for additional monitoring or altered work or additional protections to decrease the risks to the pregnancy.

1.5 TEH EXPOSURE DATA SOURCES

1.5.1 WORKPLACE IH

The practice of IH uses risk assessments and specialized surveys to collect, analyze, and apply exposure data to one individual or a group of individuals deemed to be an SEG. The resource cost of this sampling can be significant. The cost of time must be considered. Planning a sampling event, preparing instrumentation, collecting data and observing the work, and then posting the results of the sampling all take time. The second cost is the monetary cost; sampling equipment and the analysis costs can both be expensive. Because of these costs, limited numbers of samples are often collected.

The following is a practical example. A factory employs 200 workers located throughout its facility, and all have some variations in their exposure to noise. The IH office has two kits of five dosimeters for a total of ten. Noise changes from day to day as plant operations vary with daily production requirements, and a noise meter indicates levels above 85 decibels A-weighted routinely in the facility. Given this scenario, an IH would look for SEGs and would likely be sampling for many weeks and running from worker to worker documenting the work being done in a sample narrative. The lowest resource cost possible would consider the 100 workers a single SEG, and the IH would sample a minimum of ten workers for 3–10 workdays. The possibility that one SEG would adequately represent the exposures for all these workers would be highly unlikely, and for every increase in SEG, the cost in time increases. Adding more dosimeters to reduce time would be difficult due to their cost.

Under TEH, ideally, each worker not only would have his or her own exposure monitor, but when needed, exposures from non-work periods could also be measured. Obviously, new measurement methods are needed to make this possible. These methods are coming into the IHs sphere, and the next few sections will highlight examples of some of the current measurement methods. Later chapters in this volume will cover developments in low-cost, easy-to-use, and multi-analyte sensors to support more types of exposure monitoring and include each person individually.

1.5.2 Environmental and Community Health

The IH and EHS can collect some environmental exposure data in and around a traditional workplace to determine the exposure potential of the workplace apart from the operational or industrial exposures. The collection could be soil, dust, ambient air, and water samples. These samples would not represent personalized exposure data on their own; they would alert the IH to the possibility that personal sampling might be needed or that some other exposure management decisions might be necessary to reduce actual personal exposure. Much of this data is also available through monitoring and recordkeeping required under present environmental regulations. Particulate matter 10 (PM10) and PM2.5 with diameters that are generally 10 and 2.5 micrometers and smaller are collected regularly at the county and city levels (USEPA 2019) and chemical exposures through reporting under the Emergency Planning and Community Right-to-Know Act (EPCRA), specifically in sections 304 and 313. Section 304 primarily covers required reporting of hazardous substances from emergency releases. The greatest value for informing a user of TEH is the "Continuous Release Reporting" requirements where releases that are regular and ongoing are reported. Section 313 covers the Toxic Release Inventory (TRI), and facilities must report annually on more than 600 chemicals that are manufactured or used above a threshold quantity. This reporting includes how the material is released and is useful in knowing which chemicals may be present from releases in and around the population needing to have environmental exposures tabulated (USEPA 2018). The specific data files from 1987 through 2018 can be accessed at https://www.epa.gov/toxics-release-inventory-tri-program/tri-basic-data-files-calendar-years-1987-2018, and in these reports, the specific chemicals are listed with the address of the facility. The release information is sufficiently detailed to allow IHs to determine whether or not there could be some significant impact to the location or facility being evaluated by them (USEPA 2019).

Personalized sensors discussed in the next section have the advantage of being used by numerous users across an area. This data is being collected in many areas and can be available to use with the individual identification data removed, and the remaining information can be used to create exposure zones which are area environmental sensors. This can be especially advantageous in cities and towns where a small but significant portion of the community has chosen to use a sensor platform. Examples of these present usages of personalized sensors are air sampling devices provided to asthma patients for personalized air quality measurements (Patringenaru 2012) and the US Air Force study on noise monitoring (International 2017).

1.5.3 Personal Environmental Exposure Sensors
and the Internet of Things

Many exciting opportunities become available since the TEH framework allows the IH and EHS to use a host of sensors to obtain information. This volume has a chapter that provides a detailed overview of the sensor technologies that are emerging and the challenges that must be overcome to fully incorporate these sensors into healthy lifestyle practices. It is likely that workers are bringing their own sensors into the workplace and using them in their homes already, and the IHs can capitalize on these personally owned sensors to increase the amount of exposure data available to them.

Once methods are developed and standardized to meet established testing and accuracy, these personal sensors can be utilized for the collection of data which can become part of the official exposure record. In these cases, the personal sensors are often smaller and cheaper to employ than versions of the IH standard measurement equipment. Early types of sensors that fall into this lower cost and easy-to-employ class are passive monitors that rely on diffusion sampling. Newer and emerging technologies such as the silicone bands presented later in this volume take the diffusion sampler to the next level, increasing the number of analytes collected in a single sample significantly and reducing the cost to the sampler. They also reduce the time costs for the IH as they are very easy to employ, and the wearer can change to a new band at intervals which could be relevant such as work hours and non-work hours.

The advent of smart mobile devices has created other advantages that can be utilized by the IH and EHS. The personalized sensor can always be with the individual, provide real-time updates, and identify exposure location. The smart mobile device replaces the traditional monitor in every aspect except the sensor itself. This is possible because the mobile device serves as the processing power, contains the user interface, and has a custom-developed application available through the mobile device's application store. Amazingly, these high-tech devices even have some sensors onboard and can be used for measuring acceleration, vibration, or noise. Other sensors do require an add-on attachment which the IH or EHS must provide, but in effect, the individual being measured will have purchased the logic system portion of the hardware. The IH, EHS, or other occupational health professionals, such as a physician, can provide the sensor attachment, and with appropriate permissions and the application using data protection measures, personal data can arrive directly to the IH practice in real time. If the application has the ability to deliver data in real time, the IH will be able to identify when an event of significant exposure is occurring, notify the device user of the exposure, and, with input from the user, determine what activity triggered the exposure event. This greatly enhances the interpretation of the data for the IH and informs the person of specific activities and times which have a higher exposure potential.

As mentioned earlier, a number of sensors are coming to market which are being designed with a cost low enough to allow the practicing IH to have enough sensors to measure every individual. With increasing frequency, individuals are actually purchasing the entire sensor package to meet their own desire to have the information, and often these sensors come with multiple capabilities that the purchaser may not even want or use. For example, the Apple Watch Series 4 and 5 have integrated into their hardware and its operating system (version 6) an option to have continuous noise monitoring (Apple 2019). The watch continually monitors sounds in the environment and can display a real-time sound level meter. When the ambient noise exceeds a threshold (user selected between 80 and 100 dBA in 5 dBA increments), a warning is displayed, and the wearer is informed of an environment which could be hazardous. Each level is accompanied by the recommended limit in accordance with the World Health Organization's recommendation. There is not an integrating function, so it is not acting as a dosimeter, but an IH could ask a worker to set the limit at a desired setting, say 85 dBA, and ask him or her to report if the watch warned of a noisy environment. The data is collected in the health application and displays data every 2 minutes. Additionally, it has filters to show specific notifications of high noise periods. The data is sufficient for the IH to know whether or not a worker is experiencing quiet periods when not working and for how long. It will also allow the IH to learn if his worker experiences hazardous noise when not at work and the frequency of exposure. This information can be used to ensure that appropriate additional controls are implemented to keep exposure levels below the hazardous thresholds.

1.6   HEALTHCARE IS CHANGING—PERSONALIZED HEALTHCARE

Policy, competition, innovation, and consumer expectations are disrupting health-care. As the medical consumer becomes more aware, science and technology improves, and as the industrial health community realizes that one size medicine does not fit all, the prospect of individualized healthcare will have positive impacts. The individuals become more active in their healthcare while the cost to obtain more targeted results decreases due to the focused interventions that prevent and heal with laser focus.

Science and technology are rapidly changing and presenting exciting possibili-ties. More informed consumers are actively participating in their healthcare inter-ventions, the scientific communities are gaining an increased understanding of the human genome, and wearable and sensor technology with real-time diagnostics are much more affordable and available. It is a very exciting time to be in healthcare, and TEH helps to revolutionize how the IH professional provides primary prevention to identify the cause of the biological change with an emphasis on personalized health. The TEH platform can be the bridge to deliver true primary prevention for multiple populations versus just a treatment or cure once disease has gotten a foothold and improve what is currently monitored in health prevention, such as body chemistry changes or early symptoms of organ function changes.

Medical prevention efforts in effect today are not the only pathway to health. The food individuals eat, the choices they make in their daily activities, what their bodies experience externally, etc. all contribute to well-being. Personalized health is much more attainable for those alive today. For the IH and EHS to continue the present techniques and procedures used in classic medicine denies the population a chance to benefit from precision medicine which can offer truer primary prevention. TEH can be an effective tool to help achieve this goal.

1.6.1   PATIENT CENTRIC

Healthcare prior to the expansion of the internet generally placed the physician conceptually in the center of the healthcare picture. The patient would go to his or her appointment relatively uneducated and await the physician's plan of care to promote better health. Medical tests, therapeutic drugs, and diagnostic tests all were identified and ordered by the physician alone who was expected to bear the full responsibility of having the requisite medical knowledge to provide quality care or

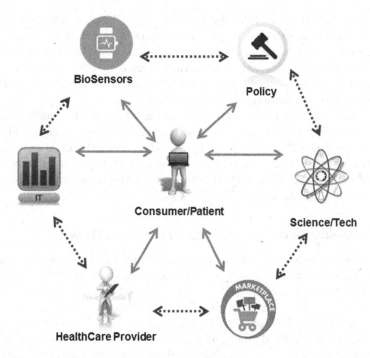

FIGURE 1.2 Patient-centric medicine is disrupting healthcare. Policy, technology, marketplace, and consumer expectations are the cause, and IHs are in a position to better support personalized healthcare.

know to refer a patient to another physician with specific expertise. Today, healthcare is moving toward a patient-driven and -centered health paradigm (see Figure 1.2). Patients use the vast amounts of data available to them to select physicians which meet their exacting requirements and can shop around to find other physicians based on patient and other third-party rating systems. The increased participation by the patient in healthcare makes the physician more likely to try to satisfy the patient even if he or she must acquiesce to some requests for diagnostic tests, pharmaceutical choices, or other options and value-based decisions that would not be requested without patient input. Where do the patients get the information to be able to influence their care? They get the information using the information technology revolution which provides vast amounts of information at their fingertips. They often come with their own information gathered from multiple sources, e.g., through biosensors such as the noise exposure information mentioned before, as well as information on body composition, dietary intake, and calories burned. They are also likely to bring the latest in science and technology information such as pollen count, air quality, water quality, the latest scientific study on what is healthful and what is harmful, and the latest medical condition along with the latest therapeutic drug which has just hit the market.

In short, patients often arrive at the medical provider's office having researched what is likely wrong with them, what tests they need, and what treatments they expect.

Patients also hear about new technology and specially developed treatments designed for them. Physicians still hold a significant amount of sway and are providing the final decisions about treatment as they have the legal ability to make the medical orders; however, the office visit just described does not place the physician in the center as he or she must tread lightly as patients may choose to switch to a provider who will meet their expectations.

As the medical consumer becomes more aware, science and technology improves and society realizes one size medicine does not fit all, the prospect of individualized healthcare will have positive impacts. Individuals will become more active in their healthcare while reducing costs due to the focused interventions that prevent disease early and heal with laser focus. TEH can move the field of industrial healthcare more quickly toward this awareness.

1.6.2   Exposure Curves: Where Does an Individual Fit In

In traditional toxicology, the method of determining the risk from exposure is to take a population, determine specific doses, and observe the elicited effects (e.g., a dose–response assessment). The effects being observed vary, but in general, changes in cell or organ function are being observed either by direct examination or through body chemistry. Ideally, there is epidemiological data from human exposure which can be used to determine dose response. It is relatively rare for this information to be available from human data except at low doses which are routinely occurring as it is unethical to expose humans just for research purposes. Higher dose exposures are only obtained from accidental exposure or from exposures prior to an under-standing of the risk. Animals are more likely the source in determining dosages in the dose–response curves, and great care is used in selecting an animal which is expected to respond similarly to a human based on the metabolic processes and physiological traits. Once the dose–response curves for the animals are obtained, some protection factors are included to account for uncertainty in the transition from animal to human (National Research Council 1994). Because these resulting dose–response curves are developed using population data, a response curve must be fit to the graph.

To facilitate an understanding of the following discussion, individuals on the curve will be called the "normal population". In fitting the curve to this normal population, there are outlying individuals which do not appear to follow the curve. As scientists, IHs and EHS understand that these outliers will occur in all samples and as a community accept the conclusion that the established exposure limit should protect the majority of the population. This "acceptance" that some individuals will not be protected has come about because there has not been any realistic way to know what makes these outlier individuals *special*.

Figure 1.3 shows a typical dose–response curve for a general exposure. In this general explanation, the exposure could be chemical, physical, or biological. There are three typical zones within the curves labeled as the *No Adverse Effect Range*, the *Increasing Effect with Increasing Dose Range*, and the *Maximum Effect Range*. The no adverse effect range occurs where there may be identified effects but not those believed to cause an adverse impact to health. It is at the end of this range, with

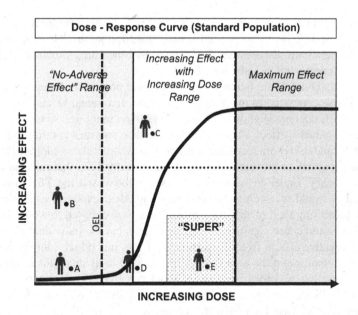

FIGURE 1.3   Dose–response curve zones and the impact of individuals as outliers.

appropriate safety factors set back, that an OEL is set. The next range on the curve is where adverse effects are increasing with increased dosage. This zone of data is often only available from animal exposure models. It is generally understood that the processes within an animal are mitigating some effects; as the dose is increased, the ability to mitigate the effects is overwhelmed. The final zone is the maximum effect range where even with increased dose no increased effect is observed. This range is considered to be the point where all mitigating effects are overwhelmed, and the maximum effect is being recorded. Individuals A through E placed on the graph as a dot (·) next to a human outline represent outliers to the normal data, and the curve represents the fit data to the population. The majority of the population falls very close to this curve and is not shown individually in this graph. The question an IH should ask is, "What are the impacts to the outliers in this data?"

Individuals A, B, and C present effects that are above the curve. Individual A has more effects for the given dose than the normal population, but these effects appear to be within the effects below the OEL threshold. It is not clear what will occur to individual A with a higher dose, but for this present discussion, the increased response is not overly concerning. Individual B is showing significant increased effect for a dose below the OEL. This individual is not being protected by the OEL; standard controls applied by today's IH will likely not prevent exposure-based disease as controls are generally not applied at 50% or less of the OEL. Individual C is showing effects greater than the normal population and would be over the OEL so controls would be recommended. It would be unclear if the standard control recommendation would be sufficient for individual C as he or she responded more significantly at a lower dose. Therefore, this individual has a chance of being protected, but it is uncertain if the

IHs efforts will be sufficient. Presently, there are individuals who are represented by points A, B, and C. These are the individuals that, despite the IHs best efforts, are likely to present with disease over time. The most concerning situation is when the exposure is represented by individual B.

Individuals D and E are below the curve and are presenting fewer effects for an increased dose compared to the normal population. Individual D has been exposed above the OEL but only slightly into the adverse effect range and would not be demonstrating an adverse effect. This individual would be provided controls to the exposure under standard IH practices, but it is not clear whether those additional controls would be necessary to prevent disease. It appears using TEH that the controls may not be necessary. Under the regulatory construct today and the TEH framework, individual D would receive protective controls for their exposure even if not beneficial in protecting their health. Individual E has been exposed to a dose far above a dose that would cause significant negative effects, but the individual clearly does not show negative effects from that exposure. These individuals can be thought of as "super" humans, and the area where this group of individuals fits is shaded and labeled. Those exposed to these doses without negative effects are not in need of the IHs or EHS support for this exposure. Individuals in this zone would be least likely to exhibit disease for jobs with significant exposure risks, or if the exposure of concern is for a personal choice, such as smoking, then their personal knowledge of how they feel would be at odds with what their provider would be telling them benefits their health.

The dose–response curve in Figure 1.3 represents one type of exposure. A further understanding of the use of this information is to begin to add new curves superimposed over each other keeping the population the same. It is conceivable that each individual in the population would be a "B" individual for some exposure curve. That is, this individual is exposed to a level considered to be low risk, but for the individual, it is a level which will likely result in disease.

1.7   THE FOURTH INDUSTRIAL REVOLUTION AND TEH

Today's society, which according to Schwab (2017) is post the first three industrial revolutions (the industrial age, the age of science and mass production, and the age of the digital revolution), has created an environment where humans are presented with numerous chemical, physical, and biological exposures on a regular basis. Not only workers but all people receive exposures. With the understanding that each person can have one or more exposures with excess risk and a high potential to end in disease, the need for exposure science services is highly likely to increase and the need for IH and EHS expertise will become more necessary. TEH as a framework aims to establish the IH profession with support from EHS as the providers of exposure services to any who need it. Many IHs will continue to serve employees primarily and account for the impacts of occupational and nonoccupational exposures, but many will also serve the non-working population and will account for any exposures which could be an increased risk individually.

Today the world is beginning the fourth revolution, and according to Vivek Wadhwa (2016), medicine is expected to advance in 10 years more than it has in the last 100 years. These advances will include paying for genomic sequencing at a price comparable to a blood test, having a true understanding of genetic proclivity to disease, and discovering the impact of the microbiome to health. These, among many other advancements in medicine, will allow medical professionals to deliver prevention and medical intervention to the masses (Wadhwa and Salkever 2017). Taking the TEH framework, this last step requires a number of developments that are underway as society begins the fourth revolution with advances in genomics, computational toxicology, the interconnections of things, and much more.

1.7.1 COMPUTATIONAL TOXICOLOGY

The Methods in Molecular Biology book series has volume 929, *What Is Computational Toxicology?* Its short definition is a perfect description to understand the core components of this subject:

> Computational toxicology is a vibrant and rapidly developing discipline that integrates information and data from a variety of sources to develop mathematical and computer-based models to better understand and predict adverse health effects caused by chemicals, such as environmental pollutants and pharmaceuticals. Encompassing medicine, biology, biochemistry, chemistry, mathematics, computer science, engineering, and other fields, computational toxicology investigates the interactions of chemical agents and biological organisms across many scales (e.g., population, individual, cellular, and molecular). This multidisciplinary field has applications ranging from hazard and risk prioritization of chemicals to safety screening of drug metabolites and has active participation and growth from many organizations, including government agencies, not-for-profit organizations, private industry, and universities.
>
> *(Reisfeld and Mayeno 2012)*

Computational toxicology (CompTox) has a number of distinct advantages over the classic toxicology described earlier because it can include human data, and it observes cellular function and connects it with genetic expression. Chapters 6 and 7 of this volume provide two example areas where exposures of concern are being identified through computational toxicology methods. This area of science promises to not only identify exposures of concern in society but also identify what genes are activated incident upon the exposure. Once the gene is activated, the molecular biological process that the gene controls is then identified. In simplified terms, the resulting cascade of additional activations and changes to cell function or output is able to be tracked and identified. In this way, we can fully understand the effects of an exposure. These effects at the cellular and gene expression level provide a more complete understanding of what generates what scientists describe as disease, namely where organ function or cellular function is negatively changed.

This understanding of the disease often uses human cells, so there is not a need to translate the results across species. There are challenges, and toxicologists have been developing new techniques to overcome the challenges as they arise, but significant new understanding of risk-based exposure and response and the mechanism of disease is impacting the knowledge base the IH and EHS use every day. If an IH or EHS expects simply to meet the law or regulation on acceptable or non-acceptable exposure, then until the law changes, the practice does not need to change. If the IH community believes disease prevention is the purpose for the profession, then adopting and using the knowledge coming from the CompTox arena is vital.

1.7.2 GENETIC EXPRESSION

CompTox and its ability to track gene expression has a valuable sister science in genetics. Geneticists are working across the globe to understand what the DNA in the human genes does specifically, not generally, and with the intent to decipher the functions of each gene identified in the Human Genome Project. The geneticists working on this identification of gene function identify the function and then move to the next gene because they estimate there are up to 25,000 human genes, and that is a lot of unfinished work (US National Institute of Health 2019). Other scientific communities use the knowledge gained by geneticists to determine if the information is beneficial in their own areas of science. The combination of geneticists identifying the gene function and CompTox determining the activation of the gene from an exposure alone assists in understanding disease and exposure levels that are more protective of the population on the whole.

An exciting part of the research which has not been discussed yet in this chapter are the genes that are not identical across the population. The genes which have differences in the sequence of DNA are called alleles. Geneticists also now understand that genes that appeared to have no active function get activated or inactivated based on external stimuli (exposure), internal stimuli (metabolomics), or by other sections of the genome once they are activated (the cascade of activated genes mentioned earlier). The alleles that each person has not only determine the physical characteristics of a person but also how the person responds to exposure. *Simply put, there are some alleles that either alone or in combination with other genes cause cells to respond to an exposure differently, and this accounts for the outlier individuals in the dose–response curves.* One of these alleles which is a single-nucleotide polymorphism (SNP) at rs7598759 demonstrated an NIHL risk with an odds (risk) ratio of 12.75 in a small population (Grondin et al 2015). A larger metanalysis of over 30 studies showed a risk ratio of 4.61 with a 95% confidence interval (Tserga et al. 2019). A risk ratio shows the increased risk that having the genetic variation increases the risk above the normal population; therefore, current understanding would place the risk to NIHL at an over four-and-a-half-fold increase (4.6 times) above the risk for a person without the genetic variation. This exciting type of science then *provides the IH and EHS the ability to identify the individuals at increased risk of disease.* As more of these alleles are identified, and their exposure-based risk factor increases or decreases, additional options to provide true primary prevention become available.

1.8 NOVEL CONTROLS ADDITIONS TO THE HIERARCHY

The hierarchy of controls available to IH is increasing, and the methods of employing the current controls are evolving as well under TEH. The exposure assessment strategies through various organizations have recommended SEGs for the last 25 years.

Using an SEG allows for treating a specific group with the same set of controls since it has exposures assumed to be similar. Having SEGs as practiced today does not account for exposures apart from the direct occupational exposures and does not account for individuals which may have the same exposure but are more susceptible to disease from that exposure due to their genetic differences. Collecting at-work exposure data will still be possible using SEG, but the IH profession using TEH will add strategies of control which account for the unique individuality of each person essentially taking the set to an N = 1.

1.8.1 Individual Exposure Health Risk Profile (IEHRP)

The Individual Exposure Health Risk Profile (IEHRP) (Chapter 2) was developed simultaneously during the development of the TEH framework to be a component of the full framework. Dr. Hartman and Dr. Oxley were specifically employed by Kirk Phillips to deliver this component of the TEH framework to the Department of Defense. Drs. Hartley and Oxley were charged with developing a method to help bring the management of the expected plethora of information into a manageable process. IEHRP is being developed as a method to combine exposure data not only from the traditional IH practice but also from genetic proclivity and data in other sources discussed in this chapter. These total exposures and clinical data from medical and diagnostic exams are being combined in this process to describe an individual's risk to the exposure. Using these multiple variables, the relative impact of the exposure to an individual can be visualized, and the IH will have a guide as to which exposures require additional controls. The protective impacts of providing a particular control compared to all the risk from exposures to the individual will be possible as well (Hartman and Oxley 2019).

1.8.2 Preexposure Prophylaxis

A new tool in the hierarchy of controls that will be available to IHs is pharmaceutical. There is at least one area of EH specialized protection against exposure which is the uptake of iodine for thyroid protection from radiation. The need for universal protection resulted in iodine being added to table salt assuring a regular daily small dose for majority of people. Therefore, the IH and the EHS are not in the habit of considering this prevention strategy as a control. A second pharmaceutical is for the protection of the body from radioactive cesium and thallium exposure in a nuclear event by reducing the biological half-life. Prussian Blue given just before or after a nuclear event is one of the IH's or health physicist's control methods, but these rare treatments have not resulted in list space in the hierarchy of control. This will change with the advent of the CompTox community's understanding of disease causation from exposures and the ensuing changes at the cellular level and the cascade of chemical process changes. The net result of these changes is the production or reduction of bioactive chemicals regulating cell and organ functions. By understanding these changes, medicine has the ability to target pharmaceutical treatments that prevent the effects from the chemical cascade. Therapies can interrupt the chemical cascade preventing the activation of the allele and breaking the chemical cascade so that the final resulting bioactive chemical is not produced or counteracts or blocks the damaging cellular process before acting in the body. Finally, pharmaceutical therapies will be able to act to increase the body's active repair mechanism at the time and location of the potential damage and mitigate harmful effects. One example which is nearing the commercial market involves prevention of NIHL. For NIHL, the allele appears to be related to the SNP rs1872328 on gene variant ACYP2, which plays a role in calcium homeostasis and increases the risk of ototoxicity activation in the body (Tserga et al. 2019). Calcium is necessary in a primary chemical process for signal transduction in the inner ear, specifically in the cochlear hair cell stereocilia mechanotransduction channels (Mammano 2011). Any therapeutic which balances these calcium levels would be protective. Audiologist and molecular biologist O'Neill Guthrie from Northern Arizona University (2019) is collaborating with a pharmaceutical company on a dietary supplement that would be protective as a preexposure prophylaxis for NIHL. His expectation is that within 3 years he will have the proper dosing and evidence that taking the drug, which is similar to a vitamin, before exposure to noise will provide protection and repair mechanism to prevent NIHL. Le Prell et al. (2019) pointed out that one of the current limitations of the prophylaxis is to determine what population would benefit from pharmaceutical interventions and to identify the factors that drive individual variability in humans. Understanding the genetic proclivity mentioned earlier is a solution to this problem. Armed with the direction by a provider that an individual has an increased genetic proclivity to NIHL, the employer or the medical community could provide a vitamin treatment that results in the risk of the individual from noise exposure returning close to the normal population.

It is exciting to think of the other preexposure prophylaxis treatments which will be possible for other types of exposure in the future. This one example of how these developing technologies are opening up new areas of research highlights how important it is that the IH profession uses the TEH framework and is ready to include these controls in the hierarchy.

1.8.3 SELF-LIMITING EXPOSURES

The discussion previously on the Apple watch and its ability to identify loud environments and notify the user of risk is an example where a person is provided the necessary information and then takes steps to reduce the exposure. Another example where recent scientific studies of NIHL can have an immediate application would be a publicly accessible kiosk where an individual could attach the headphones and the matching mobile device to a specialized monitoring system. The kiosk would then take the playlist, listening period, volume settings, and waveforms of the music (available from the internet) and set the delimiter on the volume to limit the mobile device from generating hazardous noise to the ear. Informative solutions like these are important as the youth today are experiencing NIHL prior to working age. The Centers for Disease Control and Prevention reported how recent scientific studies can have immediate applications. Its report showed, among other things, that 20% of youth have hearing loss by the age of 20. It also reported that 24% of NIHL in workers is from loud workplaces with the remaining exposures coming from non-work sources such as mowing, rock concerts, and sporting events (Harris 2017).

If genetic testing indicated increased risk to any particular exposure and this information was available at a young age to a person when selecting an occupation or making a lifestyle choice, he or she could then make informed choices to reduce exposure by avoiding the exposure entirely or choosing enhanced controls whenever the exposure is likely.

1.8.4 Nonoccupational PPE/Increased Occupational PPE

The goal of TEH is to consider work exposures and non-work exposures as equally important in providing overall protection. Using the TEH framework, the IH would understand that a worker likely has exposures away from work. Once all available data is collected, the IH should consider providing PPE which adequately addresses the total potential exposure and any genetic proclivity to disease. For instance, if the IH learns that a worker will be leaving his automobile painting job with exposure to VOCs to moonlight in a second self-owned business doing automotive repair with VOC-containing products, the IH should consider providing respiratory protection with a high enough protection factor to account for the additional post-workplace exposure. A possible preventive measure would be to provide a mask and filters for use at the moonlight position. Another possible option would be to inform the employee of the need to provide his own protection. To provide no intervention, or only intervention while in the workplace, poses more risk to the employer as disability resulting from exposure does not have to be proven to be entirely from the employer to be the responsibility of the employer for workers' compensation. The prevention of the disease is the best course of action, and providing an easy way to ensure the worker is protected 24 hours a day will, in many cases, be the lowest total cost option.

1.8.5 Durable Medical Equipment

Illness and injury from repetitive motion or acute injury occur in the joints and ligaments due to work and non-work causes. Dr. Kim and his research team from Stanford University have been researching elite athletes and have identified alleles through genome-wide association screens (GWAS) to identify DNA variants which increase the likelihood of ankle injuries (Kim et al. 2017). Jon Brazier and his team (2019) from Manchester Metropolitan University performed similar research to identify variants for increased risk to tendon and ligament injuries in rugby players. Braces and other durable medical equipment could be useful along with special training on proper movement to prevent injury for individuals with these gene variants. This research easily translates to workers or recreational sports and would provide an opportunity to prevent injury or disease. At present, a safety and health professional would need to wait for the occupational health department or family physician to identify a person with repeated injuries before recommending the regular use of a brace or wrap. With the TEH framework, the individuals with increased risk genetically could receive preexposure joint support and training from either the medical community or as a form of PPE prior to any injuries from the work-place, thereby providing true primary prevention. Giving every worker joint support would likely be too costly and would have low compliance, but providing the medical equipment to the individuals who would benefit the most could be cost-effective based on increased time on the job and reduced medical costs.

1.8.6 BLOOD CHEMISTRY TRACKING

Blood chemistry values have normal ranges which are generally well understood for monitoring changes in the body. There are some tests, though, which rely on changes from normal values to determine if there have been changes in the body. Some of these tests, while not regularly given to the population, are exposure specific. Cholinesterase testing on pesticide workers is used as a baseline test before exposure and then ongoing monitoring is used to verify if controls from exposure are working. Few individuals receive this testing unless they are expected to have work-related exposure to pesticides. Individuals with potential lifestyle exposures (e.g., gardening, vegetable-based dieting, beekeeping, living in rural areas) are those individuals who could benefit from having a baseline test especially if they are tested and learn that they have a known genetic risk to exposure to pesticides in the future.

1.9   TEH—BRINGING IT ALL TOGETHER

The primary customers for IHs at the present time are the workers, and as society moves forward in the fourth revolution, fewer and fewer workers will be in positions with large exposures over the regulatory limits or even in positions with classic industrial exposures at all. The new paradigm will be individuals who will receive as much exposure from their lifestyles, the environment, and clinically as they do in the workplace. In order to maintain relevancy to society, the IH and the EHS need to become the exposure scientists collecting and providing relevant data on the exposures to be used in primary prevention methods such as IEHRP and enhanced PPE. The IH's role will be to give individuals knowledge of the many options of controls they have so that they can reduce their exposures and the prevalence of disease. See Figure 1.4.

In its fully evolved state, TEH is a bold and innovative framework which associates exposures to the lowest common denominator—the individual's exposure—and, when possible, to the DNA ($N = 1$), enriching occupational and environmental health decisions to provide true primary prevention. Under the TEH framework, the IH and EH research communities pair with the geneticists, computational toxicologists, molecular biologists, occupational and primary care physicians, data experts using Internet of Things (IoT), and researchers to bring the latest advancements in science, technology, and informatics *to protect and advance the health and well-being of all*.

New knowledge of the relationships between individuals' genetic predispositions, epigenetic factors, and exposure to chemicals from lifestyle, occupation, and the environment can now support development of diagnostic approaches, treatment methods, and intervention strategies that consider all variables collectively. Hence, a

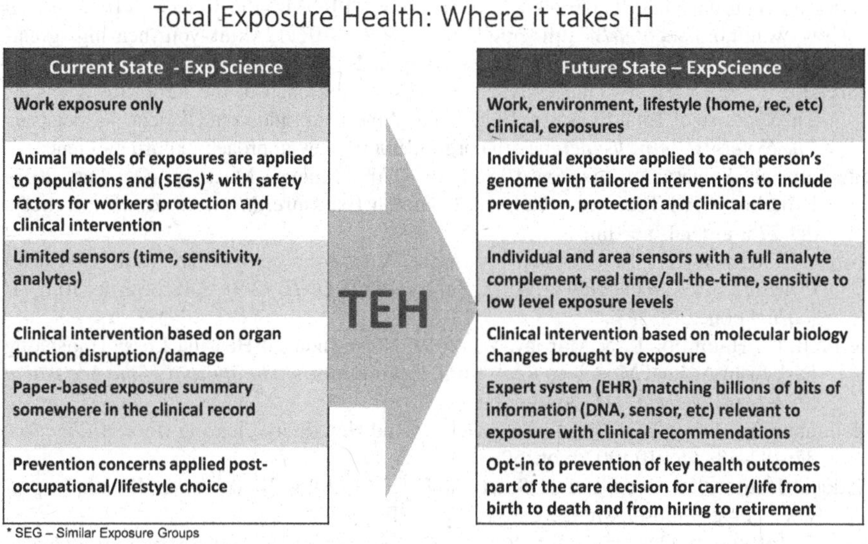

Total Exposure Health: Where it takes IH

Current State - Exp Science	Future State – ExpScience
Work exposure only	Work, environment, lifestyle (home, rec, etc) clinical, exposures
Animal models of exposures are applied to populations and (SEGs)* with safety factors for workers protection and clinical intervention	Individual exposure applied to each person's genome with tailored interventions to include prevention, protection and clinical care
Limited sensors (time, sensitivity, analytes)	Individual and area sensors with a full analyte complement, real time/all-the-time, sensitive to low level exposure levels
Clinical intervention based on organ function disruption/damage	Clinical intervention based on molecular biology changes brought by exposure
Paper-based exposure summary somewhere in the clinical record	Expert system (EHR) matching billions of bits of information (DNA, sensor, etc) relevant to exposure with clinical recommendations
Prevention concerns applied post-occupational/lifestyle choice	Opt-in to prevention of key health outcomes part of the care decision for career/life from birth to death and from hiring to retirement

TEH

* SEG – Similar Exposure Groups

FIGURE 1.4 Current and future state of exposure science with TEH.

comprehensive understanding of multiple exposures with genomic information will support a necessary paradigm shift from healthcare to health wellness by promoting more rapid identification of risks to health and well-being and enabling earlier and more tailored interventions.

Accurate calculation of disease risk factors will involve developing diagnostic systems that merge genomics to find relationships at the individual level to inform risk of disease, promote health and well-being through intervention, and mitigate these risks along with various big data from sensors, medical records, and various disparate unstructured data sets in order to understand the root causes of injury and disease and with the *TEH framework truly establish the IH and EH as the means to deliver true primary prevention healthcare.*

REFERENCES

Apple Inc. (June 3, 2019) *watchOS 6 Advances Health and Fitness Capabilities for Apple Watch* [Press Release]. Retrieved from https://www.apple.com/newsroom/2019/06/watchos-6-advances-health-and-fitness-capabilities-for-apple-watch/ (accessed 5 Jan 2020).

Bisht, M., & Bist, S. S. (2011) Ototoxicity: The Hidden Menace. *Indian Journal of Otolaryngology and Head and Neck Surgery: Official Publication of the Association of Otolaryngologists of India*, 63(3), 255–259. doi:10.1007/s12070-011-0151-8.

Brazier, J., Antrobus, M., Stebbings, G. K., Day, S. H., Heffernan, S. M., Cross, M. J., & Williams, A. G. (2019) Tendon and Ligament Injuries in Elite Rugby: The Potential Genetic Influence. *Sports*, 7(6), 138. MDPI AG.

Grondin, Y., Bortoni, M. E., Sepulveda, R., Ghelfi, E., & Bartos, A., et al. (2015) Genetic Polymorphisms Associated with Hearing Threshold Shift in Subjects during First Encounter with Occupational Impulse Noise. *PLOS ONE*, 10(6): e0130827.

Harris, R. (February 8, 2017) Shots HEALTH NEWS FROM NPR. Retrieved from https://www.npr.org/sections/health-shots/2017/02/08/514107312/think-your-hearings-great-you-might-want-to-check-it-out (accessed 5 Jan 2020).

Hartman, R., & Oxley, M. (June/July 2019) A New Approach to the Exposure Sciences: The Promise of Total Exposure Health. The American Industrial Hygiene Association. *The Synergist.* https://synergist.aiha.org/20190607-new-approach-exposure-sciences

International Society of Exposure Science 27th Annual Meeting (October 2017) Bringing It All Together – Noise, a Common Exposure. https://inses.memberclicks.net/27th-annual-meeting

Kim, S. K., Kleimeyer, J. P., Ahmed, M. A., Avins, A. L., & Fredericson, M., et al. (2017) Two Genetic Loci Associated with Ankle Injury. *PLOS ONE*, 12(9): e0185355. doi:10.1371/journal.pone.0185355

Le Prell, C., Hammill, T., & Murphy, W. (2019) Noise-Induced Hearing Loss: Translating Risk from Animal Models to Real-World Environments. *The Journal of the Acoustical Society of America*, 146, 3646–3651.

Mammano, F. (2011) Ca2+ Homeostasis Defects and Hereditary Hearing Loss. *BioFactors*, 37: 182–188. doi:10.1002/biof.150

National Institute for Occupational Safety and Health (2018) Total Worker Health. https://www.cdc.gov/niosh/twh/ (accessed 5 Feb 2019).

National Institute of Occupational Safety and Health (Nov 2015) "What Issues are Relevant to Total Worker Health?" Taken from Total Worker Health. https://www.cdc.gov/niosh/twh/faq.html (accessed 5 Jan 2020).

National Research Council (1994) *Science and Judgment in Risk Assessment.* Washington, DC: The National Academies Press. doi:10.17226/2125.

Northern Arizona University News. Research and Academics (5 Nov 2019) *NAU Audiologist Collaborates with Industry Partner to Develop Novel Therapy for Noise-Induced Hearing Loss* [Press Release]. Retrieved from https://news.nau.edu/guthrie-industry-research/#.Xgzq9C3My-o (accessed 5 Jan 2020).

Patringenaru, I. (2012) Small, Portable Sensors Allow Users to Monitor Exposure to Pollution on Their Smart Phones. *UC San Diego News.* https://ucsdnews.ucsd.edu/pressrelease/small_portable_sensors_allow_users_to_monitor_exposure_to_pollution_on_thei (accessed 5 Jan 2020).

Postelnicu, C., & Câlea, S. (2019) The Fourth Industrial Revolution. Global Risks, Local Challenges for Employment. *Montenegrin Journal of Economics*, 15(2), 195–206.

Reisfeld, B., & Mayeno, A. N. (2012) What Is Computational Toxicology? In: Reisfeld, B., & Mayeno, A. (eds) *Computational Toxicology. Methods in Molecular Biology (Methods and Protocols)*, vol. 929. Totowa, NJ: Humana Press. 3–4.

Rohé, G. H. (1898) *Text-Book of Hygiene a Comprehensive Treatise on the Principles and Practice of Preventive Medicine from an American Stand Point 3rd ed thoroughly Rev and Largely Rewritten.* Philadelphia, Davis 1901 c1899 x 553 p illus.

Schwab, K. (2017) *The Fourth Industrial Revolution.* New York: Crown Publishing Group.

Sterling, A. (15 June, 2019) Millions of Jobs Have Been Lost To Automation. Economists Weigh in On What To Do About It. *Forbes.* Retrieved from https://www.forbes.com/sites/amysterling/2019/06/15/automated-future/#63488d79779d (accessed 5 Jan 2020).

Tserga, E., Nandwani, T., Edvall, N., Bulla, J., Patel, P., Canlon, B., Cederroth, C., & Baguley, D. (2019) The Genetic Vulnerability to Cisplatin Ototoxicity: A Systematic Review. *Scientific Reports*, 9. doi:10.1038/s41598-019-40138-z

U.S. Environmental Protection Agency (2019) Air Trends. Air Quality - Cities and Counties. https://www.epa.gov/air-trends/air-quality-cities-and-counties (accessed 5 Jan 2020).

U.S. Environmental Protection Agency (2018) CERCLA and EPCRA Continuous Release Reporting. https://www.epa.gov/epcra/cercla-and-epcra-continuous-release-reporting (accessed 5 Jan 2020).

U.S. Environmental Protection Agency, Toxics Release Inventory (TRI) Program (2019) TRI Basic Data Files: Calendar Years 1987–2018. https://www.epa.gov/toxics-release-inventory-tri-program/tri-basic-data-files-calendar-years-1987-2018 (accessed 5 Jan 2020).

U.S. National Institute of Health. National Library of Medicine (2019) Help Me Understand My Genetics. https://ghr.nlm.nih.gov/primer/basics/gene (accessed 5 Jan 2020). doi:10.1371/journal.pone.0130827

Wadhwa, V. (2016) Singularity University. Singularity Hub. Medicine Will Advance More in the Next 10 Years than It Did in the Last 100. https://singularityhub.com/2016/10/26/medicine-will-advance-more-in-the-next-10-years-than-it-did-in-the-last-100/ (accessed 5 Jan 2020).

Wadhwa, V., & Salkever, A. (2017) *The Driver in the Driverless Car: How Our Technology Choices Will Create the Future* (1st ed.). San Francisco: Berrett-Koehler Publishers.

2 The Individual Exposure Health Risk Profile (IEHRP)—Developing a Risk Profile Tool beyond Dose Response

Richard Hartman
Independent Consultant

Mark Oxley
Air Force Institute of Technology

CONTENTS

2.1 INTRODUCTION

As industry continues to move toward greater degrees of automation, the concerns of workplace exposures will change as well. More and more work environments have now removed the human from the exposure or the exposure from the human. But is the workforce free from exposure-based risks as a result of the reduction in occupational exposures?

Not completely. Despite the advances to control workplace exposures, chronic diseases continue to affect workers (Sorensen et al. 2011). Why? Because the human body does not discriminate between exposures encountered at work, in the environment, or during leisure activities. But imagine the positive impact which could be made on health outcomes if there was a way to monitor, evaluate, and control or even eliminate exposures within and outside the workplace, creating a total exposure profile.

DOI: 10.1201/9780429263286-3

Total Exposure Health (TEH) is capitalizing on advancements in science, technology, and informatics to provide a framework which can be used to deliver this capability. This new approach to the exposure sciences also will associate exposures to the lowest common denominator—the individual's genes (N = 1) and monitoring for workplace, environmental, and lifestyle exposures whenever and wherever needed.

2.2 TOTAL EXPOSURE HEALTH (TEH)

After the military's experience of health consequences relating to Agent Orange exposure during the Vietnam War and the significant adverse health claims by service members deployed to the Persian Gulf War, the necessity to monitor and document exposures was codified into the National Defense Authorization Act for 1998 (Public Law 1997) whereupon the Department of Defense (DoD) was mandated to develop a deployment health surveillance system to detect, document, prevent, or minimize health problems arising as a result of occupational and environmental exposures during deployments and operations.

And while the DoD has made advances in health surveillance, the issues to collect, document, and act upon occupational and environmental health exposures while deployed remain a challenge (US Congress 2013). This is due to the nature of deployments, which are 24/7 workplaces, so the need to develop a more comprehensive view of what exposure meant beyond the typical 40-hour workweek and workplace was necessary. This meant expanding the practice of monitoring occupational and environmental exposures to include lifestyle choices.

This new way of characterizing worker well-being originated at the National Institute for Occupational Safety and Health (NIOSH) through Total Worker Health (TWH) (NIOSH 2018) as a holistic approach to worker well-being that acknowledges risk factors related to work that contribute to health problems previously considered unrelated to work.

The DoD recognized the validity of this approach but sought to realize a greater level of personalization by utilizing recent advances in the exposure sciences, genomics, sensor and data technologies, and health informatics which would aid in a more complete understanding of an individual's health risks, root causes of disease and injury, and innovative but accessible methods for primary prevention. The result is what is now referred to as Total Exposure Health (TEH).

Operationalizing TEH required partnering across multiple program areas, using traditional and emerging exposure assessment technologies (including sensors and –omics-based molecular biology), as well as leveraging a Big Data Infrastructure and Advanced Analytics.

While the near-term goal of TEH is to improve exposure characterization and understand individual variability, susceptibility, and vulnerability to cumulative exposures and risks factors, the first achievement was to demonstrate the feasibility of TEH and the ability to collect exposure data 24/7 to better understand the effects of total exposure. In the long term, TEH adds genomics and other data sets to translate these findings into clinically actionable recommendations for health prevention to improve both the health and well-being of both the workforce and their beneficiaries. Though the ultimate implementation of TEH will monitor a wide range of physical risks such as radiation and chemical exposure from the workplace and environment as well as lifestyle risks from recreational activities and diet, the first focus was on noise exposure.

2.3 NOISE EXPOSURE DEMONSTRATION PROJECT (NEDP)

Noise was the focus for this demonstration project because it is: (1) an exposure that does not discriminate by age, race, gender, and/or socioeconomic status; (2) costly (currently hearing health expenditures range from $1.5 billion to $2 billion annually for the US Department of Veterans Affairs in benefits and medical costs) (Alamgir et al. 2016); and (3) affects approximately 10% of the US population according to a 2017 report by the Centers for Disease Control and Prevention, where 40 million American adults show signs of noise-induced hearing loss (NIHL) (Carroll et al. 2012).

Noise Exposure Demonstration Project (NEDP) used sensor technology to collect total noise exposure 24 hours a day, 7 days a week. Unique to the noise monitoring devices developed for NEDP, the wearable sensor collects sound events from both ambient noise in the workplace and environment as well as in-ear sounds from ear buds used with smartphones and other devices playing digital media (such as music) with a smartphone app recording those decibel (dB) readings.

Nineteen subjects participated in this study at Moody Air Force Base, Georgia, over 10 days in June 2018. There were 12,680 noise events of 70 dB A-weighted (dBA) or above captured, with 2,968 events, or 23%, being 95 dBA or above. (A-weighted decibels are adjusted to deemphasize sounds outside of normal human hearing.) Figure 2.1 shows the average daily (24-hour) dB dose was about 75 dBA. About 10% of the subjects had total daily noise exposures under 70 dB, and 10% over 80 dB, with the majority in the middle.

High noise exposure was found at both the workplace (46%) and away from the workplace, off-duty, in the defense lexicon, (52%), and significant cumulative high-noise individual exposures were identified (3–27 hours over the 10-day study period). Geospatial "hotspot" locations of exposure were also identified across the population.

Overall, the NEDP met its objectives as a successful TEH demonstration project. The study therefore developed a low-cost noise dosimeter/sensor that monitors

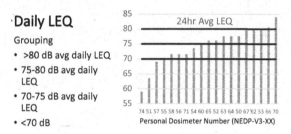

FIGURE 2.1 Daily (24-hour) equivalent continuous noise level (L_{eq}).

external and media smartphone device noise sound levels around the clock; used advanced analytics to collate multiple sensor devices, with geospatial layering; and managed participant compliance (Montgomery 2017). A summary of the NEDP is available from Yamamoto et al. (2019).

Recognizing that development of NIHL varies among populations who have been exposed to the same levels of noise, the researchers asked if there were genetic markers associated with a predisposition. A thorough review of published research within the field of genetics identified ten published studies, with small-to-modest sample sizes, which have indeed established a link between multiple genetic variants associated with NIHL. The effect is surprisingly large, with odds ratios of 5.2–22.36 indicating an elevated risk (Grondin et al. 2015).

Furthermore, within the broader United States Air Force (USAF) population, of which the NEDP participants are a subset, Figure 2.2 shows 17% of the 2,000 who have had their genes fully sequenced showed a particular gene variant, rs7598759, indicating they may be at a substantially increased risk for a hearing threshold shift—that is, of a hearing loss susceptibility due to noise.

This finding led to a new question: What if an IH or exposure scientist could take a person's cumulative, daily exposure to noise and combine this data with their genetic predisposition for NIHL to optimally protect against it? More broadly speaking, what if the IH and the care providers could predict, by aggregating big data

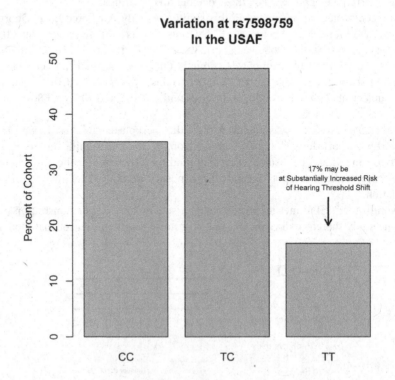

FIGURE 2.2 Gene variant associated with NIHL where the CC genotype is dominant trait and TT is the recessive trait (Phillips 2017, 2018).

and genomics, a person's susceptibility to external health risk factors—and take action to alleviate it using individualized health protocols?

The study concluded that by using an individual's medical records, it would be possible to identify pre-existing conditions that would also increase the risk of NIHL, thus bringing exposure data, genomics data, and medical record data together to describe a more holistic montage of the person's risk to a particular exposure.

This estimate/calculation of individual health risk factors involved the need for a mathematical/informatics process that could merge and analyze various data from sensors, medical records, and unstructured information as well as genomics data to identify relationships between them at the individual level called the Individual Exposure Health Risk Profile (IEHRP).

2.4 INDIVIDUAL EXPOSURE HEALTH RISK PROFILE (IEHRP)

The IEHRP integrates exposure data from both the traditional and cutting-edge emerging exposure assessment technologies (including sensors and "–omics"-based molecular biology) with clinical and genomic data. Combining the three: (1) the exposure measurement, (2) the genetic proclivity associated with the exposure, and (3) current clinical history associated with the exposure, provides a better description of the individual's risk than would a focus on any one variable. This combination originally resulted in the Individual Exposure Health Risk Index (IEHRI) defined by

$$IEHRI_1 = v_{1,1} + v_{1,2} + v_{1,3} \qquad (2.1)$$

where $v_{1,1}$ is the exposure measure, $v_{1,2}$ is the genetic proclivity to the exposure, and $v_{1,3}$ is the clinical effect per the evidence in the individual's medical record (medical history). For example, when evaluating noise, the IEHRI becomes

$$IEHRI_{(Noise)} = v_{(Noise, measure)} + v_{(Noise, genes)} + v_{(Noise, history)} \qquad (2.2)$$

Accounting for multiple exposures leads to the development of the IEHRP, which combines multiple IEHRI's for an individual, represented by equation (2.3) for (i) exposures.

$$IEHRP = (IEHRI_1, IEHRI_2, \ldots, IEHRI_i)$$
$$= \left(\left[v_{1,1} + v_{1,2} + v_{1,3} \right], \left[v_{2,1} + v_{2,2} + v_{2,3} \right], \ldots, \left[v_{i,1} + v_{i,2} + v_{i,3} \right] \right) \qquad (2.3)$$

With the IEHRP equipped to address multiple exposures, the limitations to the IEHRI became evident, which only accounted for three variables to describe an individual exposure. This was observed early in the NEDP, which revealed other variables that would affect the $IEHRI_{(Noise)}$, such as ototoxins or family history. This required the IEHRP to be modified so it could account for multiple confounding factors (Figure 2.3) and is represented by equation (2.4) with (j) confounding factors.

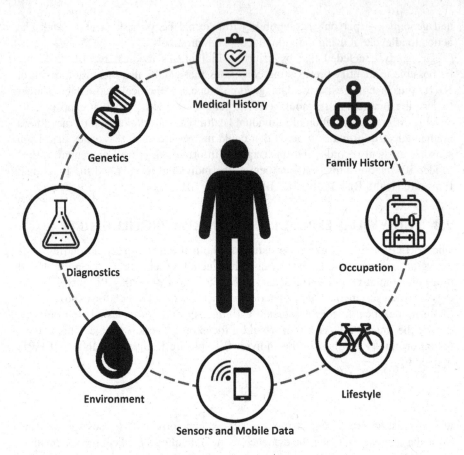

FIGURE 2.3   The IEHRI can have many variables (Phillips 2017, 2018).

$$IEHRP = \left(IEHRI_1, IEHRI_2, \ldots, IEHRI_i \right)$$

$$= \left(\left[v_{1,1} + v_{1,2} + v_{1,3} + \ldots + v_{1,j} \right], \left[v_{2,1} + v_{2,2} + v_{2,3} + \ldots + v_{2,j} \right], \ldots, \right.$$

$$\left. \left[v_{i,1} + v_{i,2} + v_{i,3} + \ldots + v_{i,j} \right] \right) \tag{2.4}$$

With the development of the IEHRP for multiple exposures and variables, two key questions still needed to be addressed: (1) Which variable ($v_{i,j}$) was the most important? That is, should some weigh more than others? and (2) How does an IH account for the variability of each variable?

To answer the first question (e.g. are genes more important than exposure measure?), the equation was enhanced with a "Weighting Factor" ($WF_{i,j}$), a numerical value that would account for importance of each variable ($v_{i,j}$). To account for the variability (confidence), the equation included a "Correction Factor" ($CF_{i,j}$), a numerical value. Combining the CF with the WF resulted in the most recent iteration of the IEHRP, equation (2.5)

$$IEHRP = \left(IEHRI_1, IEHRI_2, \ldots, IEHRI_j \right)$$

$$= \left(\left[(v_{1,1})(CF_{1,1})(WF_{1,1}) + (v_{1,2})(CF_{1,2})(WF_{1,2}) + \ldots + (v_{1,j})(CF_{1,j})(WF_{1,j}) \right], \right.$$

$$\left[(v_{2,1})(CF_{2,1})(WF_{2,1}) + (v_{2,2})(CF_{2,2})(WF_{2,2}) + \ldots + (v_{2,j})(CF_{2,j})(WF_{2,j}) \right],$$

$$\left. \left[(v_{i,1})(CF_{i,1})(WF_{i,1}) + (v_{i,2})(CF_{i,2})(WF_{i,2}) + \ldots + (v_{i,j})(CF_{i,j})(WF_{i,j}) \right] \right)$$

$$(2.5)$$

This IEHRP is for an individual, so in a group of N individuals with similar or different exposures, the expectation would be to see N distinct IEHRPs. Therefore, observing the collection of IEHRPs

$$\{ IEHRP_1, IEHRP_2, \ldots, IEHRP_N \} \qquad (2.6)$$

would be of interest.

For example, if two individuals are considered the IEHRPs set would be $N = 2$ (Figure 2.4), individual A has a high risk for noise whereas individual B has a high risk for radon. This visualization allows the provider or IH/OH professional to target and prioritize interventions based on the individual's highest risk exposure(s).

Now modify the visualized set with the same data to accommodate a policy maker, it would be apparent that noise is prevalent in both A and B, allowing the policy maker to identity the high priority exposure for either policy development/ modification or proper resourcing versus focusing on a lower priority exposure.

When fully developed, the IEHRP will provide an enhanced capability to describe individual health risks based on genetic factors and occupational, lifestyle, and environmental exposure factors, medical disposition, protective factors, and other variables that affect exposure health risk.

2.5 CONCLUSION

At the rise of the industrial revolution, Alice Hamilton pioneered the industrial hygiene profession and by building on the past knowledge and looking to the future of industry expanded began the way industrial hygienists think about exposures in the workplace. With rapid advances of science, technology, medicine, and informatics, society is on the cusp of a Fourth Industrial Revolution and is beginning to recognize the opportunity that comes with the change it brings.

IH/OH professionals and exposure scientists are well positioned to usher in this revolution in much the same way Dr. Alice Hamilton did in her time. In practice, the IH/OH professions will better understand the effects of exposures not only in the workplace and environment but also in the day-to-day activities of the

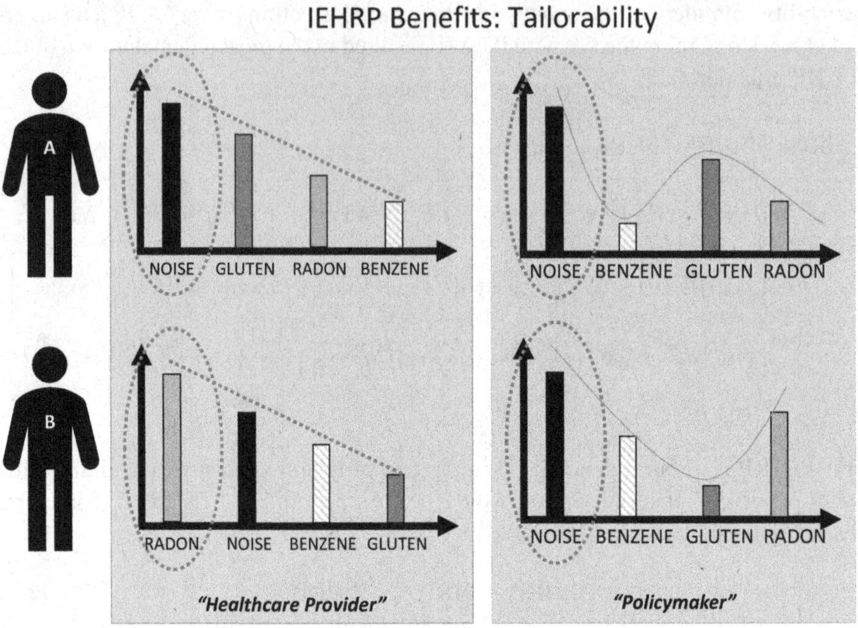

FIGURE 2.4 IEHRP data visualization for two individuals. Healthcare providers can use the visualization on the left to target interventions based on individual risks (noise for Person A and radon for Person B), while policy makers can use the visualization on the right to direct resources toward high priority risks across a population.

population. Through initiatives like TEH, the exposure communities will uncover a new understanding of the relationships between an individual's genetic predispositions, epigenetic factors, and exposures from lifestyle, occupation, and the environment to support the development of diagnostic approaches, treatment methods, and intervention strategies to truly institute primary prevention to improve worker health, performance, and productivity. The work TEH framework created by Col Kirk Phillips was placed into an end-to-end system development graphic and presented at the closing keynotes of the American Industrial Hygiene Association Fall Conference 2017 and Conference and Exposition in 2018 (Phillips 2017, 2018) (Figure 2.5).

By embracing new bold ideas as a profession, the current state of disparate exposure monitoring will be transformed, research studies, data collection, and controls into holistic and integrated systems that quantitate total exposure and inform health outcomes into precise actionable insights and initiatives for individuals and/ or similar exposure groups.

The IH/OH profession will leverage and advance genomics, sensor and data technologies, data analytics, and health informatics into a future-focused and progressive approach that represents a disruptive but necessary paradigm shift to the exposure sciences—TEH.

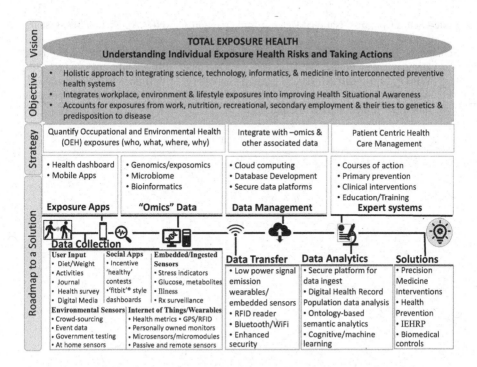

FIGURE 2.5   TEH end-to-end system development (Phillips 2017, 2018).

REFERENCES

Alamgir, H., et al.: Economic Burden of Hearing Loss for the U.S. Military: A Proposed Framework for Estimation. *Military Medicine*, 181(4): 301–306, April 2016.

Carroll, Y.I., et al.: Vital Signs: Noise-Induced Hearing Loss Among Adults – United States 2011–2012. *Morbidity and Mortality Weekly Report (MMWR)*, 66: 139–144, 2017.

Grondin, Y., et al.: Genetic Polymorphisms Associated with Hearing Threshold Shift in Subjects during First Encounter with Occupational Impulse Noise. *PLOS ONE*, 10(6): e0130827, 2015.

National Institute for Occupational Safety and Health (NIOSH): "Total Worker Health." Available at https://www.cdc.gov/niosh/twh/default.html

Montgomery, K. and R. Hartman: "Bringing It All Together – Noise a Common Exposure." *Presented at the International Society of Exposure Scientist (ISES)*, Research Triangle, NC, 18 Oct 2017.

Phillips, K.: "Total Exposure Health: A Revolutionary Way to Think of Exposure and Primary Prevention." *Presented at the American Industrial Hygiene Fall Conference 2017*, 31 Oct 2017.

Phillips, K: "Total Exposure Health: A Revolutionary Way to Think of Exposure and Primary Prevention." *Presented at the American Industrial Hygiene Conference and Exposition 2018*, 23 May 2018.

Public Law 105–85 (HR 1119): National Defense Authorization Act for Fiscal Year 1998, Subtitle F, Section 765, November 1997.

Sorensen, G., et al.: The Workshop Working Group on Worksite Chronic Disease Prevention. *American Journal of Public Health*, 101(Suppl 1): S196–S207, December 2011.

United States Congress. National Defense Authorization Act (NDAA): Section 313, January
    2013.
Yamamoto, D.P., J.W. Kurzdorfer, and K.L. Fullerton: U.S. Air Force Noise Exposure
    Demonstration Project, Final Report for December 2016 to July 2018 (AFRL-SA-
    WP-TR-2019-0010). Air Force Research Laboratory, 711th Human Performance Wing.
    Available from the Defense Technical Information Center (DTIC) at: https://apps.dtic.
    mil/dtic/tr/fulltext/u2/1071653.pdf.

3 In Pursuit of Total Exposure Health

Leveraging Exposure Science, the Omics, and Other Emerging Technologies

Sherrod Brown and Dirk Yamamoto
Wright-Patterson AFB

CONTENTS

3.1 INTRODUCTION

Evaluation of harmful exposures that could pose health threats to workers traditionally focuses on environmental and occupational exposures. Considering that the workday only accounts for approximately one-third of a worker's day, these evaluations are somewhat incomplete as they don't represent the worker's total exposure. However, how can the health of a worker be determined from only a fraction of his or her daily exposure?

DOI: 10.1201/9780429263286-4

Hazards such as first- or secondhand cigarette smoke, air pollution, and harmful contaminants in drinking water or lifestyle factors such as stress, diet, and sleep habits all affect an individual's health and subsequently their work performance. However, these stressors aren't accounted for in workplace exposure evaluations and typically are not included in an individual's clinical assessment. Not accounted for are numerous exposures from a worker's everyday lifestyle, e.g., foods and/or drugs consumed, commercial products applied to their skin, and ambient air inhaled away from the workplace. These off-duty exposures can lead to a cumulative exposure, or "total exposure," that poses a long-term threat to health. This chapter discusses exposure science and how emerging technologies may be applied to the Total Exposure Health (TEH) framework (Goff and Hartman 2018).

3.2 EXPOSURE SCIENCE: KEY PRINCIPLES USEFUL FOR TOTAL EXPOSURE HEALTH

Defined as "the study of the contact between human and physical, chemical, or biological stressors," *exposure science* seeks to understand the nature of this contact for the purpose of protecting ecologic and public health (Teeguarden et al. 2016). Exposure science has two primary goals: (1) to understand how stressors affect human and ecosystem health and (2) to prevent or reduce contact with harmful stressors or to promote contact with beneficial stressors to improve public and ecosystem health (NRC 2012). Applying exposure science principles to TEH will require the use of more tools such as sensors, biomarkers, and analytics to accomplish the goals of improving exposure characterization and identifying and understanding variability, susceptibility, and vulnerability to an individual's exposome. Doing so will, e.g., lead to a better understanding of why individuals who share duties in the same workplace have noticeably different health outcomes after experiencing the same representative occupational exposure.

First introduced by Dr. Christopher Wild (2005), the *exposome* "encompasses life-course environmental exposures from the prenatal period onwards." The Centers for Disease Control and Prevention (CDC) further defines the exposome as "the measure of all the exposures of an individual in a lifetime and how those exposures relate to health" (CDC 2014). Accordingly, each person develops his or her unique exposome ever since birth—thought of as the environmental correlation to the human *genome* (Betts and Sawyer 2016; Wild 2005). While important, particularly to the predisposition to certain diseases, researchers have determined that the genome does not play as large a role as initially expected in disease (approximately only 10%). However, the genome, in concert with the highly variable exposome, holds promise for explaining the cause of various diseases. Critical to understanding the causes, and eventually the prevention of disease, environmental hazards and their relation to diseases need to be further studied. The knowledge gained from further research of both the genome and exposome could ultimately result in more effective treatment and improved patient management under the TEH paradigm.

Wild (2012) described three overlapping domains within the exposome: (1) a general external environment (e.g., climate, stress, socioeconomic status), (2) a specific external environment (e.g., diet, occupational and environmental exposures, drugs), and finally, (3) an internal environment (e.g., DNA, metabolism, microbiome). Traditionally, occupational health evaluations have focused only on the specific external environment, with collection of samples from air, water, and other external mediums to determine potential exposures and provide risk assessments. Relying strictly on the external environment gives exposure scientists only a glimpse of the exposures affecting the overall health of an individual. Studying all three domains relies on the application of unique internal and external exposure assessment methods.

Previously, exposure science relied heavily on external exposure information for a small number of stressors, locations, times, and individuals. Now, the science is shifting to a more systematic assemblage of internal exposures of individuals in entire populations and multiple elements of the ecosystem to multiple stressors (NRC 2012). Over the past 15 years, there has been greater emphasis on the use of internal markers of exposure (i.e., biomarkers) to assist in defining exposure–response relationships. Internal measures of exposures to stressors are closer to the target site of action for biologic effects than are external measures, but the variability in the relationship between sources of stressors and effects can be greater than that when relying on external measures of exposure. Analytical methods enable detection of much lower concentrations of stressors internally and measurement of multiple stressors in single samples, but the correlation between external exposures and resulting internal concentrations is still being investigated. Thus, most biomonitoring data cannot be interpreted without far more information that can only be gained through more research. New analytical methods to quantify human biomarkers of chemical exposure have been developed for many substances, and many newly developed techniques for other chemicals are currently in the validation process (Becker et al. 2003).

3.3 HIGH-THROUGHPUT METABOLOMICS IN TOTAL EXPOSURE HEALTH

3.3.1 THE OMICS

The past few decades have seen a revolution in medical research with the rise of various *omics* technologies (see also Chapter 8, "Omics": An Introduction), and today, many biological research efforts are incorporating these high-throughput technologies into their methodologies. The suffix *omics* is used to describe a field of study in life sciences that focuses on large-scale data/information. The first of the omic technologies to gain attention, *genomics*, provided a framework useful for mapping and studying specific genetic variants contributing to various diseases. The identification of these genetic variants has allowed scientists to rationalize the development of additional *systems biology* technologies that involve integrating different omics data types—all with the goal of identifying molecular patterns associated with diseases. The *triad of omics* is comprised of *genomics*, which studies cell DNA and genetic information (genome), *proteomics*, which studies the structure and functions of proteins (proteome), and the youngest of the three, *metabolomics*, which studies the human metabolome.

3.3.2 Metabolomics

In simple terms, metabolomics looks at the unique footprint left behind after metabolism occurs and it is integral to an understanding of biological system functionality. Because of its great potential to the study of the exposome, this field is emerging as an important way of characterizing human exposures and, therefore, aiding in describing an individual's total health. This section presents the basics of metabolomics, advances in the field and advantages of high-throughput metabolomics, and how they could benefit TEH.

First introduced in 1998, the *metabolome* is the collection of low molecular weight compounds (*metabolites*), to include parts of amino acids, lipids, and organic acids present at any given time in a cell or organism that participate in metabolic reactions (i.e., metabolism). It contains the biological endpoints of genomic, transcriptomic, and proteomic perturbations, and also includes environmental (to include stress, lifestyle, and xenobiotic use) and gut microbiota influences (Johnson and Gonzalez 2012). Metabolism is the life-sustaining biochemical processes occurring in living things as a result of dissolution and nourishment, and from those processes, each individual forms a unique *metabolic profile*. Because metabolism is influenced by all the factors previously mentioned, examining the metabolic profile can provide a better representation of an organism or individual's phenotype than genomics or proteomics alone. Metabolomes become altered when an organism's biological systems are disturbed by disease, genetic mutations, or environmental factors. These altered metabolic profiles can result in large perturbations to metabolite concentrations and flux even from very subtle variations between individuals. Recently, experts in the exposure sciences have pushed to narrow the focus of the exposome to include only metabolomics (NIOSH 2019). By monitoring metabolite changes in biofluids (i.e., blood and urine), metabolomics can be used to profile individuals' responses to drug treatment or other medical therapy. Observing a set of metabolites with different concentration changes is a unique advantage to using metabolites as biomarkers. The changes in concentration can be correlated with a disease state or treatment response.

Compared to the other omics technologies that are more narrowly focused, metabolomics must interrogate a wide variety of molecules with very diverse physicochemical properties. This may explain why metabolomics is perhaps not as well developed and is highly dependent on well-defined internal standards to achieve consistent results. Although the genomics revolution brought an unprecedented ability to obtain genetic information across individuals and populations to aid in finding causes of human disease, tools for measuring the exposome have been slower to develop. However, recent technological advancements have enabled metabolomics researchers to detect the small molecules within the metabolome, quantify a large amount of those metabolites, and study their role in disease states. The science has the ability to provide a broad, agnostic assessment of the compounds existing in a biosample, rather than being limited to a chemical or class of chemicals selected in advance (Betts and Sawyer 2016). These assessments can be accomplished via two distinct detection approaches: targeted and untargeted metabolomics.

3.3.2.1 Targeted Metabolomics

Targeted metabolomics refers to the exact quantification of known, as well as expected, metabolites by employing analytical standards. The targeted approach focuses on a single analyte, a class of chemically similar analytes, or a set of analytes with chemistries similar enough to allow for their measurement in a single analysis (Metz et al. 2017). This is similar to an external exposure assessment where there is usually a targeted (i.e., known) contaminant of concern. The benefits of the targeted approach include accurate quantification of the contaminant of interest, low limits of quantification, and usually high confidence in the analyte's identification. With metabolomics capabilities, medical clinicians could periodically perform biomonitoring of the workplace employees with the goal of tracking and quantifying biomarker levels. This approach would provide a more complete assessment of workers' individual internal exposures versus only a representation of their specific external exposure.

3.3.2.2 Untargeted Metabolomics

Untargeted metabolomics simultaneously measures as many metabolites as possible in a biosample without having prior knowledge of the identity of the assessed metabolites. The untargeted approach is increasingly popular among metabolomics experts, as it allows for unknown or emerging exposures of concern to be detected. Although an advantage of the untargeted approach is that collection can be accomplished without preexisting knowledge, sample preparation and analytical methods have a direct impact on the qualitative results obtained. Due to the diversity of the metabolome, sample preparation steps, separation methods, and instrument platforms and parameters will affect the subset of the metabolites detected (Schrimpe-Rutledge et al. 2016). Datasets from untargeted studies are particularly complex, and a number of metabolites remain uncharacterized (Agin et al. 2016). When using mass spectrometry (MS) technology to analyze samples, it is likely impractical to manually inspect and interpret the thousands of peaks detected (Patti et al. 2013).

There is a significant range of platforms that can be employed to conduct metabolomics studies in biosamples. MS and *nuclear magnetic resonance* (NMR) have emerged as the most common of these available analytical platforms (Dias and Koal 2016). The high reproducibility associated with NMR, and the high sensitivity and selectivity associated with MS, make these tools superior over other analytical techniques (Emwas 2015). Various techniques within both methods of analysis offer multifaceted approaches to detect and identify a variety of metabolites. But because of its detection and quantitation sensitivity, MS is the preferred method as it allows for several hundred metabolites in a single measurement. The very diverse characteristics of small metabolites make chemical separation and detection challenging steps in the application of metabolomics. In order to separate the makeup of a mixture, MS is paired with a separation technique. These "hyphenated" analytical techniques (e.g., gas chromatography-mass spectrometry (GC-MS), liquid chromatography-mass spectrometry (LC-MS)), which combine separation technology with MS, have become highly effective tools for small-molecule analysis (Gowda and Djukovic 2014). GC-MS and LC-MS are the most popular separation techniques as both can be used to detect low-concentration metabolites. Instrument capability has slowly progressed in the number of metabolites detectable versus sensitivity, with NMR being able to detect 10^2 metabolites at $>\mu M$ (i.e., micromolar) sensitivity, GC-MS being able to detect 10^2 metabolites at $<\mu M$ sensitivity, and LC-MS being able to detect 10^3 metabolites at $<nM$ (i.e., nanomolar) sensitivity (Bradburne et al. 2015).

A relatively new and appealing technique for enhancing single-cell analysis methods is the incorporation of *ion mobility spectrometry* (IMS) with MS (Metz et al. 2017). This technique offers an improved identification of metabolites and provides an alternative to the solution-phase methods since separations are performed on the order of milliseconds in IMS, while on the order of minutes to hours in the conventional chromatographic methods. However, the potential of this integration has been hampered by the loss of sensitivity and the mismatched duty cycles traditionally associated with IMS/MS combination systems. Scientists at Pacific Northwest National Laboratory (PNNL) have developed an integrated instrument platform that overcomes these issues (PNNL 2020). The specific platform increases sensitivity and throughput by incorporating three distinct innovations: (1) an ion funnel technology, (2) ion funnel trap advancements that provide ion accumulation and precise release, and (3) a multiplexing feature for greater sensitivity with better-aligned duty cycles. The greater sensitivity derives from the technique yielding a higher signal-to-noise ratio than that produced by the conventional techniques. The new technique also increases analysis throughput because it allows ion packets to travel simultaneously through the drift region of the MS detector (PNNL 2020). Industry has further advanced the ion funnel technology by putting it on printed circuit boards, making the technology more economical. *Structures for Lossless Ion Manipulations*, or SLIM technology, can revolutionize the game of molecular and, more specifically, metabolomics studies. SLIM adds significant length—15, 20, 60 meters and more— into the typical ion path of a detector by implementing a serpentine pathway into the compactness of a small circuit board. Because the resolution of ion separations depends on the length of the drift path, the longer paths offered by SLIM provide more separation, grouping, and molecular analysis. Its developers think SLIM will "allow for a whole new universe of compounds and materials to be synthesized, purified, and collected" (PNNL 2017).

3.3.3 GROWTH OF METABOLOMICS

Ever since its introduction in the late 1990s, metabolomics has increased in popularity and applicability. It has been widely adopted as a novel approach for biomarker discovery and, in tandem with genomics, has the potential for improving the understanding of underlying causes of pathology (Trivedi et al. 2017). However, in the clinical area, the science can no longer be described as novel, as indicated by the thousands of research articles on metabolomics that are available. In 2012, it was estimated that the National Institutes of Health (NIH) would invest approximately $14.3 million, and more than $51.4 million over 5 years, to accelerate the field of research (NIH 2012). Other government bodies have followed suit, supporting metabolomics activities on the international level, which further emphasizes the promise seen in metabolomics.

Metabolomics is the omics field most closely linked to the host phenotype and, thus, can report on the status of diseases as well as the effect and response to external stimuli (e.g., drug therapy, nutrition, exercise). Even miniscule changes made to the host genome, epigenome, and proteome are easily detected in the metabolome. Some researchers are emphasizing that the metabolome can also be used to detect endogenous changes in response to environmental chemicals from one's job, diet, or other means.

Approximately 90% of deaths and disease in the United States and developed countries can be attributed to some kind of environmental exposure. When it comes to determining how these environmental exposures may contribute to disease, a major obstacle is the scarcity of publicly available information on the 80,000-plus chemicals registered for commercial use. The use of metabolomics can help, as it can provide a broad, agnostic assessment of the compounds in the respective biosample versus being limited to a preselected chemical or class of chemicals (Betts and Sawyer 2016).

Researchers have cataloged over 42,000 metabolites associated with food, drugs, food additives, phytochemicals, and pollutants (Betts and Sawyer 2016). Metabolomic studies have identified environmentally linked biomarkers related to numerous diseases, to include chronic fatigue syndrome and congenital heart defects. Three online metabolomics databases allow free access to the metabolome: DrugBank, Human Metabolome Database, and Toxic Exposome Database (Betts and Sawyer 2016). As both a bioinformatics and cheminformatics resource, DrugBank (2020) contains information on drugs and drug targets and has approximately 2,280 drug and drug metabolites. The Human Metabolome Database (2020) includes information about small molecule metabolites found in the human body and contains over 114,000 metabolite entries, with 5,702 protein sequences linked to those entries. The Toxic Exposome Database (2020), formerly the Toxin and Toxin Target Database (T3DB), is a bioinformatics resource that combines detailed toxin data with comprehensive toxin target information and contains approximately 3,670 toxins and environmental pollutants.

Although still evolving as a science compared to other more mature omics, metabolomics has found application in disease profiling, personalized medicine (e.g., drug discovery and drug assessment), toxicology, agriculture, and the environment. For its continued maturation, there are a few objectives that need to be met: (1) improvement in the comprehensive coverage of the metabolome, (2) standardization between laboratories and metabolomics experiments, and (3) enhancement of the integration of metabolomics data with other functional genomic information. The NIH (2012) funding mentioned previously was an effort to increase metabolomics research capacity by funding various initiatives in the area, to include training, technology development, standards synthesis, and data sharing capability for the field.

Founded in 2004, the Metabolomics Society (http://metabolomicssociety.org) is dedicated to promoting the growth, use, and understanding of metabolomics in the life sciences. It is a nonprofit organization with more than 1,000 members in over 40 countries, with focus on promoting the international growth and development of metabolomics, collaboration, opportunities to present research, and the publication of meritorious research (Metabolomics Society 2020). The growth of this society indicates the growing popularity of metabolomics around the world.

Whereas the data compiled from the older omics technologies is readily available and analyzed through electronic databases, a significant amount of metabolomics data is still only resident in books, journals, and other paper archives. Additionally, analytical software used in metabolomics studies is different from any software used in genomics, proteomics, and transcriptomics because of its emphasis on chemicals and analytical chemistry. Furthermore, the expanding use of metabolomics has been accompanied by a significant increase in the number of computational tools available to process and analyze the copious amounts of data it generates, with a goal of providing an automated and standardized operational platform.

3.4   THE HUMAN MICROBIOME AS A MODIFIER OF PERSONALIZED EXPOSURES

Our bodies are made up of trillions of cells and, historically, literature has suggested that each cell in our body (i.e., human cells) is outnumbered 10 to 1 by microbes (i.e., bacterial cells). In more recent history, researchers have proposed a revised ratio, such as with Sender et al. (2016) estimating that the number of bacteria in the body is on the same order as the number of human cells (i.e., 1:1 ratio). Regardless of the ratio, bacterial cells play a significant role in our health and inhabit all parts of the human body. This entire assemblage of microbes is what makes up the human microbiome. In addition, microbes play an integral role in keeping our digestive system running smoothly. However, the microbiome is more than just our partner in digestion—it is also important to boosting immunity, balancing hormone levels, preventing infection, and maintaining optimal brain function.

Passed down from mother to baby, the human microbiome is the collection of all the microorganisms on or in the human body, their genes, and the surrounding environmental conditions. Each body site of the human microbiome has a distinct microbial community. For example, the oral microbiome is recognizably different in composition and function compared to other body site microbiomes. Despite its diversity, the skin microbiome is tiny compared to the massive community inhabiting the gastrointestinal tract (gut) where there is a constant supply of nutrients. Although individually distinct, perturbations in the composition and function of a site microbiome are associated with disease at the affected site, as well as distally (NAS 2018).

3.4.1   THE MICROBIOME OF A BABY

The assembly ("colonization") of the microbiome of an infant is determined by the maternal-offspring exchange of microbiota. In fact, factors such as birth by Caesarean section (C-section), perinatal antibiotics, and dependence on formula feeding can affect this assembly process and lead to increased risk of disease (Mueller et al. 2015). In contrast to the very similar array of bacteria that a baby born vaginally inherits from the mother, the microbiome of a baby born via C-section is likely colonized by a less diverse array, mostly by skin bacteria, in addition to any bacteria picked up from the environment in which the baby is born. This disruption of bacterial transmission resulting from a C-section may increase the risk of disease.

Researchers have observed differences in the specific microbial species between C-section babies and babies delivered vaginally after 1 month, 2 years, and even up to 7 years old (Mueller et al. 2015).

The first 1,000 days of life is a critical window of early childhood growth and development, particularly for the gut microbiome. From conception to two years of age, this development period is strongly supported and influenced by rapid maturation of metabolic, endocrine, neural, and immune pathways. Adverse environmental insults experienced during this crucial period can negatively affect the trajectory of child growth, leading to malnutrition, either in the form of obesity or as undernutrition (Robertson et al. 2018).

There are two major transitions which occur sometime after delivery that accompany the establishment of stable gut microbiota, with the first occurring soon after birth during lactation and the second during the weaning period with the introduction of solid foods along with continued nursing (Robertson et al. 2018). The first transition creates a gut microbiome abundant with genes specific for the infant's digestion of milk proteins. A mother's breastmilk, which contains bacteria and prebiotic human milk oligosaccharides (HMOs), introduces new microbial communities and stimulates the maturation of the neonatal gut microbiome. In contrast, feeding an infant with formula has been found to impair the development of the neonatal immune system and alter metabolism. Breastfed babies tend to have a stable and relatively uniform gut microbiome when compared to babies fed via formula, even when only small amounts of formula are ingested. Evidence suggests that in addition to delivery via C-section and formula feeding, the use of prenatal antibiotics is another action that can compromise the microbial colonization of the newborn gut. It is suggested that these three actions be practiced prudently and followed by measures to restore the natural composition of the microbiome (Mueller et al. 2015).

The introduction of solid foods in an infant's diet activates genes in the gut that can break down complex sugars and starches in plants. This transition to solids initiates a rapid increase in the diversity of the infant microbiota and the evolving microbiome begins the resemblance of a more mature, adult-like state. Any disruption of this normal assembly of the *gut microbiome* may have considerable consequences in the development of autoimmune and metabolic pathologies (Mueller et al. 2015). However, the gut microbiome generally remains stable throughout adulthood in the absence of long-term dietary changes, disease-associated dysbiosis (i.e., gut microbial imbalance or perturbation), or the use of antibiotics (Tanaka and Nakayama 2017).

3.4.2 THE GUT MICROBIOME

Nutritionists continue to assert that a varied and balanced diet is essential for optimal health, and human microbiome researchers emphasize the importance of maintaining the diversity and proper functioning of the *gut microbiome*. Because the gut microbiota sit on the intersection between diet and host genome, they have important implications for food processing and making nutrients available to the host (programming of host metabolism). Bacteria in the gut are responsible for breaking down many of the complex molecules found in foods; the plant cellulose in fruits, vegetables, and nuts would not even be digestible without the microbiota of the gut. Such bacteria harvest energy for themselves from plant-based foods eaten and also break them down into smaller molecules for easier digestion (Microbiome Institute 2020). Perhaps the saying "you are what you eat" has scientific basis, as bacteria in the gut are somewhat of a reflection of the foods that we eat. For example, the guts of African villagers who eat high-fiber diets are dominated by plant-digesting microbiota, which are much rarer in the guts of Europeans who eat high-fat diets (Yong 2010).

Prebiotics and *probiotics* are two of the most widely studied elements in the field of gut microbiota, and specialists stress the importance of including both in our diet to help maintain the balance and diversity of the gut microbiome (ESNM 2019; Mayo Clinic 2019). Prebiotics are specialized plant fibers found naturally in fruits and vegetables and in commercial supplements. They are defined as the indigestible ingredients in food that selectively promote the growth and activity of a limited number of autochthonous bacterial species (i.e., indigenous organisms in soil) (ESNM 2019). Because they aren't digestible, prebiotics pass through the digestive system to become food for bacteria and other microbes (Mayo Clinic 2019). Excessive consumption of prebiotics, however, may lead to discomfort or abdominal bloating in some people, adding to why nutritionists say balance and variety are important. Probiotics come from bacteria traditionally used in biologically active or fermenting food (e.g., yogurt, kombucha, other bacteria-fermented foods, commercial supplements). They, too, provide a range of benefits for the body, to include the maintenance of digestive comfort and the regulation of the immune system. Probiotics can also help balance the gut microbiota when affected by poor diet, infections, some antibiotics treatments, or other external factors such as stress (ESNM 2019).

In addition to its role in the processing of foods and nutrients, the gut microbiome may also have a significant role in metabolizing environmental chemicals to which the host is exposed (Claus et al. 2016). Growing evidence suggests microbial composition of the gut is altered after an exposure. Human exposure to endocrine-disrupting chemicals has been linked to obesity, metabolic syndrome, type 2 diabetes, and others, but it is unclear how the microbiota of the gut interact with environmental chemicals and whether such interactions are relevant for human health (Claus et al. 2016).

3.5 PHARMACOKINETICS

Described as what the body does to a drug, *pharmacokinetics* (PK) is the science of the kinetics of drug *absorption, distribution, metabolism, and excretion* (ADME) (Ahmed 2015), or simply, the fate and transport of a drug into and throughout the human body. It influences the route of administration for a medication, the amount, and frequency of each dose and dosing interval. Note, however, that principles of PK extend beyond pharmaceuticals (i.e., drugs) and can be used to assess ADME of various chemicals in the body. In this section, we discuss physiologically based pharmacokinetics (PBPK) modeling, its potential benefits to metabolomics, and current shortfalls with respect to using PBPK to address gut microbiome effects.

3.5.1 Absorption, Distribution, Metabolism, and Excretion

After released from its dosage form, drugs are absorbed into the surrounding tissue, the body, or both. Once the gastrointestinal tract is reached, the microbes in the region can alter the disposition, efficacy, and toxicity of the drug (Zimmermann et al. 2019). Drug efficiency is affected both directly and indirectly by microbes. Direct effects on drugs are related to binding, degrading, or other modification of the drug, and indirect effects lead to production of microbial metabolites. A quantitative understanding of the factors that determine gut microbiome contributions to metabolism could help explain interpersonal variability in drug response and provide personalized medicine opportunities (Zimmermann et al. 2019).

3.5.2 Physiologically Based Pharmacokinetic (PBPK) Modeling

A more complex type of PK model is a PBPK model which uses a system of differential equations that are parameterized using known physiological values representing key tissue groups and organs involved in the ADME of the drug. Essentially, PBPK models describe the relationship between exposure and tissue dose (NRC 2010). PBPK modeling dates back to at least 1937, with the introduction of multi-compartmental modeling by Teorell (Jones and Rowland-Yeo 2013). Compartments represent actual portions of the body and examples include the lungs, bone, liver, kidneys, gut, and slowly perfused tissue. Such compartments are included if they serve roles in the transport, removal, or accumulation of the drug or chemical. Similar tissues are "lumped" together into a single compartment to reduce model complexity (e.g., muscle, skin, and fat lumped together to form a slowly perfused tissue compartment), unless the physiological, physicochemical, or biochemical parameters have noticeably different effects on chemical uptake and disposition (Krishnan and Andersen 2001). Compartments are connected by systemic circulation, represented by arterial and venous blood flow which facilitate *distribution*. Ordinary differential equations are developed as rate expressions, with a "mass balance" concept followed (i.e., amount of chemical entering the compartment equals the amount leaving or cleared from the compartment plus the amount physically retained within the compartment). Chemical uptake (i.e., amount physically retained) in tissue groups is modeled using applicable rates of diffusion and equilibrium partitioning (NRC 2010). *Metabolism* occurs in various tissues/organs, including the liver. *Excretion* represents the elimination of the drug/chemical, often through exhalation, excretion through the kidneys (urine) or liver (bile), with appropriate rate expressions. Subsequently, the system of differential equations is numerically solved via *in silico* (i.e., computer) to estimate drug (or chemical) concentrations in specific organs or tissues. Further details on PBPK modeling can be found in the literature (Jones and Rowland-Yeo 2013; Krishnan and Andersen 2001; NRC 2010).

Recent advances have led to a better understanding of the diversity and abundance of gut microbial species, which has resulted in a shift in research focus to exploring the effects of an individual's gut microbiome on metabolism and, more specifically, drug metabolism. It is believed that the gut microbiota and environmental chemicals interact with each other in four distinct ways: (1) upon direct ingestion, the gut microbiota metabolizes the chemical; (2) after it's conjugated by the liver, the chemical is metabolized by the microbiota; (3) the chemical interferes with the composition of the gut microbiome; or (4) the chemical interferes with the metabolic activity of the gut microbiome (Claus et al. 2016). Despite the mechanistic details captured in PBPK models, the effects of microbial metabolism are not adequately addressed. Moreover, these PBPK models do not facilitate personalization based on dietary, microbial, or genetic data.

3.6   CONCLUSIONS

The exposure science-related principles explored here, such as metabolomics, the human microbiome and gut microbiome, and PK, stand to be powerful tools for TEH. TEH is a means to integrate and provide occupational, environmental, lifestyle, and clinical exposure-related data to more effectively protect an individual's health. Employers interested in more complete health assessments stand to gain by implementing exposure science and related principles/tools.

REFERENCES

Agin, A., Heintz, D., Ruhland, E., Chao de la Barca, J.M., Zumsteg, J., Moal, V., Guachez, A.S., and I.J. Namer (2016). "Metabolomics - An Overview. From Basic Principles to Potential Biomarkers (Part 1)." *Médecine Nucléaire* **40**(1): 4–10.

Ahmed, T.A. (2015). "Pharmacokinetics of Drugs Following IV Bolus, IV Infusion, and Oral Administration." *Basic Pharmacokinetic Concepts and Some Clinical Applications.* doi:10.5772/61573

Becker, R., Brozena, S., and D. Smith (2003). "What Is Biomonitoring?" *Chemistry Business* **26**: 1–4.

Betts, K., and K. Sawyer (2016). *Use of Metabolomics to Advance Research on Environmental Exposures and the Human Exposome: Workshop in Brief.* Washington, DC: The National Academies Press.

Bradburne, C., Graham, D., Kingston, H.M., Brenner, R., Pamuku, M., and L. Carruth (2015). "Overview of 'Omics Technologies for Military Occupational Health Surveillance and Medicine." *Military Medicine* **180**(suppl_10): 34–48.

Claus, S.P., Guillou, H., and S. Ellero-Simatos (2016). "The Gut Microbiota: A Major Player in the Toxicity of Environmental Pollutants?" *Biofilms and Microbiome* 2(1603): 1–12.

Centers for Disease Control and Prevention (CDC) (2014). "Exposome and Exposomics." https://www.cdc.gov/niosh/topics/exposome/default.html (accessed 11 Jan 2020).

Dias, D.A., and T. Koal (2016). "Progress in Metabolomics Standardisation and Its Significance in Future Clinical Laboratory Medicine." *The Journal of the International Federation of Clinical Chemistry and Laboratory Medicine* 27: 331–343.

DrugBank (2020). DrugBank Webpage. https://www.drugbank.ca/ (accessed on 3 Jan 2020).

Emwas, A-H.M. (2015). "The Strengths and Weaknesses of NMR Spectroscopy and Mass Spectrometry with Particular Focus on Metabolomics Research." *Methods in Molecular Biology* **1277**: 161–193.

European Society of Neurogastroenterology & Motility (ESNM) (2019). "Gut Microbiota for Health." *Diet & Gut Microbiota.* https://www.gutmicrobiotaforhealth.com/en/about-gut-microbiota-info/about-diet-gut-microbiota/ (accessed 11 Jan 2020).

Goff, P., and R. Hartman (2018). Total Exposure Health Strategic Plan FY19–23. Department of Defense/U.S. Air Force Medical Service. https://www.slideshare.net/seniorexec/air-force-medical-service-total-exposure-health-strategic-plan (accessed 2 Apr 2020).

Gowda, G.A., and D. Djukovic (2014). "Overview of Mass Spectrometry-based Metabolomics: Opportunities and Challenges." *Mass Spectrometry in Metabolomics. Methods in Molecular Biology* **1198**: 3–12.

Human Metabolome Database (HMDB) (2020). http://www.hmdb.ca/ (accessed 3 Jan 2020).

Johnson, C.H., and F.J. Gonzalez (2012). "Challenges and Opportunities of Metabolomics." *Journal of Cellular Physiology* **227**(8): 2975–2981.

Jones, H.M., and K. Rowland-Yeo (2013). "Basic Concepts in Physiologically based Pharmacokinetic Modeling in Drug Discovery and Development." *CPT Pharmacometrics and Systems Pharmacology* **2**(8): e63.

Krishnan, K., and M.E. Andersen (2001). "Physiologically Based Pharmacokinetic Modeling in Toxicology," in *Principles and Methods of Toxicology* (4th ed., pp. 193–241). Philadelphia, PA: Taylor & Francis.

Mayo Clinic (2019). Prebiotics, Probiotics and Your Health. https://www.mayoclinic.org/prebiotics-probiotics-and-your-health/art-20390058 (accessed 6 Jun 2019).

Metabolomics Society (2020). http://metabolomicssociety.org/ (accessed 6 Jan 2020).

Metz, T.O., Baker, E.S., Schymanski, E.L., Renslow, R.S., Thomas, D.G., Causon, T.J., Webb, I.K., Hann, S., Smith, R.D., and J.G. Teeguarden (2017). "Integrating Ion Mobility Spectrometry into Mass Spectrometry-based Exposome Measurements: What Can It Add and How Far Can It Go?" *Bioanalysis* **9**(1): 81–98.

Microbiome Institute (2020). Introduction to the Human Microbiome, 2020. http://www.microbiomeinstitute.org/humanmicrobiome (accessed 6 Jan 2020).

Mueller, N.T., Bakacs, E., Combellick, J., Grigoryan, Z., and M.G. Dominguez-Bello. (2015). "The Infant Microbiome Development: Mom Matters." *Trends in Molecular Medicine* **21**(2): 109–117.

National Academies of Sciences, Engineering and Medicine (NAS) (2018). *Environmental Chemicals, the Human Microbiome, and Health Risk: A Research Strategy*. Washington, DC: The National Academies Press. doi:10.17226/24960.

National Institute for Occupational Safety and Health (NIOSH) (2019). Exposome and Exposomics. https://www.cdc.gov/niosh/topics/exposome/default.html (accessed 2 Jan 2020).

National Institutes of Health (NIH) (2012). NIH Announces New Program in Metabolomics. Retrieved January 6, 2020, from https://www.nih.gov/news-events/news-releases/nih-announces-new-program-metabolomics.

National Research Council (NRC) (2010). Committee on Acute Exposure Guideline Levels. Acute Exposure Guideline Levels for Selected Airborne Chemicals: Volume 9. Washington (DC): National Academies Press (US); 7, PBPK Modeling White Paper: Addressing the Use of PBPK Models to Support Derivation of Acute Exposure Guideline Levels.

National Research Council (NRC) (2012). *Exposure Science in the 21st Century: a Vision and a Strategy*. Washington, DC: National Academies Press.

Pacific Northwest National Lab (2017). "Biological Sciences Research Highlights." *For Robust SLIM, an R&D 'Oscar'*. https://www.pnnl.gov/science/highlights/highlight.asp?id=4786 (accessed 11 Jan 2020).

Pacific Northwest National Lab (2020). High-Throughput and Ultra-sensitive Multidimensional Analytical Platform Based on Multiplexed Ion Mobility Spectrometry/Mass Spectrometry. https://availabletechnologies.pnnl.gov/technology.asp?id=316 (accessed 3 Jan 2020).

Patti, G.J., Yanes, O., and G. Siuzdak (2013). "Metabolomics: The Apogee of the Omic Triology." *Nature Reviews Molecular Cell Biology* **13**(4): 263–269.

Robertson, R.C., Manges, A.R., Finlay, B.B., and A.J. Prendergast (2018). "The Human Microbiome and Child Growth - First 1000 Days and Beyond." *Trends in Microbiology* **27**(2): 131–147.

Schrimpe-Rutledge, A.C., Codreanu, S.G., Sherrod, S.D., and J.A. McLean (2016). "Untargeted Metabolomics Strategies - Challenges and Emerging Directions." *Journal of the American Society for Mass Spectrometry* **27**(12): 1897–1905.

Sender, R., Fuchs, S., and R. Milo (2016). "Revised Estimates for the Number of Human and Bacteria Cells in the Body." *PLoS Biol* **14**(8): 1–14.

Swanson, H.I. (2015). "Drug Metabolism by the Host and Gut Microbiota: A Partnership or Rivalry?" *Drug Metabolism and Disposition* **43**(10): 1499–1504.

Tanaka, M., and J. Nakayama (2017). "Development of the Gut Microbiota in Infancy and Its Impact on Health in Later Life." *Allergology International* **66**(4): 515–522.

Teeguarden, J.G., Tan, Y.M., Edwards, S.W., Leonard, J.A., Anderson, K.A., Corley, R.A., Kile, M.L., Simonich, S.M., Stone, D., Tanguay, R.L., Waters, K.M., Harper, S.L., and D.E. Williams. (2016). *Completing the Link between Exposure Science and Toxicology for Improved Environmental Health Decision Making: The Aggregate Exposure Pathway Framework*. Washington, DC: ACS Publications.

Toxic Exposome Database (2020). The Metabolomics Innovation Centre (TMIC). http://www.t3db.ca/ (accessed 3 Jan 2020).

Trivedi, D.K., Hollywood, K.A., and R. Goodacre (2017). "Metabolomics for the Masses: The Future of Metabolomics in a Personalized World." *New Horizons in Translational Medicine* **3**(6):294–305.

Wild, C.P. (2005). "Complementing the Genome with an "Exposome": The Outstanding Challenge of Environmental Exposure Measurement in Molecular Epidemiology." *Cancer Epidemiology Biomarkers & Prevention* **14**(8): 1847–1850.

Wild, C.P. (2012). "The Exposome: From Concept to Utility." *International Journal of Epidemiology* **41**(1): 24–32.

Yong, E. (2010). An Introduction to the Microbiome. National Geographic. https://www.nationalgeographic.com/science/phenomena/2010/08/08/an-introduction-to-the-microbiome (accessed 8 Nov 2018).

Zimmermann, M., Zimmermann-Kogadeeva, M., Wegmann, R., and A.L. Goodman (2019). "Separating Host and Microbiome Contributions to Drug Pharmacokinetics and Toxicity." *Science* **363**(6473).

4 Total Worker Health®
Bridging Worker Exposure and Well-Being

Sara L. Tamers, L. Casey Chosewood, Heidi Hudson, and Chia-Chia Chang
National Institute for Occupational Safety and Health, Centers for Disease Control and Prevention

CONTENTS

DOI: 10.1201/9780429263286-5

4.1 INTRODUCTION

The National Institute for Occupational Safety and Health (NIOSH) of the Centers for Disease Control and Prevention (CDC) defines *Total Worker Health*® (TWH) as policies, programs, and practices that integrate protection from work-related safety and health hazards with promotion of injury and illness prevention efforts to advance worker well-being (NIOSH 2018). The evolving TWH framework has wide-ranging applicability for every safety, health, and well-being issue impacting current and future workers across all occupations and industries, making it relevant to all those who focus on occupational safety and health (Tamers et al. 2019). The NIOSH Office for TWH Coordination and Research Support (Office for TWH) leads and coordinates all activities related to TWH at NIOSH and serves as a conduit for many external TWH efforts.

In this chapter, the authors first describe the main features of the TWH-integrated approach and how it compares to customary siloed approaches in occupational safety and health (OSH) or wellness programs; highlight specific issues relevant to advancing worker well-being; and offer practical, applicable examples and resources. An overview of the 1st and 2nd International Symposia to Advance *Total Worker Health*® is then provided, followed by advances in TWH research and research-to-practice. Next, the authors discuss essential and progressing work in the areas of cumulative risk assessment (CRA) and total exposure health (TEH), and how these closely align with the TWH paradigm. Finally, this chapter concludes with a review of pivotal partnership and stakeholder collaborative activities, central to all TWH endeavors.

4.2 WHAT IS TWH?

The TWH approach prioritizes a hazard-free work environment that protects the safety and health of all workers (NIOSH 2017). Simultaneously, it advocates for integration of all organizational aspects that contribute to worker safety, health, and well-being. TWH tenets focus upon safer, healthier workers, and the important contributions of work design and work organization to the well-being of working populations. It also acknowledges work-related risk factors that contribute to safety and health issues previously considered unrelated to work, such as those that extend beyond the workplace. Establishing workplace policies, programs, and practices that focus on advancing the safety, health, and well-being of the workforce is beneficial for not only the workers but also their families, communities, employers, and the United States as a whole.

4.2.1 COMPARING THE TWH APPROACH

The TWH approach is an integrated, comprehensive, holistic one that differs from the more traditional, siloed, stand-alone approaches often found in worksite wellness or OSH programs (NIOSH 2017). Unlike the TWH framework, current worksite wellness programs sometimes lack scientific rigor; focus exclusively or heavily on individual behavior change instead of addressing the nature, risks, and challenges of work itself on worker health; can be punitive and/or discriminatory; and may be designed with short-term health insurance cost savings for the employer as the primary goal.

In contrast to the TWH approach, some traditional OSH programs have solely focused on safety and health by ensuring that workers are protected from the harms, hazards, and exposures that arise from work itself. Many lack integration with other important elements vital to improving worker health, such as human resources, benefits, employee assistance programs, risk management, and occupational health services. Safety reporting and accountability may also be separated from other worker-centered services. Keeping workers safe is the foundation upon which the TWH approach is built. More than that, however, the TWH approach maintains this focus while integrating additional opportunities for workers to advance their health and well-being.

The scientific rationale behind the increased success of integrating OSH protection activities with health-enhancing ones reflects the nature of challenges facing the future workforce, which are increasingly complex, multifaceted, and wide-ranging. These challenges require all-inclusive strategies. The TWH framework supports a holistic understanding of the factors that contribute to worker well-being and focuses on the ways in which the workplace environment can eliminate or lessen risks and enhance overall worker health, beyond traditional safety and health concerns and their associated approaches. More specifically, studies have shown that implementing a TWH approach to jointly and comprehensively address work-related hazards and other exposures addresses the synergistic risks that exist, leading to improved and sustained outcomes (DeJoy et al. 1993, NIOSH 2012, Sauter 2013, Sorensen et al. 2013).

4.2.2 Issues Relevant to Advancing Worker Well-Being through Total Worker Health®

A number of work-related issues impact worker safety, health, and well-being. Some are long-standing challenges, but others have more recently evolved as a result of emerging forms of employment, changes in the demographic distribution of workers, and new technologies, modifying the nature of work and how it is performed. Figure 4.1 depicts a set of salient, but non-exhaustive, issues pertinent to enhancing worker well-being through the TWH framework. It is categorized as follows (NIOSH 2015a):

- Control of hazards and exposures
- Organization of work
- Built environment supports
- Leadership
- Compensation and benefits
- Community supports
- Changing workforce demographics
- Policy issues
- New employment patterns.

Issues Relevant to Advancing Worker Well-being
Through Total Worker Health®

Control of Hazards and Exposures
- Chemicals
- Physical Agents
- Biological Agents
- Psychosocial Factors
- Human Factors
- Risk Assessment and Risk Management

Organization of Work
- Fatigue and Stress Prevention
- Work Intensification Prevention
- Safe Staffing
- Overtime Management
- Healthier Shift Work
- Reduction of Risks from Long Work Hours
- Flexible Work Arrangements
- Adequate Meal and Rest Breaks

Built Environment Supports
- Healthy Air Quality
- Access to Healthy, Affordable Food Options
- Safe and Clean Restroom Facilities
- Safe, Clean and Equipped Eating Facilities
- Safe Access to the Workplace
- Environments Designed to Accommodate Worker Diversity

Leadership
- Shared Commitment to Safety, Health, and Well-Being
- Supportive Managers, Supervisors, and Executives
- Responsible Business Decision-Making
- Meaningful Work and Engagement
- Worker Recognition and Respect

Compensation and Benefits
- Adequate Wages and Prevention of Wage Theft
- Equitable Performance Appraisals and Promotion
- Work-Life Programs
- Paid Time Off (Sick, Vacation, Caregiving)
- Disability Insurance (Short- & Long-Term)
- Workers' Compensation Benefits
- Affordable, Comprehensive Healthcare and Life Insurance
- Prevention of Cost Shifting between Payers (Workers' Compensation, Health Insurance)
- Retirement Planning and Benefits
- Chronic Disease Prevention and Disease Management
- Access to Confidential, Quality Healthcare Services
- Career and Skills Development

Community Supports
- Healthy Community Design
- Safe, Healthy and Affordable Housing Options
- Safe and Clean Environment (Air and Water Quality, Noise Levels, Tobacco-Free Policies)
- Access to Safe Green Spaces and Non-Motorized Pathways
- Access to Affordable, Quality Healthcare and Well-Being Resources

Changing Workforce Demographics
- Multigenerational and Diverse Workforce
- Aging Workforce and Older Workers
- Vulnerable Worker Populations
- Workers with Disabilities
- Occupational Health Disparities
- Increasing Number of Small Employers
- Global and Multinational Workforce

Policy Issues
- Health Information Privacy
- Reasonable Accommodations
- Return-to-Work
- Equal Employment Opportunity
- Family and Medical Leave
- Elimination of Bullying, Violence, Harassment, and Discrimination
- Prevention of Stressful Job Monitoring Practices
- Worker-Centered Organizational Policies
- Promoting Productive Aging

New Employment Patterns
- Contracting and Subcontracting
- Precarious and Contingent Employment
- Multi-Employer Worksites
- Organizational Restructuring, Downsizing and Mergers
- Financial and Job Security

November 2015
Total Worker Health® is a registered trademark of the US Department of Health and Human Services

FIGURE 4.1 Issues relevant to advancing worker well-being through Total Worker Health®.

To impact the future of work and improve outcomes for the future workforce, it is imperative that these issues be further understood and addressed. This effort involves exploring the linkages between safety and health conditions that may not always arise from work but can be adversely affected by it both directly and indirectly.

4.2.3 WHAT TWH LOOKS LIKE IN PRACTICE

Worker well-being, which is the overall intended outcome of the TWH approach, characterizes quality of life with respect to a worker's health and work-related environmental, organizational, and psychosocial factors (Chari et al. 2018). It is increasingly being recognized as a key element that contributes to an organization's success and, hence, is also of increasing interest to employers (Vitality Institute 2016). In order to advance safety, health, and well-being, careful consideration must be given to the design of work. Jobs must be constructed to protect workers from harm while at the same time providing opportunities for skill utilization and stimulation, positive relationships, flexibility to meet the demands of life and work, and a sense of purpose and meaning (Chalofsky 2010; Day et al. 2014).

More practically speaking, organizations must prioritize multilevel, integrated approaches such as TWH to achieve marked success in preventing safety and health hazards and in promoting worker well-being and productivity. This prioritization must include continued support, commitment, and participation at all levels of leadership. Implementing a TWH approach is an ongoing, day-to-day, transformative, and participatory effort that first and foremost focuses on changes at the organizational level. Workers have a voice in the conditions of their work and are supported in voluntary participation in workplace health-enhancing offerings. Because organizations are not all alike in their size, resources, budget, needs, and workforce, various methods and strategies can help sustain a robust TWH program in any organization. These include but are not limited to

- Controlling hazards and exposures, including psychosocial ones
- Cultivating leadership norms and values that include expectations of healthy supervision, respect for workers, and responsible business decision-making
- Implementing organizational and management policies that offer workers more flexibility and control over their schedules and greater work-life balance
- Building environments that support and maintain safety and health
- Ensuring fair compensation and affordable benefits that recognize and reward workers and enhance worker health
- Creating policies and environments that are inclusive and supportive of workers' diversity
- Using participatory approaches to reorganize or redesign work with reasonable demands
- Providing supervisors with skill-building, training, tools, and resources to motivate, engage, and empower workers and to help nurture and navigate employee-to-employee and supervisor-to-employee relations
- Offering workers opportunities for career advancement, continual learning, and professional development.

Evidence-based templates of TWH programs in practice across varied occupations and industries are publicly available (CPH-NEW 2019; CWHWB 2012; NIOSH 2015, 2016c, 2016d, 2018b; OHWC 2014) and serve as useful tools and resources.

4.3 THE 1ST AND 2ND INTERNATIONAL SYMPOSIA TO ADVANCE *TOTAL WORKER HEALTH*®

To introduce TWH to those with a stake and interest in OSH and worker well-being, and to provide a scientific sharing forum for those already immersed, the Office for TWH held the 1st and 2nd International Symposia to Advance *Total Worker Health*® in 2014 and 2018, respectively, at the National Institutes of Health (NIH) (NIOSH 2018a). The theme of the first symposium was simply "Total Worker Health," and these were its goals:

- Showcase current research that advances the concept of TWH
- Connect stakeholders who share an interest in TWH

- Provide resources and strategies for practitioners working to improve the health, safety, and well-being of workers
- Inform a future research agenda to expand the evidence base for TWH.

The theme of the second symposium was "Work & Well-Being: How Safer, Healthier Work Can Enhance Well-Being," and these were its goals:

- Reaffirm TWH dedication and commitment to the safety and health of workers by prioritizing safety in all jobs
- Redesign the organization of work to promote a workplace environment that optimizes healthy opportunities through leadership, management, and supervision
- Reveal new strategies to redesign work to improve worker well-being through new links and solutions for work and chronic disease risks
- Introduce novel research methods and interventions for advancing TWH.

Both symposia brought together numerous partner organizations and more than 350 national and international scientists and practitioners representing academia, labor, industry, nonprofit organizations, and government. Participants and speakers featured those from human resources, employee benefits, employee assistance, workplace health, health promotion, organized labor, workers' compensation, disability management, emergency response, public health, health policy, health economics, organizational and occupational health psychology, industrial hygiene, and related disciplines. The conference explored areas relevant to the TWH approach, such as TWH frameworks, research methods, integrated approaches, implementation, and evaluation. Practical toolkits were presented for the fields of construction, transportation, agriculture, firefighting and first response, manufacturing, health care, and law enforcement and corrections. Topics focused on the changing workforce, new employment patterns, physical/built environments, community/workplace supports, small businesses, vulnerable populations, organizational policies and practices, healthy leadership, ways to enhance the work-life continuum and work design, advances in return-to-work policies, disability and rehabilitation management, work stress and psychosocial factors, obesity, musculoskeletal conditions, mental health, fatigue, and violence.

Subsequent International Symposia to Advance *Total Worker Health®* are planned. These will continue to build off the previous ones and reflect the growth, development, and evolution of TWH, along with engagement from even more national and international partners and stakeholders.

4.4 ADVANCES IN RESEARCH

Much has been accomplished in TWH research, and future research will continue to build the evidence base and address existing gaps, as was made evident at the first two International Symposia to Advance *Total Worker Health®*. A seminal literature review in 2015 by Anger et al. (2015), which examined outcomes related to both OSH and well-being, found only 17 articles that met those criteria; the researchers concluded that additional research, particularly in the intervention research space, was warranted. These conclusions were mirrored by those from an independent panel of an NIH Pathways to Prevention Workshop, published that same year (NIH 2015). The independent panel looked at known benefits and harms of integrated research interventions, characteristics of effective ones, and factors influencing their degree of effectiveness. In doing so, they also highlighted the need for increased transdisciplinary research and for studies examining the psychosocial work environment and optimization of working conditions.

4.4.1 NATIONAL TOTAL WORKER HEALTH® AGENDA

To advance TWH research and other related domains of the field, the NIOSH Office for TWH published the first National Occupational Research Agenda (NORA) in TWH, entitled National *Total Worker Health*® Agenda (NIOSH 2016b). Aligned with NIOSH tradition, the goal of the National *Total Worker Health*® Agenda was to encourage and stimulate varied stakeholders committed to concomitantly protecting workers from hazards in the workplace and advancing their well-being. These stakeholders include OSH practitioners, wellness professionals, labor organizations, employers, workers, researchers, educators, health care providers, and policy makers. The National *Total Worker Health*® Agenda's four strategic goals, each supported by a number of intermediate and activity/output goals, are in the domains of research, practice, policy, and capacity-building and reflect stakeholder comments, peer-reviewed evidence (Cherniack et al. 2010; Hymel et al. 2011; Sorensen et al. 2011), and findings from two central TWH workshops (IOM 2014; NIH 2015):

1. Research: Advance and conduct etiologic, surveillance, and intervention research that builds the evidence base for effectively integrating protection from work-related safety and health hazards with promotion of injury and illness prevention efforts to advance worker well-being.
2. Practice: Increase the implementation of evidence-based programs and practices that integrate protection from work-related safety and health hazards with promotion of injury and illness prevention efforts to advance worker well-being.
3. Policy: Increase adoption of policies that integrate protection from work-related safety and health hazards with promotion of injury and illness prevention efforts to advance worker well-being.
4. Capacity building: Build capacity to strengthen the TWH workforce and TWH field to support the development, growth, and maintenance of policies, programs, and practices that integrate protection from work-related safety and health hazards with promotion of injury and illness prevention efforts to advance worker well-being.

Realization of these goals by partners over the next decade (2016–2026) will better safeguard the safety, health, and well-being of workers, support overall workforce vitality, and foster US economic prosperity.

4.4.2 TOTAL WORKER HEALTH® RESEARCH METHODOLOGY WORKSHOP

Motivated by the described research gaps, in 2017, the NIOSH Office for TWH and the Healthier Workforce Center of the Midwest convened the *Total Worker Health®* Research Methodology Workshop, which assessed methodological and measurement issues for TWH intervention research. The objectives of this workshop were sever-alfold. Per prior expert recommendations, the first intent was to expand research and evaluation design options to include a range of rigorous methodologies and develop a core set of measures and outcomes to incorporate in all integrated intervention studies (NIOSH 2015). The second was to apply and develop rigorous, standardized methods for TWH interventions, as outlined in the National *Total Worker Health®* Agenda (NIOSH 2016b). The third was to fill gaps in the TWH intervention research space, as advocated by Anger et al. (2015) and Feltner et al. (2016), by focusing on methodological and measurement issues and creating and prioritizing common and comparable TWH-relevant measures and outcomes. Tamers et al. (2018) published the workshop findings, summarizing TWH research methodological and measurement approaches currently in use and novel ones that experts believe have the potential to advance the field through rigorous and repeatable TWH intervention research (Tamers et al. 2018).

4.4.3 WORKER WELL-BEING FRAMEWORK

The need to focus on and develop measures that comprehensively assess worker well-being and, in turn, advance the TWH scientific evidence base has gained increasing attention. To this end, the NIOSH Office for TWH partnered with the RAND Corporation to develop a framework for worker well-being (Chari et al. 2018). Using multidisciplinary literature reviews and an expert panel, a worker well-being model with five major domains was created:

1. Workplace physical environment and safety climate
2. Workplace policies and culture
3. Health status
4. Work evaluation and experience
5. Home, community, and society.

The framework conceptualizes worker well-being as a subjective and objective phenomenon that is inclusive of experiences both within and beyond the work context. This effort lays the foundation for subsequent well-being measurement activities and will provide useful tools, such as a worker well-being survey instrument (under development), that will prove pivotal in helping to better measure and advance worker well-being.

4.4.4 CENTERS OF EXCELLENCE FOR TWH

Though NIOSH leads the TWH program and conducts associated research, TWH research and related activities are conducted predominantly by six NIOSH-funded Centers of Excellence for TWH (Figure 4.2): Healthier Workforce Center of the

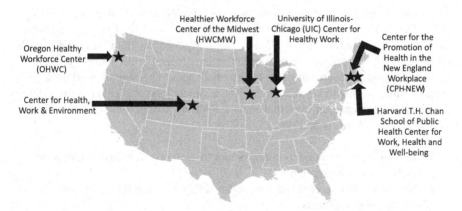

Centers of Excellence for *Total Worker Health*®

FIGURE 4.2 Locations of Centers of Excellence for Total Worker Health®.

Midwest (University of Iowa); Center for the Promotion of Health in the New England Workplace (University of Massachusetts Lowell and University of Connecticut); T.H. Chan School of Public Health's Center for Work, Health, and Well-Being (Harvard University); Oregon Healthy Workforce Center (Oregon Health and Science University); Center for Health, Work & Environment (University of Colorado); and Center for Healthy Work (University of Illinois–Chicago) (NIOSH 2018b). These academic institutions are uniquely qualified to be among the top leaders in TWH research, and they are conduits for research-to-practice efforts that hold promise to impact the safety, health, well-being, and productivity of the US workforce. They use multidisciplinary research projects—including intervention-focused research, outreach and education, and evaluation activities—to improve our understanding of which evidence-based solutions work.

4.5 RESEARCH TO PRACTICE

As the interests of researchers and practitioners in varied disciplines (such as OSH, medicine, psychology, and public health) have converged, awareness has increased of the potential for work to contribute positively to safety, health, and well-being (Chari et al. 2018; Day et al. 2014; Hymel et al. 2011; NIOSH 2016a; Sauter & Hurrell 2017) and for this to be reflected through practical application. Although the scientific evidence base is still evolving, the uptake of the TWH concept has gained substantial traction among leaders and practitioners in OSH and other related fields who are interested in using, adopting, and adapting knowledge, interventions, and resources within the workplace. To respond to this demand, the NIOSH Office for TWH and its partners have developed practice-based tools, promising practices, and frameworks to guide the development and expansion of organizational cultures of safety, health, and well-being (NIOSH 2016c, 2016d). Many more such TWH resources are available than this chapter allows mentioning. Below, the authors highlight two.

4.5.1 Fundamentals of Total Worker Health® Approaches

A practice-oriented document published by the NIOSH Office for TWH in 2016, *Fundamentals of Total Worker Health® Approaches: Essential Elements for Advancing Worker Safety, Health, and Well-Being* (familiarly known as *Fundamentals*), is designed to help organizations identify and address job-related factors that may be contributing to health challenges. This unique workbook provides organizations with key practical self-assessment tools and guidance to develop actionable implementation steps that apply a TWH approach. *Fundamentals* focuses on five defining elements of TWH:

1. Demonstrating leadership commitment to worker safety and health at all levels of the organization
2. Designing work to eliminate or reduce safety and health hazards and promote worker well-being
3. Promoting and supporting worker engagement throughout program development
4. Ensuring the confidentiality and privacy of workers during program design and implementation
5. Integrating relevant systems to advance worker well-being.

4.5.2 Hierarchy of Controls Applied to NIOSH Total Worker Health®

To link traditional OSH and TWH approaches, the NIOSH Office for TWH created a model to augment the traditional hierarchy of controls and provide a conceptual framework for prioritizing efforts to advance worker well-being. The Hierarchy of Controls Applied to NIOSH *Total Worker Health®* (Figure 4.3) guides researchers and practitioners in implementing workplace safety and health policies, programs, and practices that both protect workers and advance their health and well-being by

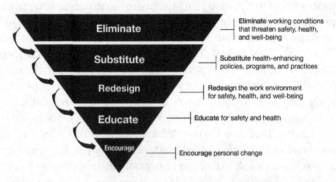

FIGURE 4.3 Hierarchy of Controls Applied to NIOSH Total Worker Health®.

improving the conditions of their work. The emphasis on addressing system-level or environmental determinants of health before individual-level approaches is a key tenet of the TWH approach.

4.6 DETERMINING OVERALL RISK AND EXPOSURE FOR WORKER SAFETY, HEALTH, AND WELL-BEING

Today's environmental, public, and occupational health professionals have a greater understanding of the health risks associated with multiple stressors encountered, either simultaneously or in sequence, over the life span of individuals. They can also better estimate not only the additive or exponential impact of individual stressors but also the interaction between and among risk factors. Below, we highlight two approaches closely aligned with the TWH framework designed to assess overall risk and exposure.

4.6.1 CUMULATIVE RISK ASSESSMENT

The US Environmental Protection Agency defines cumulative risk as the combination of risks posed by aggregate exposures (exposure by all routes and pathways and from all sources of each given agent or stressor) to multiple agents or stressors (EPA 2003). Application of CRA principles in the work setting should result in better understanding of complex exposures and health risks experienced by workers, with the potential to inform more effective controls and improvements in safety and health risk management overall. Such an approach, which parallels the TWH framework, may be especially important for helping employers prioritize the risks facing workers and for aligning strategies that address occupational as well as personal and community risks (Fox et al. 2018). The application of CRA approaches can also result in added appreciation of more complex exposures and, where applicable, assist in assigning or attributing proportions of risk across multiple domains. This has the potential to improve overall safety and health risk management, increase its efficiency, and provide greater insight into the connectedness of work and non-work risks that may lead to earlier detection, screening, and intervention for disease (Fox et al. 2018).

This said, because of the power dynamics of the workplace, employers addressing personal risk factors may inadvertently create additional issues by placing greater onus on workers as more responsibility shifts to controlling risks outside the workplace. The potential for discrimination against certain workers due to personal, genetic, or behavioral risk factors may increase; in addition, employer intervention into personal life carries risks around privacy and autonomy. Supplementary health evaluations, screenings, and monitoring may also result, as risk factors are more readily recognized. Therefore, caution should be taken to ensure that these additional burdens do not outweigh the potential benefits that may accrue for workers through this broadened approach (Fox et al. 2018). The TWH paradigm emphasizes the need to address and modify aspects of the work organization and work itself for improved worker safety, health, and well-being, and is counter to any approach that would shift that responsibility onto the worker or blame the worker for any personal health challenges.

4.6.2 Total Exposure Health

TEH is an approach that assesses workers' exposure to all hazards at work (environmental and lifestyle) and integrates these with wellness efforts to better safeguard workers' long-term health (Zielhuis 1985). Exposure, as similarly gauged and evaluated in the TWH framework, is by nature broad and encompassing, accounting for legacy physical and chemical hazards as well as those seen in the evolving economy. Work stress, work organization, less formal and less secure employment arrangements, shifts in benefits provided, emerging technologies, and global and competitive demands all represent growing areas of risk to worker health and well-being. Within the context of TWH, TEH represents the cumulative lifetime experience of risk conditions, influences, and circumstances that impact an individual worker's health and well-being. It recognizes the potential of well-designed work and secure employment as sources of gain for health and well-being.

Although recognition of and action upon the origins of exposure are important factors to consider, TWH interventions do not artificially divide these between work and non-work. Rather, they recognize the interaction and influences of each on the other and look for integrated solutions to safeguarding work and well-being in a holistic way. This approach also recognizes the frequent uncertainty as to the absolute attribution of exposures or the full causality of outcomes.

In the characterization of total exposure over a lifetime, workplace exposures provide significant contribution to overall health, including important influence on disability and life span. Most workers in the United States vastly underestimate the risks they face related to their work exposures, especially in the.domains of motor vehicle accidents, cardiovascular disease, cancer, and respiratory health (Takala et al. 2012). Additionally, each worker brings in her or his own unique exposure history and physiological makeup to work each day, including genetic and epigenetic (the interaction between environmental influences and genetics) factors. These differences in predispositions mean that some workers may be more susceptible than other workers to adverse health outcomes from workplace exposures.

4.6.3 TWH, CRA, and TEH

The TWH program, as envisioned by NIOSH, promotes a more integrated approach to worker safety and health and is complementary to the CRA and TEH approaches. As illustrated in this chapter, the TWH framework integrates multiple efforts to advance the health of workers, from the traditional control of workplace hazards and exposures to addressing work organization, compensation and benefits, work-life management, organizational culture and leadership, and the community and built environments (NIOSH 2015). The focus on prevention, inherent in the CRA and TEH strategies, emphasizes system-level or environmental determinants of health before moving to evaluation of individual-level approaches. This is also a crucial tenet of the TWH approach and is fully aligned with traditional industrial hygiene and OSH priorities, as shown on the traditional hierarchy of controls.

The TWH approach advocates that workers are entitled to a fair and complete assessment of the risks and exposures they face during all periods of employment.

This important transparency of the health consequences of work should drive all developments around CRA and TEH estimates and related interventions as well. Workers should have access to comprehensive risk and exposure information from the very beginning of employment and periodic updates, particularly if the facts change over time. Such information should be used in negotiations around conditions of work, hours, shift requirements, wages, and other compensation for higher-hazard duties.

Evaluating total risk and exposure may be daunting in its complexity and immensity, but this does not change the significance of the task and should not impede its pursuit, nor deter organizations from prioritizing it in the workplace. Although more research is needed, emerging CRA models and work in the area of TEH hold valuable promise and currently provide frameworks for the assessment of multiple risk factors emanating from various domains. Ideally, these will enable employers and workers to develop more effective controls and prevention strategies, bridging exposure and well-being—the very mission of TWH.

4.7 PARTNERSHIP AND STAKEHOLDER INVOLVEMENT

Partners and stakeholders across occupations and industries, both domestically and internationally, have been heavily engaged in the development and growth of the TWH approach. As discussed earlier in this chapter, to move the field forward, the National *Total Worker Health*® Agenda set TWH goals to be met over the coming years in large part by external parties, recognizing that stakeholder ownership is needed to maximize progress in the TWH field. This aligns with NIOSH's history and commitment of having tripartite involvement in all its activities. Undeniably, achieving worker safety, health, and well-being requires buy-in, ownership, and action by existing and new stakeholders. Thus, it is fitting to conclude this chapter with these important relationships. The next section particularly emphasizes two TWH partnership groupings and highlights several significant TWH collaborative activities.

4.7.1 NIOSH TWH Affiliates

In addition to the NIOSH-funded Centers of Excellence, the NIOSH TWH Affiliate program serves as an invaluable effort in promoting and increasing capacity by conducting TWH research, translation, and training activities. Although they receive no funding from NIOSH, the NIOSH TWH Affiliates are leaders in the TWH field and conduct myriad activities that help support and move forward the TWH approach, each in a unique way. The NIOSH Office for TWH established this network (of now 45 Affiliates) to recognize not-for-profit, labor, academic, and government organizations that are advancing the TWH framework.

The academic NIOSH TWH Affiliates conduct research that contributes to the goals of the National *Total Worker Health*® Agenda and to our knowledge and understanding about exposures to physical and psychological safety and health hazards, worker well-being, and organization of work. They are also among the leaders in the United States providing TWH training to students and professionals from a diversity of disciplines, thereby building the future TWH workforce. Employer NIOSH TWH Affiliates partner with researchers to provide living laboratories for evaluating workplace policy and practice interventions. By putting research findings into practice, they apply the TWH framework to their workforce, facilitate uptake of TWH recommendations and guidance, and share lessons learned from which promising practices can be developed. Not-for-profit NIOSH TWH Affiliates, such as regional employer coalitions, provide opportunities for organizations to learn from one another about strategies for evaluating exposure and improving worker health. Labor union NIOSH TWH Affiliates serve as the worker voice and share the priorities and experiences of workers in the planning, implementation, and evaluation of TWH activities. Professional association/society NIOSH TWH Affiliates are important in translating, communicating, and sharing TWH messages with their members, who are professionals in a variety of fields, including industrial hygiene, safety, and medicine. Finally, industry association NIOSH TWH Affiliates reach a vast audience of organizations with a shared interest. They help translate materials, train practitioners, and identify promising practices within industries or sectors.

Though NIOSH is greatly engaged with external entities, it is encouraging that many partnerships take place exclusively among external stakeholders. For instance, one of the NIOSH TWH Affiliates (the SAIF Corporation, a workers compensation provider in Oregon), one of the six Centers of Excellence for TWH (the Oregon Healthy Workforce Center), and the Oregon Occupational Safety and Health Administration created an alliance with a goal of drawing on the strengths of each organization to expand the knowledge and application of TWH principles beyond the workplace (35). This alliance will use data to identify workplace exposures, provide guidance for recognizing and preventing industry-specific hazards, share information about the TWH approach, and encourage adoption of TWH strategies in the work environment.

4.7.2 COLLABORATIVE ACTIVITIES

By increasing the public's awareness and understanding of the interplay between workplace exposures and health, more innovation and adoption can occur to promote worker well-being. In addition to the need and merit of developing external partnerships as discussed thus far, strategic partnerships are useful for increasing the TWH knowledge base through co-sponsorship of workshops and meetings and collaborations on other activities and outputs.

One seminal example is a public workshop, *"Total Worker Health*®: Promising and Best Practices in the Integration of Occupational Safety and Health Protection with Health Promotion in the Workplace," which the NIOSH Office for TWH and the National Academy of Medicine convened to identify existing and best practices in small, medium, and large workplaces (IOM 2014). Workshop discussions and panel recommendations led to a summary report identifying steps for going forward, such as prioritizing leadership recognition of the importance of TWH in organizational culture and strategy.

Additionally, the NIOSH Office for TWH teamed up with Gallup to analyze the Sharecare Well-Being Index to explore the relationship between well-being and working conditions. The findings derived from these shared activities resulted in new knowledge about associations between workforce participation and healthy worker biases, skill utilization and employee health, and trust in the work environment and cardiovascular health (Alterman et al. 2019; Fujishiro 2017; Johnson et al. 2017; Stiehl et al. 2019).

Another instance of the long-lasting impact, benefit, and forward momentum garnered by developing these collaborations is exemplified well by the NIOSH Office for TWH's co-sponsorship of the 2015 NIH Pathways to Prevention Workshop *Total Worker Health®*: What's Work Got to Do With It?, with the NIH's Office of Disease Prevention and National Heart, Lung, and Blood Institute (NHLBI), mentioned previously. With over 700 registered attendees, this workshop partnership provided the opportunity to engage new, diverse audiences about the TWH framework, and it became the largest TWH event to date. Working in partnership with NIH leveraged new resources, created novel and significant initiatives, and translated into subsequent joint ventures. To this point, the workshop led to a review of the literature that identified research gaps, which in turn led to a convened independent panel that issued vital recommendations to move the TWH research base forward (Curry et al. 2015; Feltner et al. 2016). Two of those recommendations were later addressed in the *Total Worker Health®* Research Methodology Workshop, noted earlier, and additional collaborative endeavors are being planned.

Finally, a concluding, central illustration of the significant role of partners and stakeholders is in addressing existing gaps in TWH workforce development. The Centers of Excellence for TWH, NIOSH-funded Education and Research Centers (ERCs), and NIOSH TWH Affiliates are frontrunners responding to the need to develop, train, and grow practitioners who are knowledgeable and skilled in the TWH framework. These entities have worked intimately with the NIOSH Office for TWH to initiate the process of identifying core competencies, engaging other stakeholders, developing curricula, integrating the TWH framework in existing OSH or health education programs, and creating new programs. Universities that currently have or are developing TWH-relevant certificates are Northern Kentucky University (Alterman et al. 2019); Oregon and Portland State Universities, in collaboration with the SAIF Corporation; the University of Colorado (Johnson et al. 2017); the University of North Carolina–Chapel Hill; and Western Kentucky University.

4.8 CONCLUSION

The TWH framework is a responsive constellation of policy enhancements, leadership, and management practices and programs that create a robust culture of safety, as well as greater health opportunities, through healthier work design and improved workplace strategies. The TWH approach champions efforts that are voluntary and participatory in nature, and places emphasis on organizational and system-wide factors as the starting point for improvements rather than focusing first on individual behavior change efforts (Chosewood and Tamers in press). As TWH principles are applied, worker centricity in design and implementation are paramount. To holistically assess and intervene for worker protection, those concerned with the safety, health, and well-being of workers must appreciate the totality of risks and exposures borne by workers. Doing so requires a seamless, integrated interplay between multiple parties responsible for the safety and health outcomes of all workers, which is fundamental to the development of the TWH approach.

REFERENCES

Alterman T, Tsai R, Ju J, Kelly K. Trust in the Work Environment and Cardiovascular Disease Risk: Findings from the Gallup-Sharecare Well-being Index. *International Journal of Environmental Research and Public Health*. 2019;16:230.

Anger WK, Elliot DL, Bodner T, et al. Effectiveness of Total Worker Health Interventions. *Journal of Occupational Health Psychology*. 2015;20:226–247.

Center for Work Health & Well-Being. SafeWell Practice Guidelines: An Integrated Approach to Worker Health. http://centerforworkhealth.sph.harvard.edu/resources/safewell-resources (accessed February 5, 2019). 2012.

Chalofsky N. *Meaningful Workplaces: Reframing How and Where We Work*. San Francisco, CA: Jossey-Bass; 2010.

Chang CC. TWH Exclusive: New Alliance in Oregon Aims to Promote TWH Statewide. TWH in Action! https://www.cdc.gov/niosh/twh/newsletter/twhnewsv6n2.html (accessed February 5, 2019). 2017.

Chari R, Chang CC, Sauter SL, et al. Expanding the Paradigm of Occupational Safety and Health: A New Framework for Worker Well-being. *Journal of Occupational Environmental Medicine*. 2018;60(7):589–593.

Cherniack M, Henning R, Merchant J, et al. Statement on National WorkLife Priorities. *American Journal of Industrial Medicine*. 2010;54: 10–20.

Chosewood CL, Tamers SL, eds. Patty's Industrial Hygiene: An Introduction to Total Worker Health® for Today's Industrial Hygienist (7th ed). Somerset, NJ: Wiley and Sons (in press).

Curry S, Bradley C, Grossman D, Hubbard R, et al. NIH Pathways to Prevention Workshop Total Worker Health®: What's Work Got to Do with It? https://prevention.nih.gov/sites/default/files/documents/twh/twh-final-report-2016.pdf. 2015.

Day A, Kelloway E, Hurrell J, eds. Workplace Well-being: How to Build Psychologically Healthy Workplaces. Hoboken, NJ: Wiley-Blackwell, 2014.

DeJoy D, Southern D. An Integrative Perspective on Work-site Health Promotion. *Journal of Occupational Medicine*. 1993;35:1221–1230.

Environmental Protection Agency. Framework for Cumulative Risk Assessment. http://cfpub.epa.gov/ncea/cfm/recordisplay.cfm?deid=54944, EPA/600/P-02/001F. National Center for Environmental Assessment, Risk Assessment Forum, U.S. Environmental Protection Agency. Washington, DC. 2003.

Feltner C, Peterson K, Palmieri Weber R, et al. The Effectiveness of Total Worker Health Interventions: A Systematic Review for a National Institutes of Health Pathways to Prevention Workshop. *Annals of Internal Medicine*. 2016;165:262–269.

Fox MA, Spicer K, Chosewood LC, Susi P, et al. Implications of Applying Cumulative Risk Assessment to the Workplace. *Environment International*. 2018;115:230–238.

Fujishiro K. "Doing What I Do Best": The Association between Skill Utilization and Employee Health with Healthy Behavior as a Mediator. *Social Science & Medicine*. 2017;175:235–243.

Hymel PA, Loeppke RR, Baase CM, et al. Workplace Health Protection and Promotion: A New Pathway for a Healthier--And Safer--Workforce. *Journal of Occupational Environment Medicine*. 2011;53:695–702.

Institute of Medicine. *Promising and Best Practices in Total Worker Health: Workshop Summary*. Washington, DC: The National Academies Press. http://www.iom.edu/Activities/Environment/TotalWorkerHealth/2014-MAY-22.aspx. 2014.

Johnson CY, Rocheleau CM, Lawson CC, et al. Factors Affecting Workforce Participation and Healthy Worker Biases in U.S. Women and Men. *Annals of Epidemiology*. 2017;27:558–562. e552.

National Institute for Occupational Safety and Health. 1st and 2nd International Symposia to Advance Total Worker Health®. https://www.cdc.gov/niosh/TWH/symposium.html (accessed February 5, 2019). 2014, 2018.

National Institute for Occupational Safety and Health, Caruso C, Geiger-Brown J, et al. NIOSH Training for Nurses on Shift Work and Long Work Hours. DHHS (NIOSH) Publication No. 2015–115, Cincinnati, OH. www.cdc.gov/niosh/docs/2015-115/.

National Institute for Occupational Safety and Health. Centers of Excellence. https://www.cdc.gov/niosh/twh/centers.html (accessed February 5, 2019). 2018.

National Institute for Occupational Safety and Health. Healthy Work Design and Well-being Program. https://www.cdc.gov/niosh/programs/hwd/default.html (accessed February 19, 2019). 2016.

National Institute for Occupational Safety and Health. Issues Relevant to Advancing Worker Well-being through Total Worker Health. https://www.cdc.gov/niosh/twh/pdfs/TWH-Issues-4x3_10282015_final.pdf (accessed February 5, 2019). 2015.

National Institute for Occupational Safety and Health. National Occupational Research Agenda (NORA)/National Total Worker Health® Agenda (2016–2026): A National Agenda to Advance Total Worker Health® Research, Practice, Policy, and Capacity. Cincinnati: OH, U.S. Department of Health and Human Services, Centers for Disease Control and Prevention, National Institute for Occupational Safety and Health, DHHS (NIOSH) Publication 2016–114. 2016.

National Institute for Occupational Safety and Health. Promising Practices for Total Worker Health. https://www.cdc.gov/niosh/twh/practices.html (accessed February 5, 2019). 2016.

National Institute for Occupational Safety and Health. Research Compendium; The NIOSH Total Worker Health™ Program: Seminal Research Papers 2012. Cincinnati, OH: U.S. Department of Health and Human Services, Centers for Disease Control and Prevention, National Institute for Occupational Safety and Health, DHHS (NIOSH) Publication No. 2012–146. 2012.

National Institute for Occupational Safety and Health. Total Worker Health. https://www.cdc.gov/niosh/twh/ (accessed February 5, 2019). 2018.

National Institute for Occupational Safety and Health. Total Worker Health Tools: Let's Get Started. https://www.cdc.gov/niosh/twh/letsgetstarted.html (accessed February 5, 2019). 2016.

National Institute for Occupational Safety and Health. What Is Total Worker Health? https://www.cdc.gov/niosh/twh/totalhealth.html (accessed February 5, 2019). 2017.

National Institutes of Health and National Institute for Occupational Safety and Health. Pathways to Prevention Workshop: Total Worker Health: What's Work Got to Do with It? https://prevention.nih.gov/programs-events/pathways-to-prevention/workshops/total-worker-health (accessed February 22, 2018). 2015.

Oregon Healthy Workforce Center. COMPASS Resources. https://www.ohsu.edu/xd/research/centers-institutes/oregon-institute-occupational-health-sciences/oregon-healthy-workforce-center/projects/compass/resources/index.cfm (accessed February 5, 2019). 2014.

Sauter SL. Integrative Approaches to Safeguarding the Health and Safety of Workers. *Industrial Health*. 2013;51:559–561.

Sauter SL, Hurrell J. Occupational Health Contributions to the Development and Promise of Occupational Health Psychology. *Journal of Occupational Health Psychology*. 2017;22:251–258.

Sorensen G, Landsbergis P, Hammer L, et al. Preventing Chronic Disease in the Workplace: A Workshop Report and Recommendations. *American Journal of Public Health.* 2011;101 Suppl 1:S196–S207.

Sorensen G, McLellan D, Dennerlein JT, et al. Integration of Health Protection and Health Promotion: Rationale, Indicators, and Metrics. *Journal of Occupational Environmental Medicine.* 2013;55:S12–18.

Stiehl E, Jones-Jack NH, Baron S, Muramatsu N. Worker Well-being in the United States: Finding Variation across Job Categories. *Preventive Medicine Reports.* 2019;13:5–10.

Takala J, Hamalainen P, Saarela KL, et al. Global Estimates of the Burden of Injury and Illness at Work in 2012. *Journal of Occupational Environmental Hygiene.* 2014;11:326–337.

Tamers SL, Chosewood LC, Childress A, et al. Total Worker Health((R)) 2014(-)2018: The Novel Approach to Worker Safety, Health, and Well-being Evolves. *International Journal of Environmental Research Public Health.* 2019;16.

Tamers SL, Goetzel R, Kelly KM, et al. Research Methodologies for Total Worker Health®: Proceedings from a Workshop. *Journal of Occupational and Environmental Medicine.* 2018;60:968–978.

The Center for the Promotion of Health in the New England Workplace (CPH-NEW). Total Worker Health for Employers. https://www.uml.edu/Research/CPH-NEW/Worker/ (accessed February 5, 2019).

Vitality Institute. Reporting on Health: A Roadmap for Investors, Companies, and Reporting Platforms. www.thevitalityinstitute.org/healthreporting (accessed September 3, 2018). 2016.

Zielhuis RL. Total Exposure and Workers' Health. *The Annals of Occupational Hygiene.* 1985;29:463–475.

5 Industrial Hygiene
A Foundational Role in Total Exposure Health

Dirk P. Yamamoto
Wright-Patterson Air Force Base

CONTENTS

DOI: 10.1201/9780429263286-6

5.1 INTRODUCTION

Total Exposure Health (TEH) has origins as a US Air Force and Air Force Medical Service concept (see Chapter 1). To summarize, TEH recognizes that an individual, and his/her health, is influenced by more than just an occupational exposure. The health outcomes of each of us are, in theory, influenced by our occupational, environmental, and lifestyle-related exposures. In addition, our genetic profile can leave each of us predisposed for certain health outcomes, good or bad. TEH is individual-centric, due to the differences in exposure and genetic profile. It empha-sizes that *sensor technology*, i.e., sampling and measurement, will be increasingly important to assess such a large set of exposures. It is theorized that when individual-centric exposure and genetic data are merged, more *personalized healthcare* is pos-sible and will increase the well-being of individuals through prevention and other interventions.

Interestingly, *industrial hygiene* (IH) professionals have extensive skills related to assessment of occupational exposures and, arguably, many environmental expo-sures. These skills stand to be very important to TEH, with its holistic approach on assessing exposures around the clock. More specifically, industrial hygienists have practical skills in instruments with sensors aboard, designed to quantify exposures. Industrial hygienists stand to play a foundational role in TEH, and this chapter will cover the basics of the profession and will conclude with further discussion on how IH professionals can help with TEH and some challenges that might occur.

5.2 WHAT IS INDUSTRIAL HYGIENE?

5.2.1 DEFINITION OF INDUSTRIAL HYGIENE

Traditionally focused on occupational exposures, i.e., those exposures occurring in an employer's workplace, IH is a long-standing profession designed to protect worker health. The term *industrial hygiene* was likely first coined in the early 20th century, but examples of professionals looking out for the health of industrial workers dates back many centuries. Hazards faced by workers are generally classified as chemi-cal, biological, or physical stressors. Examples of stressors include chemical vapors, gases, mold, asbestos noise, and ionizing radiation. Stressors can pose a hazard via various pathways, including inhalation, ingestion, and dermal absorption.

The American Industrial Hygiene Association (AIHA®) defines "industrial hygiene" as a "science and art devoted to the anticipation, recognition, evaluation, prevention, and control of those environmental factors or stresses arising in or from the workplace which may cause sickness, impaired health and wellbeing, or signifi-cant discomfort among workers or among citizens of the community" (AIHA 2019). The profession is often summarized by the *industrial hygiene decision framework*, which has tenets of *anticipation, recognition, evaluation, and control* (AREC) of occupational and environmental hazards. In more recent history, a fifth tenet, *confirm*, has been added to represent the importance of validating that exposure assessments of those exposures remain correct (Jahn et al. 2015).

5.2.2 OSHA Compliance

Additionally, the practice of IH is integral to compliance with safety and health regulatory bodies, such as the US Department of Labor's Occupational Safety and Health Administration (OSHA). As a result of the Occupational Safety and Health (OSH) Act of 1970, OSHA was created to assure safe and healthful working conditions by setting and enforcing standards, and by providing training, outreach, education, and other assistance (OSHA 1970). Known as the General Duty Clause, section 5(a)(1) of the OSH Act states that each employer "shall furnish to each of his employees employment and a place of employment which are free from recognized hazards that are causing or are likely to cause death or serious physical harm to his employees" (OSHA 1970). Industrial hygienists and safety professionals work to ensure employers are in compliance with OSHA and, in doing so, help protect workers under those employers. Further discussion on OSHA appears in Section 5.3.3.4.

5.3 HISTORY OF INDUSTRIAL HYGIENE

5.3.1 Early Names in IH

Centuries before the term "industrial hygiene" was even coined, there were numerous examples of professionals concerned about the health of industrial workers. Perhaps the earliest records of occupational disease were from Hippocrates, who around 370 BCE documented his observations regarding lead poisoning (Perkins 1997). In 50 CE, Pliny the Elder, a Roman author, philosopher, and army commander, recommended the use of animal bladders as pseudo-industrial "respirators" to protect against inhalation of toxic dusts from mining operations. In 1556, *De Re Metallica*, by Georgius Agricola (1494–1555), was published posthumously (Perkins 1997). It was believed to be the first comprehensive book on the mining industry based on field research and observation ("the scientific approach") (Hoover and Hoover 1950). In the book are detailed descriptions of industrial processes, prevalent diseases, types of accidents, and preventive measures including rudimentary ventilation systems (i.e., "engineering controls") (Blunt et al. 2011). With detailed hand-drawn pictures of mining and metallurgy, Agricola's book remained the only authoritative reference on mining and metallurgy for over 200 years.

Other notable names important to the history of IH (and occupational medicine) include Paracelsus, Ramazzini, and Percivall Pott. In 1567, Paracelsus ("Father of Toxicology") described mercury poisoning in extensive detail (Anna 2011). Later in 1713, Bernardino Ramazzini published what is believed to be the first book on occupational diseases, *De Morbis Artificum Diatriba* (Discourse on the Disease of Workers) (Blunt et al. 2011; Perkins 1997). In his book, Ramazzini described diseases of certain types of workers, such as seafarers, soldiers, salt workers, lawyers, and others. His descriptions included details on the conditions and hazards associated with the various diseases, along with principles to prevent disease (Perkins 1997). Ramazzini is credited with having the intuition to ask the important question, "what is your trade?" to better understand worker exposures and resulting diseases. In 1775, Percivall Pott, an English surgeon, deduced that scrotal cancer among

English chimney sweeps (a.k.a. Chimney sweepers' carcinoma) was due to exposure to soot from coal combustion (Anna 2011).

Dr. Alice Hamilton (1881–1972) is widely regarded as a pioneer in both IH and occupational medicine. Although a physician, she is often regarded as being the first industrial hygienist as she pioneered and vigorously promoted *hygiene in industry* (Perkins 1997). During her career, Hamilton studied diseases associated with lead, mercury, carbon monoxide, aluminum, beryllium, cadmium, chromium, benzene, methanol, carbon disulfide, and synthetic rubber exposures. One of her greatest contributions was her study of "phossy-jaw", the extremely disfiguring disease of the human jawbone due to exposure to phosphorus during the manufacturing of matches (Perkins 1977). Her book, *Exploring the Dangerous Trades* (Hamilton 1943), chronicles many of her occupational health findings during her career and remains a classic publication for the IH profession.

5.3.2 ACADEMIC PROGRAMS AND ABET

The first academic program for IH was developed at Harvard University in 1918 and, coincidentally, is the university where Dr. Alice Hamilton became the first female faculty member (Blunt et al. 2011). With the increased emphasis on IH and worker protecting came an increase in the number of IH-related academic programs during at least the first half of the 20th century. There are currently 19 undergraduate- and graduate-level IH programs accredited by ABET, as of October 2019 (ABET 2019a) and note also that there are likely dozens of other programs for IH or IH-related degrees which are not ABET accredited. Well regarded around the world, ABET is an ISO 9001-certifed, nonprofit, nongovernmental agency that accredits programs in applied and natural science, computing, engineering, and engineering technology (ABET 2019b). Being accredited by ABET signifies that an academic program meets certain quality standards with regard to what students experience and learn. ABET relies on over 2,200 experts from industry, academia, and government to serve as program evaluators, commissioners, board members, and advisors for accreditation of academic programs (ABET 2019b). With assistance from member societies related to specific degree programs, ABET has established specific accreditation criteria against which individual academic degree programs are evaluated. For IH and similarly-named programs, AIHA serves as the member society which helps oversee the accreditation criteria for IH academic programs.

5.3.3 PROFESSIONAL ORGANIZATIONS

5.3.3.1 · American Conference of Governmental Industrial Hygienists (ACGIH®)

As the IH profession grew during the early 1900s, two major societies emerged in support of the profession of IH and its practitioners. On June 27, 1938, the National Conference of Governmental Industrial Hygienists was convened in Washington D.C. with a limit of two representatives per governmental agency accepted as a member. In 1946, the organization changed its name to the American Conference of Governmental Industrial Hygienists (ACGIH®) and membership was expanded to all IH personnel in select US governmental agencies, along with governmental IH professionals in other countries. Today, ACGIH remains a nonprofit scientific organization dedicated to the advancement of occupational and environmental health with over 3,000 members (ACGIH 2019b). Membership has expanded to be inclusive of all professionals in IH, occupational health, environmental health, and safety in the United States and abroad. Regarding its organizational content, ACGIH currently has nine committees focused on various health and safety topics to advance the IH profession and support its membership. ACGIH is well known for its exposure guidelines, called Threshold Limit Values (TLVs®) and Biological Exposure Indices (BEIs®) (ACGIH 2019a, 2019b), which are used by IH professionals worldwide. The organization has many publications and educational courses to support the IH profession and also co-sponsors the well-regarded *Journal of Occupational and Environmental Hygiene* (*JOEH*) with the AIHA. Further details on ACGIH are available at their website, www.acgih.org.

5.3.3.2 American Industrial Hygiene Association (AIHA®)

The second major professional society for IH is the AIHA®, which was founded in October 1939. AIHA is a "nonprofit organization serving professionals dedicated to the anticipation, recognition, evaluation, control, and confirmation of environmental stressors in or arising from the workplace that may lead to injury, illness, or affect the well-being of workers and members of the community". AIHA provides a wide variety of education, training, working groups, committees, publications, and services such as laboratory accreditation to benefit the profession of IH. AIHA has nearly 8,500 members in the industrial, consulting, academic, and government sectors (AIHA 2019). Its annual American Industrial Hygiene Conference and Expo (AIHce EXP) is a premier destination to share new ideas and learn new strategies to protect worker health. Signature publications, such as *The Occupational Environment: Its Evaluation, Control, and Management* (Anna 2011) and *A Strategy for Assessing and Managing Occupational Exposures* (Jahn et al. 2015), are important educational and reference tools for industrial hygienists. Further details on AIHA are available at their website, www.aiha.org.

5.3.3.3 Board for Global EHS Credentialing (BGC®)

In 1959, the AIHA Certification Committee recommended a separate board be created for the certification of industrial hygienists, which led to the creation of the American Board of Industrial Hygiene (ABIH®). ABIH was founded in 1960, as an independent not-for-profit organization dedicated to protecting the public through the certification of IH professionals with the Certified Industrial Hygienist (CIH®) credential. The first exams for certification were administered in 1963. Today, eligibility requirements for applicants include certain academic degree, coursework, and experience requirements before being eligible to take the exam. The CIH is an ANSI ISO/IEC-accredited credential, currently held by over 6,800 diplomates worldwide (ABIH 2019). In 2019, ABIH was rebranded as the Board for Global EHS Credentialing (BGC®), which is the new larger organizational name to represent a growing line of credentials focused on environmental, health, and safety. These credentials include the CIH®, Qualified Environmental Professional® (QEP®),

Environmental Professional In-Training® (EPI®), and the new Certified Professional Product Steward™ (CPPS™) credential. The mission of BGC is "To be the leader in offering credentials that elevate the technical and ethical standards for professionals practicing the science of protecting, managing, and enhancing the health and safety of people and the environment" (BGC 2019).

5.3.3.4 Occupational Safety and Health Administration (OSHA)

The OSH Act of 1970 created both the OSHA and the National Institute for Occupational Safety and Health (NIOSH). Officially established a year later (1971), OSHA is an agency of the US Department of Labor, created to ensure safe and healthful working conditions for working men and women by setting and enforcing standards, along with providing training, outreach, education, and assistance (OSHA 2019). As discussed previously, the General Duty Clause, section 5(a)(1) of the OSH Act, requires that the employer provide "a place of employment which are free from recognized hazards that are causing or are likely to cause death or serious physical harm to his employees" (OSHA 1970). To understand the positive impact of OSHA, recognize that in 1970, there were an estimated 14,000 US workers killed on the job, as compared to only 4,340 killed in 2009 (OSHA 2019).

Beyond the General Duty Clause, OSHA issues many standards (i.e., "regulations") for a wide variety of workplace hazards. These standards are published in Title 29 of the Code of Federal Regulations (CFR), under four major categories of General Industry, Construction, Maritime, and Agriculture and are available at the OSHA webpage, www.osha.gov (OSHA 2019). Examples of IH-related standards are 29 CFR 1910.134 Respiratory Protection, 29 CFR 1910.146 Permit-Required Confined Space, 29 CFR 1910.1001 Asbestos, and 29 CFR 1910.1027 Cadmium. These standards describe the general requirements to maintain compliance, with some standards being hazardous substance-specific and others being program-specific. As a program-specific standard, 29 CFR 1910.134 Respiratory Protection is fairly comprehensive, with enough discussion possible that a separate text was authored (Racz et al. 2018). Note that in the absence of a specific standard for a hazard, employers are still required to comply with the General Duty Clause, i.e., keep their workplace free of serious recognized hazards (OSHA 2019). Related to standards, OSHA adopted its first permissible exposure limits (PELs) in 1971 and these were based on the 1968 ACGIH TLVs® (AIHA 2019).

5.3.3.5 National Institute for Occupational Safety and Health (NIOSH)

As mentioned previously, the OSH Act of 1970 also created the NIOSH. NIOSH was established as a research agency focused on the study of worker safety and health, along with empowering employers and workers to create safe and healthy workplaces (NIOSH 2019a). After its creation in 1970, NIOSH was transferred to the Centers for Disease Control (CDC; now, Centers for Disease Control and Prevention) from the then Health Service & Mental Health Administration. In 1974, the NIOSH (and OSHA) Standards Completion Program was the basis for 387 new standards (NIOSH 2019a). In 1977, the first nine NIOSH Education and Research Centers (ERCs) were awarded to major universities across the United States (note: as of October 2019, there are now 18 ERCs). These ERCs help translate scientific knowledge into practice through various education, training, and outreach programs. In 1978, the first edition of the *NIOSH/OSHA Pocket Guide to Chemical Hazards* was published (NIOSH 2019a) and, today, this publication is commonly referenced for its information on chemical properties and hazards. Over the years since its creation, NIOSH has developed numerous documents and other knowledge products covering health risks related to chemicals.

5.4 TODAY'S INDUSTRIAL HYGIENE

5.4.1 ANTICIPATION-RECOGNITION-EVALUATION-CONTROL-CONFIRM

IH is described as the science and art of AREC of occupational and environmental hazards which otherwise may lead to injury, illness, impairment, or otherwise adversely affect human health and well-being (Ficklen et al. 2019). Discussed previously, this IH decision framework of AREC, which now includes a fifth tenet of *confirm*, is well known to industrial hygienists and represents the ordered set of principles that health and safety professionals follow as they mitigate hazards and reduce exposures to the industrial workforce. To protect workers, and to comply with OSHA standards, an industrial hygienist is trained to *anticipate* and *recognize* the potential for exposures to specific hazards (e.g., chemicals, gases, noise, biological agents, radiation) in a workplace and then *evaluate* the exposures before determining how best to *control* the exposures. Periodically, the IH should *confirm* that exposures remain properly controlled. A summary of AREC is shown in Figure 5.1.

Increasingly, industrial hygienists are called upon to assist with nonoccupational exposure issues. Examples of such exposures include mold remediation after flood damage to homes, indoor air quality (indoor environmental quality) problems, and

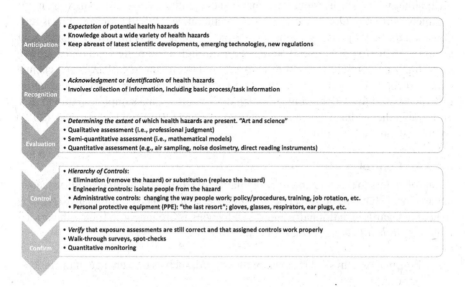

FIGURE 5.1 Classic industrial hygiene decision framework: AREC of occupational and environmental hazards.

exposures to various environmental pollutants which may jeopardize the health of the community. Industrial hygienists specialize in identifying which chemical, biological, and physical agents pose hazards to the human ("anticipation" and "recognition"), then can perform exposure assessments ("evaluation"), and can determine appropriate protective measures ("controls") to mitigate the risk to those hazards.

5.4.1.1   Anticipation

"Anticipation" is the expectation of potential health hazards in the workplace and depends on the industrial hygienist having knowledge of a wide variety of potential health hazards. Further, a skilled IH will have knowledge of the latest scientific developments, emerging technologies, and any new or evolving regulatory requirements (Ficklen et al. 2019), in order to fulfill the tenet of anticipation.

5.4.1.2   Recognition

"Recognition" is the acknowledgment or actual identification of health hazards in the workplace and typically includes some sort of collection of information (Ficklen et al. 2019), such as basic process/task information. The difference between "anticipation" and "recognition" is subtle, with the difference being "expectation" versus "identification". Often, the terms anticipation and recognition are used together, e.g., "the anticipation **and** recognition of occupational and environmental hazards", as they commonly occur concurrently.

5.4.1.3   Evaluation

"Evaluation" is the examination of a work task or process to determine the extent of which health hazards are present (Ficklen et al. 2019). This includes assessments that are qualitative (i.e., professional judgment) and quantitative (e.g., air sampling, noise dosimetry, direct-reading instruments). A "quantitative" skill like air sampling is fundamental to the IH profession, and a simplified description is the use of a calibrated sampling pump to pull a fixed volume of air through a sampling media (i.e., "active sampling") appropriate to capture a specific contaminant (e.g., hazardous chemical). A second common type of sampling is "passive sampling", such as through a diffusion-based (or badge) sampler which does not rely on a sampling pump to pull air through the media. The reader is referred to Anna (2011) and Ficklen et al. (2019) for more details on sampling.

5.4.1.4   Control

"Control" refers to the adjustment or regulation of work tasks or processes to meet an occupational standard or guideline and, in general, to reduce or eliminate exposures to health hazards. Traditionally, industrial hygienists are taught to follow the prioritized *hierarchy of controls* (Ficklen et al. 2019):

1. Elimination: physical removal of the hazard, such as by a change of the task or process
2. Substitution: replacing the hazard with a nonhazardous or less-hazardous solution

3. Engineering controls: isolate people from the hazard; includes implementation of industrial ventilation systems
4. Administrative controls: changing the way people work; includes use of management involvement, policy, training, job rotation, preventive maintenance, and housekeeping procedures
5. Personal protective equipment (PPE): "the last resort"; includes devices (e.g., protective gloves, safety glasses/goggles, chemical protective clothing, industrial respirators, hearing protection devices) designed to protect individual workers from exposures to hazards.

Elimination, substitution, and engineering controls are always the preferred solutions, as they provide a more reliable line of defense. Conversely, PPE is always the "last resort", as it is usually deemed most prone to failure of the three types of controls. For example, nitrile gloves can tear, chemically protective clothing can succumb to permeation and penetration of chemicals through the material or at its seams, the respirator-to-face seal can be compromised by unshaven faces, and hearing protection devices (i.e., "foam plugs") can be incorrectly inserted into the ear canal. With PPE, the wearer can lack the necessary training or become complacent, leading to improper use which can compromise the protection provided.

5.4.1.5   Confirm

Added to the IH decision framework in more recent history (now, ARECC), "confirm" represents the principle that the IH needs to verify that assigned controls are working properly (Ficklen et al. 2019). Implemented controls are prone to failure—e.g., ventilation systems can have degraded performance due to failing motors, workers can become lackadaisical regarding cleaning/housekeeping procedures, and PPE can fail due to reasons described in the paragraph above. Periodic walk-through surveys, "spot-checks", and quantitative ventilation system checks are techniques used to confirm that assigned controls are, indeed, controlling the hazards.

5.4.2   Exposure Assessment: A Core Function of Industrial Hygiene

5.4.2.1   Exposure Assessment—Defined

Exposure assessment is the process of defining *exposure profiles* and judging the acceptability of exposures to workers. It is considered a core function of the IH profession (Ficklen et al. 2019) and is an overarching term used to represent the work performed to quantify or otherwise characterize the exposure to the worker. If referring to the IH decision framework (i.e., AREC), *exposure assessment* process is synonymous with the *evaluation* tenet, which was described earlier.

5.4.2.2   Comprehensive Exposure Assessment—More than Compliance

In more recent years, the AIHA® has coined the term *comprehensive exposure assessment* (CEA) to represent the migration of the IH profession from being strictly "compliance" focused, where often the maximum-risk (i.e., worst-case) worker is purposely selected for exposure assessment, to a more comprehensive approach, where the goal is to characterize "all exposures for all workers on all days"

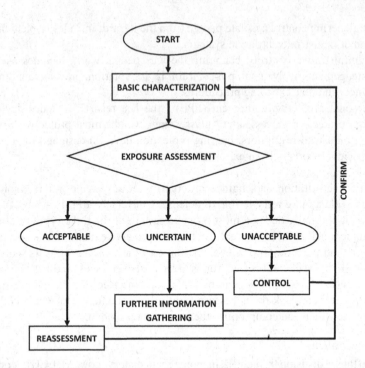

FIGURE 5.2 The AIHA® Exposure Assessment Model. Adapted from Mulhausen and Damiano (2011).

(Mulhausen & Damiano 2015). Fundamental to this shift was the development of the AIHA *exposure assessment model* (Figure 5.2), which summarizes the *basic characterization*, *exposure assessment*, and determination of *acceptability or unacceptability* (Mulhausen & Damiano 2015). CEA, a cyclical model, is now commonly used across the IH profession and effectively covers the entire IH decision framework of AREC discussed earlier.

In Figure 5.2, the exposure assessment model starts by first defining the *exposure assessment strategy*, including defining the decision criteria to be used to determine exposure acceptability. *Basic characterization* represents a series of activities focused on gathering of information regarding the workplace, workforce, industrial processes, and industrial hazards. Exposure assessment is an elaborate set of activities, including establishing *similar exposure groups* (SEGs), defining *exposure profiles*, and comparing the exposure profile (and any statistical uncertainty) to an appropriate *occupational exposure limit* (OEL) (and any statistical uncertainty around the OEL). Process, task, agent, and job classification information is used to help establish an SEG, which is a way to group workers in order to aid in efficient characterization of workplace exposure profiles. Essentially, a small subset of the SEG can be sampled with the results (i.e., exposure profile) being representative of the entire SEG.

Next, the industrial hygienist compares the exposure profile to the OEL and decides whether the exposure is *acceptable*, *uncertain*, or *unacceptable*. This is typically done using a *decision statistic*, e.g., the 95th percentile compared against an OEL.

If acceptable, then the industrial hygienist should conduct periodic re-evaluation. If uncertain, further information gathering should be conducted, to include prioritized exposure monitoring (e.g., sampling) or gathering more information on the health effects of hazards. If unacceptable, the *hierarchy of controls* should be used to mitigate risk of exposure. Finally, the industrial hygienist should periodically *confirm* that the exposure assessment is accurate and controls are effective.

In Table 5.1 is a summary of the key components of the Exposure Assessment Model. The reader is referred to *A Strategy for Assessing and Managing Occupational Exposures* (4th ed.) (Jahn et al. 2015) for details on conducting exposure assessments following the Exposure Assessment Model.

TABLE 5.1

Key Components of the AIHA® Exposure Assessment Model and Their Descriptions

Component	Description
Basic characterization	• "Anticipation" and "Recognition" • Walk-through surveys of workplaces • Gathering data: workplace and workforce information, hazard information

Exposure assessment	• "*Evaluation*"
	 • Establish SEGs: groups of workers performing similar tasks/processes; assumes exposure profile will be similar for an entire SEG
	 • Define the exposure profile: magnitude and variability of exposures for the SEG
	   • Qualitative exposure assessment: "professional judgment" and experience
	   • Semi-quantitative: reliance on mathematics-based exposure modeling
	   • Quantitative: reliance on measured exposure data via air sampling pumps, noise dosimeters, direct-reading instruments, etc.
	 • Select an appropriate OEL
	 • Compare exposure profile and its uncertainty to the OEL and its uncertainty

Determine acceptability	• "*Control*"
	 • Decide whether the exposure profile is "Acceptable", "Uncertain", or "Unacceptable"
	 • Acceptable:
	   • Use the decision criteria to determine whether the exposure profile is acceptable
	   • Reassessment: If acceptable, then plan for periodic re-evaluation of the exposures, including possible routine monitoring (e.g., sampling)
	 • Uncertain:
	   • If unsure whether the exposure profile is acceptable or unacceptable
	   • Further information gathering: Do prioritized exposure monitoring (e.g., sampling) or gather more information on the health effects to improve confidence in the exposure judgment
	 • Unacceptable:
	   • Control: Implement prioritized control strategies for any exposure profiles deemed unacceptable

Adapted from Ficklen et al. (2019) and Mulhausen and Damiano (2011).

5.5   THE FUTURE OF INDUSTRIAL HYGIENE AND TOTAL EXPOSURE HEALTH

5.5.1   Industrial Hygienists: Ready for Total Exposure Health

Today, the IH profession remains largely focused on compliance, with the AREC of hazards limited to the workplace and during work hours. But arguably, the principles of IH are important as a basis for TEH, as the AREC skills of industrial hygienists can readily be applied for exposures occurring after hours (i.e., outside the traditional work-shift). An example of IH skills being applied on "24/7" exposures is the study, "US Air Force Noise Exposure Demonstration Project", where a novel noise sensor (dosimeter) was coupled with a smartphone app to transmit around-the-clock occupational, environmental, and lifestyle-related noise exposure data to a "cloud" platform (Yamamoto et al. 2019). For many people, occupational exposures play the most dominant role in total exposure; for others, especially those with little to no occupational exposure, the relative contributions of environmental and lifestyle exposures can dominate. Regardless of how much contribution there is, the IH skills related to anticipation, recognition, evaluation, control, and confirm of occupational and environmental hazards will be useful to help characterize both workplace and "after hours" exposures.

In addition, IHs are skilled at evaluating/assessing exposures to hazards and typically know which quantitative technique (i.e., sampling or real-time measurement) to apply to a given hazard. TEH presents some challenges as being able to assess exposures to a much wider variety of hazards over a much larger population, which suggests that access to lower cost and accurate sensor technology available in plentiful quantities (e.g., "novel sensors" or Internet of Things—IoT technology) may be important. Although IHs may not be leading the actual development of new/novel sensors, it might be expected that they are heavily involved in discussions on what sensors are important to develop and guidelines on parameters such as sensitivity, specificity, and accuracy. Examples of such sensors include small/low-cost photoionization detector (PID) technology for volatile organic compound measurement, noise meter smartphone/smartphone "app" technology, and particulate matter sensors.

With the training and experience they have, IHs are also very skilled at how to control or mitigate the effects of exposures to occupational and environmental hazards. They are very experienced with using the *hierarchy of controls,* which suggests consideration of control techniques in the order of elimination, substitution, engineering controls, administrative controls, and finally, reliance on PPE ("the last resort"). There is a compelling argument that if assessment of 24/7 exposures is important, then the logical next question to address is how to *control* such exposures. Industrial hygienists are well versed in controlling of exposures. Determining simple controls, such that PPE, might be important to mitigate the effects of environmental- or lifestyle-based exposures.

5.5.2   Challenges for Industrial Hygienists in Fulfilling TEH

Several questions come to mind when thinking about the role of the industrial hygienist in a TEH context. For example, can an IH function without exposure limits being available to assess exposures to perhaps thousands of chemicals of interest to

TEH? Currently, there are many sources for exposure limits (e.g., OSHA, NIOSH, ACGIH, AIHA), but the total number of accepted peer-reviewed, toxicology-based exposure limits is somewhat limited to several hundred chemicals, with around 2,000 chemicals either regulated by a government statute or having an OEL (Laszcz-Davis et al. 2014). With TEH (and emphasis on "total"), there would be need for a much larger set of exposure limits (or, *guidelines*) to compare with sample results. Laszcz-Davis et al. (2014) describe an entire hierarchy of OELs, ranging from quantitative health-based OELs, working provisional OELs (e.g., set by the employer), and hazard or occupational exposure banding (OEB). OEB, which has been used by the pharmaceutical industry and some major chemical companies over the past several decades, is designed to quickly and accurately assign chemicals into specific categories (i.e., bands) corresponding to a range of exposure concentrations designed to protect human health. These bands are assigned based on toxicity of the chemicals and resulting adverse health effects (NIOSH 2019b). As TEH introduces the idea of assessing exposures "24/7", perhaps there will be a fundamental need for new exposure limits (or, "guidelines") and tools such as OEB may play an important role.

REFERENCES

ABET. (2019a) ABET-Accredited Programs. Retrieved October 14, 2019, from http://main. abet.org/aps/Accreditedprogramsearch.aspx.

ABET. (2019b) About ABET. Retrieved November 7, 2019, from https://www.abet.org/about-abet/.

American Board of Industrial Hygiene® (ABIH®). (2019) ABIH Webpage. Retrieved November 6, 2019, from www.abih.org/about-abih/index.

American Conference of Governmental Industrial Hygienists (ACGIH®). (2019a) *2019 TLVs® and BEIs®, based on the Documentation of the Threshold Limit Values for Chemical Substances and Physical Agents & Biological Exposure Indices.* Cincinnati, OH: ACGIH®.

American Conference of Governmental Industrial Hygienists (ACGIH®). (2019b) About ACGIH. Retrieved October 14, 2019, from https://www.acgih.org/about-us.

American Conference of Governmental Industrial Hygienists (ACGIH®). (2019c) *Guide to Occupational Exposure Values.* Cincinnati, OH: ACGIH®.

American Industrial Hygiene Association (AIHA®). (2019) AIHA Webpage. Retrieved January 18, 2019, from https://www.aiha.org/about-ih/Pages/default.aspx.

Anna, D.H. (Ed.). (2011) *The Occupational Environment: Its Evaluation, Control, and Management* (3rd ed.), Volume #1. Fairfax, VA: AIHA®.

Board for Global EHS Credentialing (BGC®). (2019) BGC Webpage. Retrieved November 13, 2019, from https://ehscredentialing.org/.

Blunt, L.A., Zey, J.N., Greife, A.L., & Rose, V.E. (2011) History and Philosophy of Industrial Hygiene. In D.H. Anna (Ed.), *The Occupational Environment: Its Evaluation, Control, and Management* (3rd ed., pp. 3–24). Fairfax, VA: AIHA®.

Ficklen III, C.B. (Ed.), Fleeger, A.K., & Lillquist, D.L. (2019) *Industrial Hygiene Reference and Study Guide* (4th ed.). Falls Church, VA: AIHA®.

Hamilton, A. (1943) *Exploring the Dangerous Trades.* Boston, MA: Little, Brown and Company (reprinted by American Industrial Hygiene Association, Fairfax VA, 1995).

Hoover, H.C., & Hoover, L.H. (1950) *De Re Metallica.* Translated from the original work of Georgius Agricola, published posthumously in 1556. New York: Dover Publications, Inc.

Jahn, S.D., Bullock, W.H., & Ignacio, J.S. (Eds.). (2015) *A Strategy for Assessing and Managing Occupational Exposures* (4th ed.). Falls Church, VA: American Industrial Hygiene Association.

Laszcz-Davis, C., Maier, A., & Perkins, J. (2014) The Hierarchy of OELs: A New Organizing Principle for Occupational Risk Assessment. In *The Synergist* (pp. 27–30). Falls Church, VA: American Industrial Hygiene Association.

Mulhausen, J., & Damiano, J. (2015) Establishing the Exposure Assessment Strategy. In Jahn, S.D., Bullock, W.H., & Ignacio, J.S. (Eds.), *A Strategy for Assessing and Managing Occupational Exposures* (4th ed.). Falls Church, VA: American Industrial Hygiene Association.

National Institute for Occupational Safety and Health (NIOSH). (2019a) NIOSH Webpage. Retrieved October 14, 2019, from https://www.cdc.gov/niosh/about/default. html#about%20niosh.

National Institute for Occupational Safety and Health (NIOSH). (2019b) Occupational Exposure Banding. Retrieved November 15, 2019, from https://www.cdc.gov/niosh/topics/oeb/default.html.

Occupational Safety and Health Administration (OSHA). (1970) Public Law 91–596, OSH Act. Retrieved August 18, 2019, from https://www.osha.gov/laws-regs/oshact/completeoshact.

Occupational Safety and Health Administration (OSHA). (2019) OSHA Webpage. Retrieved June 26, 2019, from https://www.osha.gov/about.html.

Perkins, J. (1997) Industrial Hygiene—Historical Perspective. In *Modern Industrial Hygiene* (pp. 11–28). New York: Van Nostrand Reinhold.

Racz, L., Yamamoto, D.P., & Eninger, R.M. (Eds.). (2018) *Handbook of Respiratory Protection- Safeguarding Against Current and Emerging Hazards*. Boca Raton, FL: CRC Press.

Yamamoto, D., Kurzdorfer, J.W., & Fullerton, K.L. (2019) U.S. Air Force Noise Exposure Demonstration Project. Report #AFRL-SA-WP-TR-2019-0010. Retrieved October 14, 2019, from Defense Technical Information Center (DTIC), https://apps.dtic.mil/dtic/tr/fulltext/u2/1071653.pdf.

Section II

---

*Advances in Toxicology
and the -Omics*

6 Personalizing Environmental Health for the Military— Striving for Precision

Christopher E. Bradburne
Johns Hopkins University

CONTENTS

6.1 THE NEED FOR PRECISION IN MILITARY ENVIRONMENTAL HEALTH

Military service members see a broad range of operating environments, with a range of known and unknown chemical and immunological challenges during deployments. High-profile chronic health conditions have been associated with toxic agents, such as Agent Orange in Vietnam, but there are also those with no clear cause, such

DOI: 10.1201/9780429263286-8

as Gulf War Syndrome. These cases did more than just cause health issues—they also resulted in enormous costs, lost time and productivity, and the degradation of trust in the military to protect its own. Better understanding of causes and effects could have provided better options for preventive medicine, personal protection, and other means of risk mitigation. Likewise, better understanding of individual susceptibilities, proximity and duration of exposures, and extenuating factors could have provided additional avenues to protect those most vulnerable.

Current advances in both environmental health and precision medicine offer some intriguing possibilities. A goal of the environmental/occupational health field is to identify health risks and minimize their impact on workers. Goals include identifying, characterizing, and mitigating threats; implementing preventive and protective strategies, detection with health surveillance and diagnostic tools; and providing treatment where needed. Scientific approaches have historically focused on reducing threats to single chemical causes, using established epidemiological tools population statistics to predict individual risks. While useful for sources and exposures of high or sustained effect, these approaches can collapse for exposures with more moderate effect and/or multifactorial causes and when trying to estimate individual risks and susceptibilities. It is difficult to overstate the need for better individual tracking and susceptibility characterization to environmental threats; generally, the more that is known about the source and the individual, the better (Figure 6.1). Knowledge of 'personalized' susceptibility and individual exposures can illuminate health threats that might otherwise be invisible in population health data. Such information can identify toxicological sources and health effect modifiers and provide more precise actionable information for decision makers, health care providers, and researchers.

Most strategies for connecting active health effects with sources are retrospective. For example, for an acute exposure that results in a health effect, an epidemiological investigation may involve 'tracing back in time' an individual's geo-temporal activities to co-localize them with a source. Similar actions may be taken for chronic exposures, but it may be years before associations and other affected individuals are identified, if ever. Characterizing the threat from toxicological sources would benefit from better tools which allow precise measurements of components, geographic outlay, functionalization, and persistence. For the individual, better understanding of genetic susceptibility, individual risk factors, geographic proximity, and

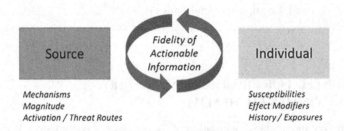

FIGURE 6.1 'Knowledge is power': The more known about a hazard source, the individual, and their overall interaction, the better decisions can be made by individuals, decision makers, and stakeholders.

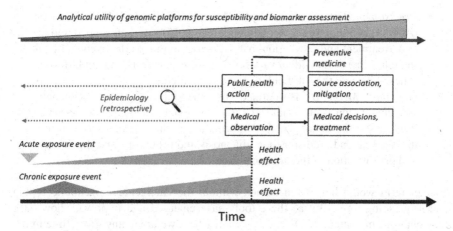

FIGURE 6.2 Temporal nature of tools and actions for precision (genomic) environmental health. Actionable information for precision environmental health is developed using retrospective investigation techniques and a constantly changing genomic toolset. For population studies, GWAS done with earlier genomic technologies may miss variants that are predictive of susceptibility to an exposure event. For individual exposures, genomic tools used for detection of exposure-linked adducts or biomarkers may be inadequate.

duration of exposure would also be useful. Many studies have been done to associate toxicological health effects in populations and associate them with genetic markers. However, the analytic utility (i.e., the ability of the technology to detect true genomic markers) can shift over time as the technologies shift in their ability measure sources of genetic variation (Figure 6.2).

One particular challenge is dealing with the constant change in technology and interpretation of impacts for precision medicine. The genomics and other 'omics' technologies present an array of new tools and techniques to characterize individual susceptibility and a range of biomarkers (Bradburne & Lewis 2018). However, interpretation can change over time as tools improve, meaning that an understanding of 'where we have been' is just as important as 'where we are going'. This chapter will attempt to shed light on the history and trajectory of precision (genomic) medicine tools for determining genetic susceptibility to environmental toxicants and review a framework for how comprehensive risk outlooks can be developed which combine genomic and environmental diagnostic approaches.

6.2 FROM PAST TO PRESENT: THE CHANGING LANDSCAPE OF PRECISION MEDICINE

6.2.1 TECHNOLOGY AND MEDICINE

Technology is constantly changing over time, which can create both excitement and frustration in a technology-dependent field, such as medicine. An example is the genomic tool evolution over the past few decades that has created the field of 'precision medicine'.

- *Precision medicine* is defined by the American College of Medical Genetics (ACMG) board of directors (Adler & Stead 2015) as '… an approach to disease treatment and prevention that seeks to maximize effectiveness by taking into account individual variability in genes, environment, and lifestyle'. It has at its core the sub-field of genomic medicine.
- *Genomic Medicine* is defined by the Clinical Pharmacogenetics Implementation Consortium (CPIC) (National Academies of Sciences 2014) as '… the use of genomic information and technologies to determine disease risk and predisposition, diagnosis and prognosis, and the selection and prioritization of therapeutic options'.

Neither term would have been coined without the emergence of genomic typing and sequencing tools. But as these tools have emerged and improved, how have they changed medicine, and how can we tell where we are at any given time in the medical landscape? Does a genomic test from 2010 provide the same efficacy as a genomic test from 2020?

6.2.2 GENETICS VERSUS GENOMICS

Historically, the field of *genetics* is very different than the newer field of genomics. Genetics started >150 years ago with Gregor Mendel, who described patterns of inheritance that followed simple mathematic rules. These 'Mendelian traits' are described as phenotypes that can be localized to individual genetic loci. However, the majority of common traits in higher organisms and humans are complex (e.g., tied to more than one locus) and do not follow Mendelian patterns of inheritance. For example, most chronic diseases come about through some level of inherited genetics and environmental exposures. Therefore, the field of genetics has evolved to rely on heavy mathematical inference, with little understanding of individual molecular mechanisms. The heyday of quantitative genetics was in the 1900s–1930s, when statisticians such as Ronald Fisher described quantitative descriptions of inheritance that are still used to this day in agriculture and animal breeding, such as linear mixed models, the infinitesimal model, and others (Bradburne & Lewis 2017).

In the 1990s, the new field of *genomics* offered to change that paradigm. Genomics emerged with the advent of the human genome project, which in 2001 generated a draft sequence of one person (Bradburne et al. 2015) and later went on to characterize population genetic variation between tens of global human ethnic populations. The mapping of the human genome and the contrasting of individual differences offered to provide the 'roadmap' to understanding molecular mechanisms, by tying individual genomic variants or groups of variants to traits and diseases. The workhorse of tying genetic loci to traits was the Genome-Wide Association Study (GWAS), which genotyped control and trait/disease groups and looked to identify genetic variants that could be statistically associated with the trait/disease. By 2011, there had been ~1400 GWAS on 380 traits and diseases (De Castro et al. 2016). The National Human Genome Research Institute (NHGRI) published a strategic roadmap the same year that predicted impactful contributions from basic human genomic sciences to begin to significantly advance the science of medicine and improve the effectiveness of health care over the next 10 years (De Castro et al. 2016).

6.2.3 GENOMICS AND THE OVERPROMISE OF GWAS

While the advancements have been exciting, there have also been unrealized expectations. From 2001 to 2015, the primary workhorse of genotypic variation has not been genomic sequencing, but rather, single-nucleotide polymorphism (SNP) genotyping arrays. SNP genotyping arrays are an older technology (developed between the late 1990s and early 2000s) and have generated almost all of the hundreds of GWAS-defined trait associations curated by the NHGRI and the European Bioinformatics Institute (EBI) (US National Library of Medicine 2019). However, SNPs are not very predictive for most traits and phenotypes. There are several reasons for this: (1) SNPs do not represent all of the variations of the human genome. In fact, they are less than half of the variations by most estimates (National Human Genome Research Institute 2019). Other forms of genomic variation include insertions and deletions (INDELS), copy number variants (CNVs), segmental duplications, and others. These 'structural variants' are not readily assayable by standard SNP array technologies. (2) SNPs do not account for much of the heritability of most complex traits (Fisher 1918). The highest estimated heritability that can be explained by SNPs for a non-Mendelian, complex disease is age-related macular degeneration (~50% from 5 SNPs), which has made it a prime candidate for several focused gene therapy treatments currently underway (Venter et al. 2001), but most other complex diseases are not this straightforward. (3) Genetics (SNPs, etc.) does not account for the majority of the heritability of most human chronic diseases (Green & Guyer 2011). In fact, most have a larger environmental, causative component.

6.2.4 SEQUENCING AND 'OMICS' TECHNOLOGY ADVANCEMENTS

It is important to note the issues with genotyping technologies over the past two decades and how these affect our current practice of genomic medicine. The majority of the thousands of GWAS have been done with SNP arrays, which means they did NOT look for non-SNP variation such as INDELS, CNVs, and other structural variants. Interestingly, most commercial SNP genotyping since the 2000s did include array-based CNV typing capabilities, but because of the variability in CNV morphologies *in vivo*, these have not been useful. In fact, curation of CNV variant calls generated from these chips over the last two decades was discontinued by the National Human Genome Research Institute-European Molecular Biology Laboratory (NHGRI-EMBL) SNP variation databases in early 2018.

The original draft human genome from 2001 represents a higher quality construct than most of the individual genomes that came after it, as it was done by an accurate but very low-throughput and painstaking technology called Sanger sequencing. High-throughput Illumina sequencing technologies emerged in 2007 and have controlled most of the genomic sequencing market (~90%) from 2010 to 2019. However, this technology relies on breaking up genomes into pieces between 50 and 300 base pairs (bps), in order to sequence and requires large *in silico* resources and complex approaches to reconstruct the genome. Since much of the human genome is comprised of low-complexity regions (e.g., two base pair repeats such as ATATATATATAT…), a typical moderate-quality human genome construct only comprises 20%–30% of the actual human sequence. A related approach, exome sequencing, provides even less—typically targeting only the expressed regions of the human genome, or about 1%–2%. As most SNPs associated with complex diseases and traits are NOT caus- ative and not in the expressed protein regions (Buniello et al. 2019), it is reasonable to assume that missing variation in structural variants may also be an important piece of the puzzle, and those are still largely uncategorized in global populations and in disease phenotypes.

More recently, new and disruptive 'long-read' technologies have emerged, highlighted by the Oxford Nanopore (OxNan) single-molecule sequencers. These sequencers can read thousands, to hundreds of thousands bps, alleviating much of the shortfalls of the *in silico* reconstruction. Quality has lagged (typically Q10 or less, or 1 error in 100 bps), so resolving SNPs has been difficult. However, the new- est upcoming platform forecasts read qualities comparable to Illumina (<Q30, or 1 error in 10,000 bps (Sudmant et al. 2015)); hence, they could revolutionize GWAS by providing both SNPs and structural variants.

6.2.5   The 'Great GWAS Do-over'?

As older GWAS have been done with early, less capable platforms, this implies that the DNA measurements of many GWAS may need to be redone in order to obtain struc- tural variants and SNPs in low-complexity genomic regions. Prime candidates for reassessment would be studies in which the sum of the statistically significant SNPs does not reach the level of known genetic heritability measured in monozygotic twins. An example would be type 2 diabetes. This complex trait has ~42 SNPs that have been associated with it through GWAS. Interestingly, most SNP risk is cumulative (Manolio et al. 2009). Essentially, one can potentially sum the risk (i.e., odds ratio) of each SNP associated with a complex trait or disease and compare to the level of heri- tability as measured by $H^2 = Var\ (G)/Var\ (P)$, where H = Heritability, G = Genetics, and P = Phenotype. The difference between the two may provide a measure of how much variability is remaining that is heritable but has not been accurately measured by SNP arrays. In other words, this 'missing heritability' (Fisher 1918) could very likely be comprised of structural variants missed by SNP arrays, which could be measured by OxNan and other long-read sequence typing technologies.

Of final note is the advancement in computational power to be able to assess genomic information and find variants or more complex multi-locus haplotypes. Because of the significant *in silico* resources required for genomic bioinformatics, most analysis approaches and algorithms are designed to sacrifice rigor for speed and memory conservation (Chen et al. 2010). Analysis can become very computationally intensive when doing pairwise epistatic computations of just SNPs. As an example, a four-way combination of a modest collection of 30 million SNPs could take 2.4×10^{20} CPU hours per phenotype. The advent of ultra-high-speed computing, such as the Summit supercomputer at Oak Ridge National Labs (ORNL), provides the oppor- tunity to more robustly evaluate the data. A team led by Dan Jacobson at ORNL has pioneered the use of Ricker wavelets to comprehensively mine large genomic datasets for new features. Briefly, Ricker wavelets provide a coefficient for every scale and translation of a genomic dataset (Rappaport 2016) by a brute force evaluation of all possible permutations of the data. As greater computational power allows more robust analyses of genomic data, such as Ricker wavelets, more features may be discerned in higher complexity genomic data to allow new associations to be made. This will become increasingly important as more and more layers from other 'omics' technologies are added to complex trait phenotypes (Raychaudhuri et al. 2009).

6.2.6 Incorporating the Changing Landscape of Genomics into the Clinic over Time

Ultimately, the utility of genomic information will change over time as genomic assessment improves, variation studies are expanded, population traits and disease cohorts are better characterized, and clinical interpretation is improved. Figure 6.3 shows the continuum of improving laboratory characterization of individual genomes and how that will be reflected and assessed in downstream interpretation and clinical reporting. Assessment of the utility of genomic information can be divided into three categories:

1. *Analytic validity*: Does the test for the allele work in the laboratory?
2. *Clinical validity*: Does the test for the allele work and provide actionable information in the clinic?
3. *Clinical utility*: Does providing the results in the clinic have a net positive benefit?

Across each of these areas, health informatics is a foundation providing storage and analyses environments, interoperability, and caching and retrieval in medical records. Several large university health systems, such as Vanderbilt and Johns Hopkins, are beginning to establish health informatics data analytics capabilities encompassing all of these areas (e.g., electronic health records—EHRs, 'omics', and others) to perform corporate and academic assessment of all patient data. This application of data science tools to health system data at scale will likely be important to clinical utility assessment in the future.

6.3 PRECISION BEYOND GENOMICS: ENVIRONMENT, EXPOSURES, AND SOCIAL BACKGROUND

While genomics captures a portion of risk of complex chronic disease over one's lifetime, it cannot be properly captured without lifetime cumulative environmental interactions: Risk $= G + E$, where $G =$ Genetics and $E =$ Environment. Assessing lifetime risk requires defining population health risk factors, controlling for cumulative or confounding factors, and measuring, as best as possible, the quantitative summary exposure. One such effort to do this is the 'Global Burden of Diseases, Injuries, and Risk Factors (GBD) Study' (Robison 2018). Each year, the GBD collaborator group

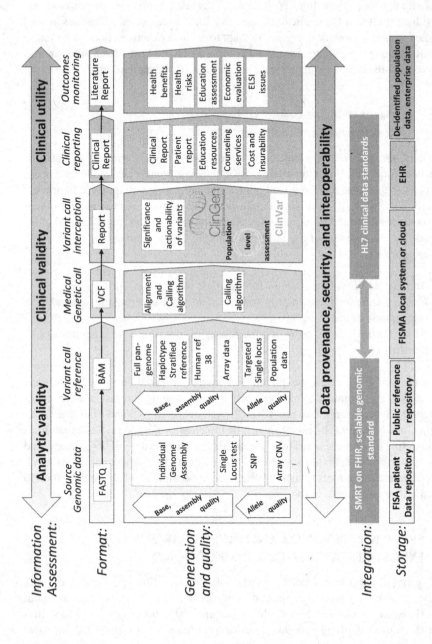

FIGURE 6.3 Provision and quality assessment of actionable genomic information over time. This framework illustrates how improving genomic resolution for individuals, populations, and disease cohorts can impact the clinic and be assessed in the academic literature.

publishes quantitative risk estimations for behavioral, occupational, and metabolic risks for 195 countries. While useful for calculating population-level risk, it can be difficult for estimation of individual-level risk. For precision medicine, efforts are underway to define, measure, and interpret individual environmental interactions using health and population records, and clinical measurements. This effort can best be summed up in characterizing the 'exposome'.

- The National Institute for Occupational Safety and Health (NIOSH) defines the *exposome* as the measure of all the exposures of an individual in a lifetime and how those exposures relate to health (Dudbridge 2013; NIOSH 2019).

The exposome can be divided into three categories (Bradburne & Lewis 2018): The *general external exposome* represents an individual's social, economic, psychological, and geographic background. The *specific external exposome* is an external event or events, such as a toxicological exposure, particular diet, radiation event, or lifestyle factors, such as smoking. The *internal exposome* represents the body systems affected by the external exposomes. These include organ systems, gut microflora, adducts, oxidative stress, and others.

Within the exposome, three classes of biomarkers can be described. The first class is *biomarkers of susceptibility*. These would include genetic variants tied to increased risk of susceptibility to a toxicant or exposure. The second class is *biomarkers of exposure*, which describe a marker, such as a DNA adduct, whose presence indicates an exposure event. Examples include adducts that are indicative of aflatoxin exposure, such as the presence of AFB-1 guanine in urine or blood. Interestingly, the presence of AFB-1 guanine in urine is typical of an 'acute' exposure to aflatoxin in the past 24 hours. It can persist for months in blood, however, so its presence there is more indicative of a chronic exposure event. The last class is *biomarkers of effect*. These are markers whose magnitude is indicative of the level of exposure effect. An example is bladder cell micronuclei which can be observed in urine using a simple assay. In general, the higher the proportion of micronuclei, the more the amount of arsenic that the subject may have ingested from a contaminated water source (Bradburne & Lewis 2018).

6.3.1 GETTING MORE PERSONAL: THE MICROBIOME AS AN INTERFACE

At the interface of nearly all human systems with the environment is the microbiome. Mucosal lung, skin, gastrointestinal tract, mouth, vaginal, and cochlear surfaces all contain microbiomes that interface chemical exposures. These communities can modify drug interactions, activate (or de-activate) xenobiotics, and induce inflammatory responses by the presence or absence of key taxa (termed dysbiosis). Efforts are underway to define normal versus abnormal microbiota conditions for various health effects, including for environmental exposures. Gut microbiota alone have been shown to affect obesity, depression, quality of life, and can be heritable (Breitwieser et al. 2017). Specific taxa can be used for biomarkers or as sentinels for exposures, but it is not well understood how to incorporate them into overall measures of quantitative risk.

6.3.2 MODELS OF RISK AND EXPOSURE

There are two basic ways to establish evidence that can inform actionable information. The first is establishing mechanisms that can be assessed, or even detected, which inform the presence and progression of a disease resulting from an exposure. An example of this is the use of a diagnostic to detect a biomarker indicative of a disease, such as the detection of lactate dehydrogenase (LDH) circulating in blood for melanoma or a variety of other pathologies (Weighill et al. 2019). For exposure research, many mechanisms are either not known or they do not have a direct diagnostic test. One solution for this is the development of 'Adverse Outcome Pathways', or AOPs (Bradburne & Lewis 2018). This involves classing mechanistic toxicological effects that are common to particular chemical exposure. For example, a molecular initiating event could be chemical absorption on the skin, followed by intermediate steps such as cellular interactions, cellular effects, and organ-level effects, and lastly, the adverse outcome such as skin inflammation. By using an AOP, even if the offending chemical or exposure is not known, one can look at the mechanistic effects and make some inference of the exposure and the treatment.

The second way to build actionable information for exposures is to develop quantitative risk measurements. In genomic medicine and exposure science, there are some basic statistical tools that can be used to calculate risk. *Odds ratios* are used to measure the effectiveness of a particular diagnostic test (e.g., a genomic assay or a serum biomarker test). It is the probability of a test being positive if a patient has a disease, versus the odds of a test being positive if a patient does not have a disease. *Absolute risk* is the probability of a health effect occurring under specific conditions, while *relative risk* is the likelihood of a health effect occurring in a group of people compared to a separate group of people with different backgrounds or in different environments. The GBD group utilizes relative risk as the primary method for calculation of global disease burden. The quantitative measurement utilized is the summary exposure value (SEV), which represents the continuous relative risk accumulated over time.

Using this methodology, the GBD provides a quantitative measure of risk-attributable burdens in life years, which are adjusted to remove the influence of pre-existing disability as a confounding factor (disability-adjusted life years, or DALYs). The 2017 GBD report claims to quantitate risks that combined add up to 61% of all deaths and 48% of DALYs worldwide, represented in categories such as unsafe water, air pollution, lead exposure, and others.

6.3.3 LIKELIHOOD RATIO (LR)

Likelihood ratios (LRs) have utility in combining quantitative risk from a disparate source, such as from the SEV, with the pre-existing risk from genetic variants. An LR can be defined as the ratio of the probability that a result is correct to the probability that the result is incorrect. A positive LR = sensitivity/(1 − specificity), whereas a negative LR = (1 − sensitivity)/specificity. LRs have been used for over 100 years to provide confidence that the risk for a disease resulting from a test is 'overlayed' onto the pre-existing risk. For example, in the nomogram in Figure 6.4, if a pre-test probability for

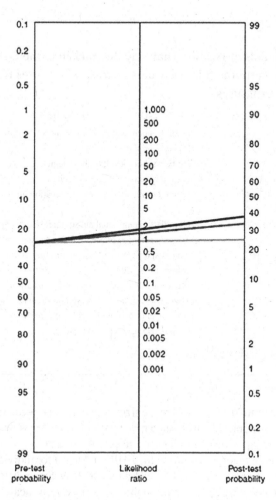

FIGURE 6.4 Application of LRs from a genetic test to inform risk for a chronic disease. A nomogram showing the relationship between the pre- and post-test probabilities when applying an LR.

a disease or trait is 25% and the LR is 1, indicating no change in risk, the probability remains at 25%. However, if the LR is 2, indicating a higher probability that the outcome is correct, the resulting (post-test) probability is ~40%. In the same way, genomic risk scores for variants have adopted LRs to predict pre- and post-test probabilities. This may provide a seamless way to obtain a quantitative, combinatory risk score between risk generated from exposure science and risk generated from genetic variants.

6.3.4 SOCIAL DETERMINANTS OF HEALTH (SDOH)

It is well known that overall chronic disease risk does not come from the presence or absence of a variant or an exposure alone, but rather, is placed over a background of lifestyle, demographic, and economic factors that influence health effects and disease

TABLE 6.1

Social Determinants of Health* That May Be Tracked in the EHR and Could Eventually Be Incorporated into Chronic Disease Risk Scores for Environmental Exposures

SDOH* Domains	Metrics
Alcohol use	Drink frequency; binge (six or more) drinking frequency
Depression	Malaise; hopelessness
Education	Highest school level; highest degree
Financial-resource strain	Difficulty in meeting basic needs
Income (neighborhood median household income)	Entered or median income for location through census data
Intimate-partner violence	Humiliation/emotional abuse; fear; sexual exploitation; violence
Physical activity	#Days/week of exercise; duration of each exercise period
Race or ethnic group	Non-Hispanic White, Hispanic/Latino, Asian; self-identification
Residential address	Address, zip code
Social connection/isolation	Frequency of social contact; religious affiliation and attendance, frequency; organization attendance, frequency
Stress	Anxiety and inability to feel comfortable, rest, or sleep
Tobacco use	Cumulative use; repetitive use

Modified from Bradburne and Lewis (2018).

outcomes. This information has been recognized for years to be predictive in the public health arena. For example, it is well known that variables such as your education level, ethnicity, and even zip code can influence lifespan. Efforts are now underway to collect this information, incorporate it into the EHR, and use it for individualized patient health care. Table 6.1 shows typical SDOH data (Adler & Stead 2015; Bradburne & Lewis 2018) that are being collected through surveys in various health care systems.

6.4 PRECISION MEDICINE AND ENVIRONMENTAL HEALTH FOR THE MILITARY

6.4.1 The Million Veterans Program

The primary study for associating environmental and occupational hazards with active duty service members is the Million Veteran Program (MVP). The pool of study subjects represents the best look at the phenotypes for long-past chronic exposures. The MVP has also been coupled with a similarly-themed civilian effort, the All of Us study. Study goals and integration of All of Us and MVP scientific goals, and resources are reviewed in National Academies of Science (2014). The military will be able to utilize this cohort for GWAS studies, and pre- and post-exposure samples are available for biomarker discovery in the Department of Defense Serum Repository (Bradburne & Lewis 2017). Tracking resources are available to associate exposure sources with geographic locations, and an effort is underway to establish an Individual Longitudinal Exposure Record (ILER) for each service member (Bradburne et al. 2015; National Academies of Sciences 2014). These efforts and resources should allow opportunities to associate sources with health effects, establish population GWAS studies to determine individual genomic susceptibility, evaluate serum samples for biomarkers of exposure and effect, and incorporate SDOH for a more comprehensive and quantitative understanding of risk of individuals and groups to environmental and occupational exposures.

6.4.2 ETHICAL, LEGAL, AND SOCIAL ISSUES (ELSI)

Determining individual genetic susceptibility in a military service member has been considered since the 1960s and 1970s when individual Mendelian genetic tests were utilized (De Castro et al. 2016). Military populations share most of the same ethical, legal, and social issues as civilian populations, with a significant exception for the military as the insurer is also the health care provider, and any clinical test for genetic susceptibility is establishing what could be a pre-existing risk that could impact insurability or even service status. The primary action taken by the military at this time has been to adopt, as policy, The Genetic Information Non-discrimination Act (GINA). GINA states that a service member cannot be discriminated against based on this genetic information (De Castro et al. 2016). However, an important distinction is that GINA is not *law* for DoD personnel (as it is for civilians), but only *policy*, which perhaps leaves it easier to change in the future.

6.5 OUTLOOK

Personalized environmental health for the military is emerging as genomic medicine emerges, providing new tools to associate exposed populations with genetic markers and discover new biomarkers of exposure and biomarkers of effect. Many of the tools for incorporating genomic medicine into medicine and preventive medicine use techniques for estimating quantitative risk that are amenable to incorporating environmental health risk. Lastly, grouped ontologies of toxicologic effect and direct mechanistic correlative biomarkers are on the horizon for direct interrogation using emerging genomic tools. These should provide better resolution for association studies, preventive medicine, and source mitigation in the future.

REFERENCES

Adler, N., Stead, W.W. "Patients in context—EHR capture of social and behavioral determinants of health," *New England Journal of Medicine*, vol. 372, pp. 698–701, 19 February 2015.

Bradburne, C., Graham, D., & Kingston, H.M., et al. "Overview of 'omics technologies for military occupational health surveillance and medicine," *Military Medicine*, vol. 180, no. suppl_10, pp. 34–48, 2015.

Bradburne, C., & Lewis, J.A. "Personalizing environmental health: At the intersection of precision medicine and occupational health in the military," *Journal of Occupational and Environmental Medicine*, vol. 59, no. 11, pp. e209–2214, 2017.

Bradburne, C., & Lewis, J.A. The U.S. Military and the Exposome. In: Dagnino S., Macherone A. (eds) *Unraveling the Exposome - A Practical View*, pp. 63–85. Cham: Springer Nature, 2018.

Breitwieser, F.P., Lu, J., & Salzberg, S.L. "A review of methods and databases for metagenomic classification and assembly," *Briefings in Bioinformatics*, vol. 18, pp. 1125–1136, 23 September 2017.

Buniello, A., MacArthur, J.A.L., & Cerezo, M., et al. "NHGRI-EBI GWAS Catalog of Published Genome-Wide Association Studies, Targeted Arrays and Summary Statistics 2019". [Online]. Available: https://www.ebi.ac.uk/gwas/ [Accessed 9 September 2019].

Chen, W., Stambolian, D., & Edwards, A.O., et al. "Genetic variants near TIMP3 and high-density lipoprotein–Associated loci influence susceptibility to age-related macular degeneration," *Proceedings of the National Academy of Sciences of the United States of America*, vol. 107, no 16, pp. 7401–7406, 20 April 2010.

De Castro, M., Biesecker, L.G., & Turner, C., et al. "Genomic medicine in the military," *NPJ Genomic Medicine*, vol. 1, p. 15008, 2016.

Dudbridge, F. "Power and predictive accuracy of polygenic risk scores," *PLoS Genetics*, vol. 9, no. 3, p. e1003348, 21 March 2013.

Fisher, R. "The correlation between relatives on the supposition of Mendelian inheritance," vol. 52, no. 2, p. 3990433, 1918.

Green, E.D., Guyer, M.S., and the National Human Genome Research Institute. "Charting a course for genomic medicine from base pairs to bedside," *Nature*, vol. 470, pp. 204–213, 2011.

Manolio, T.A., Collins, F.S., & Cox, N.J., et al. "Finding the missing heritability of complex diseases," *Nature*, vol. 461, pp. 747–753, 8 October 2009.

National Academies of Sciences. "Recommended Core Domains and Measures," in Capturing Social and Behavioral Domains and Measures in Electronic Health Records: Phase 2, NAS, 2014, pp. 227–236.

National Human Genome Research Institute. "Genomics and Medicine," [Online]. Available: https://www.genome.gov/health/Genomics-and-Medicine [Accessed 9 September 2019].

National Institute for Occupational Safety and Health (NIOSH). "Exposome," [Online]. Available: https://www.cdc.gov/niosh/topics/exposome/ [Accessed 9 September 2019].

Rappaport, S.M. "Genetic factors are not the major causes of chronic diseases," *PLoS One*, vol. 11, no. 4, p. e0154387, 22 April 2016.

Raychaudhuri, S., Plenge, R.M., & Rossin, E.J., et al. "Identifying relationships among genomic disease regions: Predicting genes at pathogenic SNP associations and rare deletions," *PLoS Genetics*, vol. 5, no. 6, p. e1000534, 26 June 2009.

Robison, K. "Omics! Omics!," November 2018. [Online]. Available: http://omicsomics. blogspot.com/2018/11/nanopore-community-meeting-2018-clive.html [Accessed 9 September 2019].

Sudmant, P., Rausch, T., & Gardner, E.J., et al. "An integrated map of structural variation in 2,504 human genomes," *Nature*, vol. 526, pp. 75–81, 1 October 2015.

U.S. National Library of Medicine. "Genetics Home Reference," 2019. [Online]. Available: https://ghr.nlm.nih.gov/primer/precisionmedicine/definition [Accessed 9 September 2019].

Venter, J.C., Adams, M.D., & Myers, E.W., et al. "The sequence of the human genome," *Science*, vol. 291, no. 5507, pp. 1304–1351, 2001.

Weighill, D., Macaya-Sanz, D., & DiFazio, S.P., et al. "Wavelet-based genomic signal processing for centromere identification and hypothesis generation," *Frontiers in Genetics*, vol. 10, p. 487, 2019.

7 *In Silico* Identification of Protein Targets for Chemical Neurotoxins Using ToxCast *In Vitro* Data and Read-Across within the QSAR Toolbox

Yaroslav G. Chushak, Jeffery M. Gearhart, and Heather A. Pangburn
Wright-Patterson Air Force Base

Hannah W. Shows
Wright State University

CONTENTS

7.1   INTRODUCTION

Every day humans are exposed to thousands of manufactured chemicals. Some of these chemicals, such as organic solvents or pesticides, can interact with neurological proteins in the brain and cause neurotoxic effects leading to headaches, altered sensation or motor skills, impaired memory and cognitive functions, behavioral problems,

DOI: 10.1201/9780429263286-9

even paralysis and death. The neurotoxicity of chemicals greatly depends on their interactions with neurological targets. The recently introduced adverse outcome pathway (AOP) framework links these molecular interactions (Molecular Initiating Event) with a series of key events on different biological levels that result in an adverse outcome effect (Vinken 2013). Within the AOP framework, neurotoxicity can be defined as an adverse effect on the functioning of the nervous system (Bal-Price et al. 2015).

With the recent advances made in the field of *in vitro* high-throughput screening (HTS), it is now possible to screen the biological activity of large chemical libraries in a cost-efficient and timely manner. In 2006, the US Environmental Protection Agency (EPA) initiated the ToxCast program to develop and evaluate *in vitro* biochemical and cell-based assays for screening thousands of chemicals at multiple concentrations in the high-throughput mode (Dix et al. 2007). In Phase II of the program, approximately 1,800 compounds were tested in ~900 HTS assays. The chemicals in the library included pesticides, commercial compounds, and some failed pharmaceuticals. In 2008, the ToxCast program was merged with a large multiagency Tox21 collaboration. Under this new program, ~8,400 chemicals were screened in ~70 HTS assays (Tice et al. 2013). These *in vitro* screenings generated an enormous volume of data which is publicly available at https://www.epa.gov/chemical-research/toxicity-forecaster-toxcasttm-data. Although ToxCast and other *in vitro* screening programs provide a significant amount of information about the biological activities for thousands of chemicals, a great deal of information for millions of chemicals remains missing. Computational methods together with the HTS data offer a great opportunity to partially address this data gap and identify molecular targets and other endpoints for chemical toxins of interest.

According to the European Chemical Agency (ECHA) guidance on information requirements and chemical safety assessment, two computational methods— (quantitative) structure–activity relationship [(Q)SAR] and grouping of chemicals with read-across—can be used for evaluating intrinsic properties of chemicals (European Chemical Agency 2016). Both methods are based on the similarity principle, i.e., that similar molecules have similar properties and the biological activities are defined by molecular structure (Patlewicz and Fitzpatrick 2016). (Q)SAR methods are statistical in nature as they try to correlate the molecular descriptors of chemicals with their properties. Furthermore, these methods are global in their scope as they build models for all chemicals in the training dataset and make predictions for a wide range of chemicals within the applicability domain. QSAR modeling was applied to develop predictive models based on ToxCast HTS data. Some of the models were successful (Liu et al. 2015; Mansouri and Judson 2016; Mansouri et al. 2016), while other QSAR models yielded low predictive performance (Novotarskyi et al. 2016; Thomas et al. 2012).

Grouping of chemicals into a category and read-across is another important technique for data gap filling in chemical hazard assessment. This approach is local in scope as its predictions are based on the properties of a small set of similar chemicals. *The OECD Guidance on Grouping of Chemicals* defines a chemical category as a group of chemicals whose physicochemical and toxicological properties are similar or follow a regular pattern as a result of structural similarity (Organization for Economic Co-operation and Development 2014). The similarities may be based on common functional groups, common modes or mechanisms of action, common constituents or chemical classes, etc. Read-across is a technique to predict the unknown properties of chemicals of interest based on the known properties of chemicals in the same chemical group (European Chemical Agency 2016). Grouping of chemicals and the read-across technique are implemented in several freely available tools such as QSAR Toolbox (Dimitrov et al. 2016), Toxmatch (Gallegos-Saliner et al. 2008), and ToxRead (Gini et al. 2014). QSAR Toolbox is a software platform developed by the Organisation for Economic Co-operation and Development (OECD) in collaboration with the ECHA, intended to be used to fill data gaps in hazard assessment of chemicals. QSAR Toolbox v.3.5 has a database with about 200,000 chemicals provided by governmental and commercial institutions. Furthermore, it allows access to import custom databases and use data for hazard assessment. The main aim of the present study was to explore the application of the QSAR Toolbox and data from ToxCast HTS assays to identify and predict molecular interactions of chemical neurotoxins with their targets.

Recently, activities of 86 compounds from the ToxCast library were tested in neuronal cultures on multi-well microelectrode arrays (MEAs) (Valdivia et al. 2014). Activities of these compounds on MEAs were compared with their activities on 20 ToxCast binding assays that measured the interaction of chemicals with 8 different ion channels. In our approach, we identified 123 proteins from ToxCast HTS assays that are related to neurological functions. This set of proteins includes ion channels, G protein-coupled receptors, nuclear receptors, transporters, and enzymes as potential neurological targets. The developed approach was evaluated by predicting neurological targets for pyrethroids and comparing the predicted results with ToxCast screening data.

7.2 MATERIALS AND METHODS

7.2.1 ToxCast Compound Dataset

The Tox21/ToxCast dataset released in October 2015 consists of 9,076 chemicals tested in 1,193 cellular and biochemical assays (US Environmental Protection Agency 2016). These assays were developed across multiple human and animal cell lines by several providers, including Attagene, Inc. (marked as ATG), BioSeek (BSK), NIH Chemical Genomics Center (Tox21), and NovaScreen (NVS), among others. However, not all chemicals were tested in all of the assays. The majority of biochemical assays related to the activity of neurological proteins, such as ligand-gated ion channels and G protein-coupled receptors, were screened in the NovaScreen assay platform. Therefore, for our analysis, we selected a subset of 1,077 chemicals that were all screened in NVS assays. Furthermore, we reduced this subset by eliminating mixtures and compounds without the molecular description of their structure in the SMILES (Simplified Molecular Input Line-Entry System) format. As a result, the final subset contained 1,050 chemicals that were screened in 656 ToxCast HTS assays.

7.2.2 Bioactivity Data Associated with Neurotoxicity

The Tox21/ToxCast HTS assays targeted 342 different proteins. Using the Gene Ontology (GO) database, we have identified that 123 of these proteins have neurological functions. To identify proteins that are related to neuronal functions, we used three terms in the GO search: "neurological," "synapse," and "axon." This search identified 2,499 unique proteins related to neurological functions, and 123 of these proteins were screened in 216 ToxCast assays. Data from these assays were imported into the QSAR Toolbox and used in further analysis. The chemical concentration at half maximum efficacy AC50 (in µM) was used to identify chemical–assay activities. Two sets of data were generated: one set coded with a "1" for active compounds and a "0" for inactive compounds was used for classification, while a second dataset containing AC50s for only active compounds was used for prediction of AC50 values for unknown chemicals of interest.

7.2.3 Performance Evaluation

To evaluate the performance of ToxCast HTS assays on chemical neurotoxins, compounds with known protein interactions from two databases were used: DrugBank (DB) (https://www.drugbank.ca/) and Ki database from the Psychoactive Drug Screening Program (PDSP) (https://kidbdev.med.unc.edu/databases/kidb.php).

The DB database combines detailed drug data with comprehensive drug-target information containing 8,261 drugs and 4,338 nonredundant proteins that are linked to these drug entries (Wishart et al. 2008). Twenty-nine chemicals from the DB database were screened in selected ToxCast assays and were used to evaluate the activity of neurological proteins in ToxCast screening.

The PDSP Ki database, which is funded by the US National Institute of Mental Health Psychoactive Drug Screening Program, serves as a data warehouse for published and internally derived Ki, or affinity, values for a large number of drugs and drug candidates at an expanding number of G protein-coupled receptors, ion channels, transporters, and enzymes (Roth et al. 2000). Currently it has ~60,000 Ki values. Seventeen chemicals from that database were tested on their targets in selected ToxCast HTS assays and were used to evaluate the performance of ToxCast assays.

Another database, the Toxin and Toxin Target Database (http://www.t3db.ca/), also provides mechanisms of toxicity and target proteins for toxins. However, ToxCast HTS data are already included in this database for chemical–protein associations. Therefore, this database information was not used for evaluation of ToxCast screening assays to avoid bias.

7.2.4 Software

Data processing and management were performed using SQLite v.3 SQL database engine (https://www.sqlite.org/). Grouping of chemicals into a category and read-across was performed within OECD QSAR Toolbox v.3.5. The compounds were grouped by organic functional groups and by structural similarity.

7.3 RESULTS AND DISCUSSION

In the presented approach, we used 1,050 chemicals from the ToxCast dataset that were screened in 656 ToxCast high-throughput assays. Among the 342 different proteins that were screened in the ToxCast HTS assays, there are 123 proteins with neurological functions identified according to the Gene Ontology database. The distribution of active chemicals for these proteins was exceptionally skewed, with some proteins exhibiting >450 active chemicals, regressing to some with only two (Figure 7.1). The top 22 neurological proteins with more than 100 active chemicals are shown on the inset in Figure 7.1.

The estrogen receptor (ESR1), well known for its promiscuous interactions with structurally diverse chemicals that can potentially cause a range of adverse outcome effects, demonstrated the highest number of interacting chemicals (453) (Ng et al. 2014). ESR1 is associated with several nervous system diseases including migraine (Chai et al. 2014) and Alzheimer's disease (Bertram et al. 2007). Recent studies indicate that ESR1 antagonists play a crucial role in neuroinflammation and neurodegeneration (Chakrabarti et al. 2014). Two other proteins with more than 300 active chemicals are HLA class II histocompatibility antigen (HLA-DRA) with 414 active chemicals and C-C motif chemokine (CCL2) with 386 active chemicals. HLA-DRA is associated with Parkinson's disease (Ahmed et al. 2012) and multiple sclerosis (International Multiple Sclerosis Genetics Consortium 2007), while CCL2 is involved in a variety of neuroinflammatory (Conductier et al. 2010) and neurodegenerative (Bose and Cho 2013) diseases. Furthermore, these three proteins have 184 common active chemicals, e.g., bisphenol B, DDT (dichlorodiphenyltrichloroethane), and

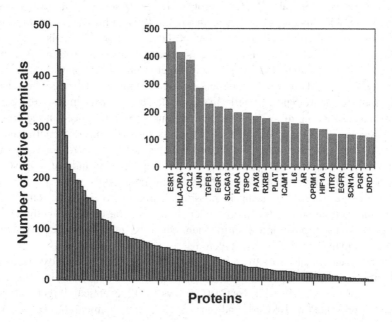

FIGURE 7.1 Distribution of the number of active chemicals for neurological proteins. The inset shows 22 proteins with more than 100 active chemicals.

PFDA (perfluorodecanoic acid). On the other end of the spectrum where there is low chemical–protein interaction, 16 neurological proteins have less than 10 active chemicals, which corresponds to less than 1% of screened compounds. Among the proteins with a low number of active chemicals detected by the ToxCast HTS assays are such important neuronal proteins as GABA receptors (GABRA5, GABRA6, GABBR1), glutamate receptors GRIK1 and GRM5, glycine receptor GLRA1, and voltage-gated calcium ion channel CACNA1B. The low number of active chemicals for these proteins limits the predictability for these proteins for new unknown chemicals.

As previously mentioned, neurological proteins were screened in 263 ToxCast high-throughput assays. In the ToxCast screening protocol, initially all chemicals were screened in each assay at a single concentration of 25 µM (10 µM for CYP assays) to identify active chemical–assay combinations in which the mean assay signal differed by at least 30% from the DMSO control signal (Sipes et al. 2013). Next, for active chemical–assay pairs, each chemical was run in eight-point serial dilutions starting from a top concentration of 50 µM down to 0.023 µM to estimate the AC50s. We generated two sets of data for neurological proteins from the ToxCast dataset: one set for classification of compounds as active or inactive and another set for prediction of AC50 values which were subsequently imported into the QSAR Toolbox to identify and predict molecular interactions of chemical neurotoxins with their targets.

We evaluated the performance of the ToxCast HTS assays on neurological proteins by using chemical neurotoxins with known mechanisms of action from the two databases: Drug Bank and Ki databases from the PDSP. Twenty-nine chemicals from the DB database were screened in ToxCast assays on neurological protein targets. The results of the comparison of drug-target pairs from DB and ToxCast screening are shown in Table 7.1. Only proteins that were screened in ToxCast assays are represented in this table. Chemicals in rows 1–19 were found to have all of their targets from DB represented in the ToxCast database. For chemicals in the rows 20–22, only some DB chemical–target pairs were reproduced in ToxCast screening, and for chemicals in the rows 23–29, their targets were not present in the ToxCast screening. Overall, there are 46 chemical–protein interactions between the selected compounds and neurological proteins in the DB database. Thirty-three of these interactions, corresponding to ~72% of the interactions, were reproduced in the ToxCast HTS screening. ESR1 is a target for seven of the screened drugs in the DB database, and it was identified as a target for all selected chemicals in the ToxCast screening. The androgen receptor (AR) interacts with six drugs in DB, and the progesterone receptor (PGR) interacts with five drugs; all these interactions were also identified in ToxCast screening. Among the 13 missing chemical–protein pairs, four of them involve interactions of prostaglandin-endoperoxide synthase PTGS2 with common analgesics such as aspirin or acetaminophen. Only one interaction of celecoxib with PTGS2 was identified in ToxCast screening.

Seventeen chemicals from the Ki database were screened in the ToxCast assays, and their neurological targets are shown in Table 7.2. In rows 1–9, all DB chemical–target pairs were represented in ToxCast; in rows 10–12, chemical–target pairs were partially represented in ToxCast; and in rows 13–17, all chemical–target pairs were not present in the ToxCast screening.

TABLE 7.1

Chemicals from the DrugBank Database That Were Screened in ToxCast HTS Assays Together with Their Targets and Number of Neurological Targets in ToxCast Assays

Name	CAS	DB Targets	Number ToxCast Targets
1. Celecoxib	169590-42-5	PTGS2;	9
2. Nilutamide	63612-50-0	AR;	4
3. Tamoxifen	10540-29-1	ESR1;	17
4. Retinoic acid	302–79-4	RARG; RXRB; RXRG;	17
5. Diethylstilbestrol	56-53-1	ESR1;	34
6. Flutamide	13311-84-7	AR;	10
7. Caffeine	58-08-2	ADORA1; ADORA2A; PDE4A;	6
8. 17-Methyltestosterone	58-18-4	AR;	4
9. 17beta-Estradiol	50-28-2	ESR1;	6
10. Testosterone propionate	57–85-2	AR;	11
11. Estrone	53-16-7	ESR1;	7
12. Norethindrone	68-22-4	PGR;	7
13. Norgestrel	797-63-7	AR; ESR1; PGR;	5
14. Mifepristone	84371-65-3	PGR;	23
15. Reserpine	50–55-5	SLC18A2;	16
16. Genistein	446–72-0	ESR1;	11
17. Haloperidol	52–86–8	DRD1; DRD2; HTR2A;	38
18. 5,5-Diphenylhydantoin	57-41-0	SCN1A;	3
19. 3,5,3'-Triiodothyronine	6893-02-3	THRA;	12
20. Theophylline	58-55-9	ADORA1; ADORA2A; PDE4A;	2- ADORA1, ADORA2A
21. Spironolactone	52-01-7	AR; CACNA1A; CACNA1B; PGR;	13- AR, PGR
22. Progesterone	57–83-0	ESR1; OPRK1; PGR;	10- ESR1, PGR
23. Valproic acid	99-66-1	SCN1A;	2
24. Butanoic acid	107–92–6	BCHE;	1
25. Acetaminophen	103–90–2	PTGS2;	1
26. Aspirin	50-78-2	EDNRA; PTGS2;	8
27. Theobromine	83-67-0	ADORA1; ADORA2A;	5
28. Indomethacin	53–86-1	PTGS2;	2
29. Sulfasalazine	599-79-1	PTGS2;	6

Rows 1–19: all DB chemical–target pairs were represented in ToxCast; Rows 20–22: chemical–target pairs were partially represented in ToxCast; and Rows 23–29: all chemical–target pairs not present in the ToxCast screening.

TABLE 7.2

Chemicals from the PDSP Ki Database That Were Screened in ToxCast HTS Assays Together with Their Targets and Number of Neurological Targets in ToxCast Assays

Name	CAS	PDSP Targets	Number ToxCast Targets
1. Haloperidol	52–86–8	ADRA1A;ADRA1B; ADRA2A;ADRA2C; ADRB2;CCKBR; CHRM1;CHRM2; CHRM3; CHRM4; CHRM5;DRD1; DRD2;DRD4;HRH1; HRH2;HTR1A; HTR2A;HTR2C; HTR3A;HTR6;HTR7; OPRD1;OPRK1; OPRM1;SLC6A3; SLC6A4;	37
2. Volinanserin	139290-65-6	ADRA1A;ADRA1B; ADRA2A;ADRA2C; DRD1;DRD2;DRD4; HRH1;HTR2A;HTR2C; HTR6;	26
3. Diphenhydramine hydrochloride	147-24-0	CHRM1;CHRM2; CHRM3;CHRM4; CHRM5;HRH1;	29
4. Forchlorfenuron	68157-60-8	HTR1A;	20
5. Pyrimethamine	58-14-0	CHRM1;	27
6. 17beta-Estradiol	50-28-2	ESR1;	6
7. Theophylline	58–88–9	ADORA1, ADORA2A,	2
8. Methadone	1095-90-5	SLC6A4, OPRD1, OPRK1, OPRM1	25
9. Nicotine	54-11-5	CHRNA2, CHRNA7	3
10. Progesterone	57–83–0	HTR3A;PGR;	8- PGR
11. Enadoline	124378-77-4	OPRD1;OPRK1; OPRM1; ·	4- OPRK1
12. Dicofol	115–32-2	SLC6A3;SLC6A4;	8- SLC6A3
13. Naphthalene	91-20-3	ADRA2A;ADRA2C;	5
14. Celecoxib	169590-42-5	SLC6A3;	9
15. Quercetin	117–39-5	DRD4	13
16. Reserpine	50–55-5	HTR1A, HTR2A, HTR2C, DRD1, DRD2, DRD3,	16
17. Cyclohexylamine	108–91–8	ADORA1;	0

Rows 1–9: all DB chemical–target pairs were represented in ToxCast; Rows 10–12: chemical–target pairs were partially represented in ToxCast; and Rows 13–17: all chemical–target pairs not present in the ToxCast screening.

Although only 17 chemicals from the Ki database were screened in the ToxCast assays, there are 74 chemical–protein interactions. The majority of these chemical–protein pairs represent interactions of two drugs—haloperidol and volinanserin—with their targets. Haloperidol, which is used to treat schizophrenia and other psychoses, has five protein targets in the DB database (only three of them were used in the ToxCast screening), but it has 27 protein targets in the PDSP database. In the ToxCast screening, haloperidol was active on 37 neurological protein targets, which indicates the very high activity of this drug having potential side effects. Volinanserin was tested in clinical trials as a potential antipsychotic drug, but it was never advanced to the market place. It interacts with 11 protein targets in the PDSP database and has 26 interactions in the ToxCast screening assays. Among the chemicals whose protein interactions were not identified in the ToxCast screening, celecoxib and reserpine are also present in the DB database. The anti-inflammatory drug celecoxib interacts with prostaglandin synthase PTGS2 in DB, and this interaction was captured in ToxCast screening. However, its interaction with the sodium-dependent dopamine transporter SLC6A3 from the Ki database was not observed. The antipsychotic drug reserpine has the synaptic vesicular amine transporter SLC18A2 listed as a target in DB, which was identified in ToxCast, while in PDSP, it interacts with serotonin and dopamine receptors that were not observed in the ToxCast screening. Overall, out of 73 chemical–protein interactions between the selected compounds and neurological proteins in the Ki database, 58 chemical–protein pairs that correspond to 80% of interactions were identified in the ToxCast screening assays.

The neuronal activities of 86 compounds from the ToxCast library were recently examined in primary cortical cultures with MEAs (Valdivia et al. 2014). The changes in the weighted mean firing rate were used as indicators of chemical activities on neuronal networks. The effects of tested chemicals on spontaneous neuronal activity in MEAs were compared with their activities on 20 ToxCast assays that measured the interaction of chemicals with ion channels. Pyrethroids were among the classes of chemicals that affected neuronal activity in MEAs. The primary mechanism of pyrethroid neurotoxicity is proposed to be via their effects on the sodium channels of nerve cells (Vijverbert and van den Bercken 1990). However, only one of the six studied pyrethroid compounds—allethrin—showed activity in the ToxCast ion channel assays, while all but permethrin were active in MEA measurements (Valdivia et al. 2014). This indicates the presence of different mechanisms of toxicity for pyrethroids. We selected chemicals from this group to evaluate the predictive capability of the proposed approach.

The first step in the read-across approach is to identify a group of chemicals from the ToxCast screening database that belongs to the same class as a studied compound. There are several ways to perform a similarity search in the QSAR Toolbox ("Category Definition"). We used two terms, "pyrethroids" and "esters," to identify pyrethroids in the ToxCast database. The search recognized 12 compounds that are shown in Figure 7.2. Two different types of pyrethroids are recognized based on differences in their structure and the symptoms of poisoning (Vijverberg and van den Bercken 1990). Structures of four of the selected compounds include a cyano group, and these chemicals belong to the Type II pyrethroid group. The remaining chemicals that lack a cyano group belong to the Type I pyrethroid group.

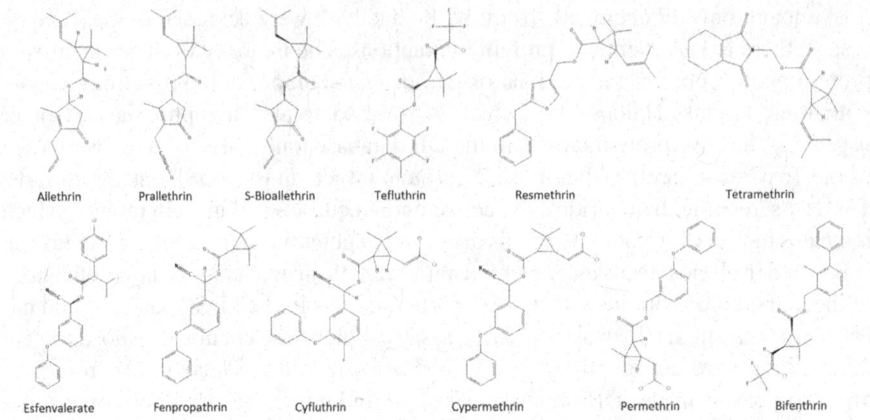

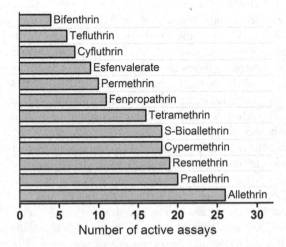

FIGURE 7.2 Pyrethroid compounds from ToxCast database that were used in the current study. Four compounds (esfenvalerate, fenpropathrin, cyfluthrin, and cypermethrin) have a cyano group and belong to Type II pyrethroids; the remaining compounds belong to Type I pyrethroids.

The majority of pyrethroids are active in 10–20 ToxCast HTS assays with neurological proteins (Figure 7.3). However, allethrin shows very high activity as it is active in 26 assays, while bifenthrin is only active in four assays and tefluthrin in six assays. This is a clear indication that some compounds in the pyrethroid group have unique structural features that are reflected in their distinctive activities. As for neuronal targets, the ATG_DR5_CIS assay that targeted retinoic acid receptors

FIGURE 7.3 Number of active assays with neurological proteins for pyrethroids from the database of chemicals.

RARA, RARB, and RARG exhibited activity for 10 of the 12 pyrethroids examined. Another assay that also targeted RARA—ATG_RARa_TRANS—has seven active compounds, indicating that retinoic acid receptors are targeted by pyrethroids.

Another potential target of pyrethroid compounds is the dopamine transporter SLC63. Two assays that targeted human and guinea pig transporters—NVS_TR_hDAT and NVS_NVS_gDAT—have nine and five active pyrethroids, respectively. Among the neuronal proteins with only one or two active chemicals are GABA receptor GABRA1, which is affected only by allethrin, and muscarinic cholinergic receptors CHRM1 and CHMR3, which are affected by prallethrin. Since we can only make predictions for protein targets that are affected by a group of chemicals and not just by a single chemical, we selected a set of 14 ToxCast assays with five or more active pyrethroids to assess the predictive capability of the proposed approach. Eight of the studied assays are cell-based assays and the effect of chemicals was investigated by measuring the activity of proteins or changes in the protein expression level. Five of the biochemical assays measured protein–ligand binding while in one assay enzymatic activity was measured to evaluate activity of chemicals.

The predictions for pyrethroids were based on the activity of five nearest neighbor chemicals, and data from target chemicals was not used in the prediction. For four compounds—allethrin, S-bioallethrin, prallethrin, and fenpropathrin—activity in only one of the studied assays was incorrectly predicted. On the other hand, activities for tetramethrin and for bifenthrin in seven and five assays, respectively, were incorrectly predicted. Tetramethrin is the only compound among the studied pyrethroids that has an imide group that potentially explains the high number of incorrect predictions. Bifenthrin, as mentioned before, showed extremely low activity in the ToxCast screening, as it was active with neurological proteins only in four assays (see Figure 7.3). The summary of classification predictions for pyrethroid compounds is presented in Table 7.3. Overall, there are 168 chemical–protein pairs: 89 are active, and 79 are inactive. Eighty-three percent of active interactions, 73 of 89 interactions in the ToxCast database, were correctly predicted using our approach. We also correctly predicted 60 inactive chemical–protein pairs, which corresponds to a 76% hit rate.

Table 7.4 shows the predicted AC50 values (in mg/L) for a set of five pyrethroid compounds in comparison with the ToxCast screening results. For cyfluthrin, we

TABLE 7.3

Summary of the Classification Prediction of Pyrethroid Activity

	Predicted		
ToxCast	Active	Inactive	Hit Rate
Active	73	16	83%
Inactive	19	60	76%
Accuracy	79%	79%	

TABLE 7.4

Comparison of the Predicted AC50 Values (in mg/L) with the ToxCast Screening Data for a Set of Pyrethroid Compounds

Assays	Cyfluthrin		Permethrin		Cypermethrin		Fenpropathrin		Tetramethrin	
	ToxCast	Predicted	ToxCast	Predicted	ToxCast	Predicted	ToxCast	Predicted	ToxCast	Predicted
ATG_DR5_CIS	1.05	1.62	2.55	2.51	3.55	2.4	1.74	1.13	Inactive	0.963
ATG_ERE_CIS	Inactive	5.84	9.13	4.59	5.6	5.6	2.79	5.36	Inactive	Inactive
ATG_ERa_TRANS	Inactive	Inactive	8.6	6.97	9.72	8.05	6.81	5.32	Inactive	Inactive
ATG_RARa_TRANS	Inactive	2.62	Inactive	2.95	3.23	3.35	3.75	2.64	Inactive	2
BSK_3C_HLADR	Inactive	Inactive	2.32	3.67	Inactive	5.68	Inactive	6.61	6.64	5.13
BSK_3C_MCP1	Inactive	Inactive	Inactive	Inactive	Inactive	Inactive	Inactive	Inactive	2.93	6.3
BSK_4H_MCP1	2.87	5.47	Inactive	Inactive	2.88	5.19	Inactive	Inactive	Inactive	3.67
BSK_SAg_MCP1	2.94	6.78	Inactive	Inactive	Inactive	Inactive	Inactive	Inactive	4.93	4.42
NVS_ENZ_hBACE	1.59	4.06	16.0	4.04	Inactive	Inactive	0.778	3.6	7.8	3.82
NVS_GPCR_h5HT7	Inactive	6.23	8.77	5.02	3.35	6.91	10.4	4.18	Inactive	Inactive
NVS_GPCR_hDRD1	Inactive	Inactive	4.21	6.95	Inactive	Inactive	Inactive	Inactive	19.9	3.83
NVS_GPCR_mCCKA	Inactive	Inactive	Inactive	Inactive	8.58	8.66	6.48	7.46	Inactive	6.88
NVS_TR_hDAT	0.953	2.91	Inactive	4.14	3.75	4.68	4.25	1.66	Inactive	1.68
NVS_TR_gDAT	Inactive	Inactive	Inactive	Inactive	4.91	8.14	6.83	6.02	Inactive	5.86

Fourteen assays with five or more active pyrethroids were selected for evaluation.

correctly predicted activity in 11 out of 14 assays. The predicted AC50 values for cyfluthrin are in good correlation with those observed experimentally. Activity predictions for permethrin yielded incorrect results for two assays while only a few predicted AC50 values were in agreement with those measured in ToxCast assays. In several *in vitro* assays, permethrin shows very low activity, with AC50 values in the range of 8.6–16.0 mg/L. This is in agreement with the low potency of permethrin, which showed no effect on neuronal network activity measured using the MEA technique (Valdivia et al. 2014). The predicted values are based on the values measured for a group of similar chemicals. As a result, the predicted AC50 values for permethrin in these assays are lower compared with the observed. For cypermethrin, only BSK_3C_HLADR assay activity was incorrectly predicted, while predicted AC50 values show, in general, a good correlation with the measured ones. Although tetramethrin is active in 16 neurological assays, it is active only in five of the assays selected for the evaluation. As mentioned before, classification incorrectly predicted activity of tetramethrin in seven of the ToxCast assays. Predicted AC50 values also showed mixed accuracy compared with the ToxCast data. These results indicate that it is currently difficult to predict activity of a compound that has different structural and activity properties compared with the other chemicals in the same group.

7.4 CONCLUSIONS

The neurotoxicity of chemicals greatly depends on their interactions with neurological targets. We used ToxCast *in vitro* HTS data and the OECD QSAR Toolbox to identify and predict AC50 values for the interaction of chemical neurotoxins with their protein targets. The developed approach was evaluated by predicting chemical–protein interactions for a set of pyrethroid compounds. The classification prediction results showed 79% accuracy while AC50 predictions demonstrated mixed accuracy compared with the ToxCast screening data. Several observed challenges of the proposed approach need to be highlighted.

Grouping of chemicals. The first and most critical part in the read-across prediction is finding similar chemicals in the database. There is no unique way for grouping chemicals into a category. Therefore, the same chemical can belong to different groups based on the similarity criteria (Shah et al. 2016). We used two terms to identify pyrethroids in the ToxCast database, "pyrethroids" and "esters." However, 12 pyrethroid compounds that were identified showed very different activities in the ToxCast assays. For example, allethrin is active in 26 assays, while bifenthrin is active only in four assays and tefluthrin is active in six assays. Furthermore, this set of pyrethroids contains eight Type I and four Type II pyrethroids classified according to eliciting different symptomology. Clearly, the difference in the chemical structure of these chemicals resulted in their different activities. One way to improve the similarity is to subcategorize the list of chemicals based on structural similarity on a chemical-by-chemical basis.

Low activity of chemicals. In some cases, a chemical showed low activity in a ToxCast assay with multiple points above the baseline, but the AC50 value could not be calculated from the dose–response data (Sipes et al. 2013). In such cases, chemicals were marked as "inactive" in the ToxCast database, making it difficult to identify the active/inactive boundary for chemicals with low activity.

The number of active/inactive compounds in the classification dataset should be similar. The ATG_DR5_CIS assay has 10 active pyrethroids out of 12 and several assays have 9 active pyrethroids. It is impossible to predict inactive compounds for ATG_DR5_CIS (like tetramethrin and bifenthrin) when ten neighbors are active in the assay. The same is true also for assays that have just one to three active compounds. Therefore, these assays were not considered in the current approach. In this case, a different grouping schema needs to be applied that will identify a different set of similar chemicals.

Descriptors and applicability domain. The QSAR Toolbox allows the use of a different set of molecular descriptors for read-across prediction. Special attention is needed when selecting descriptors to be sure that they show correlation with the AC50 values and the tested chemical is within the applicability domain for the selected descriptors. Another approach is to use trend analysis, which can improve the predicted results when the chemical is outside the applicability domain for the selected descriptor. However, that approach was not used in the current study.

Our results demonstrate that ToxCast *in vitro* screening data and the QSAR Toolbox can be used to identify neurological targets and predict AC50 values for chemical neurotoxins that have similar chemicals in the ToxCast database. This approach can be combined with MEA measurements to link molecular interactions to cellular response. Very recently, MEA techniques were used to evaluate the effect of a set of pyrethroids on spontaneous activity of cortical neuronal networks (Krishnan and Prakhya 2016). Besides the weighted mean firing rate, authors also measured other burst parameters such as mean burst duration and mean interspike interval in burst. In the present study, we show that pyrethroids affect multiple protein targets that can result in complex neurological responses. Therefore, it is of interest to investigate the correlation of molecular interactions with the multiple endpoints in MEA measurements. Such a combined *in vitro/in silico* approach would allow us to connect the MIE with cellular response of chemical neurotoxins.

7.5   CONFLICT OF INTEREST

There are no conflicts of interest to declare.

7.6   ACKNOWLEDGMENTS

This research was funded by the Defense Health Program under the RSAAC project 17-003 and by the 711th Human Performance Wing. The views expressed in this chapter are those of the authors and do not necessarily reflect the official policy or position of the Air Force, the Department of Defense, or the U.S. Government.

The text for this chapter is reprinted with permission from the following publication:

Y.G. Chushak, H.W. Shows, J.M. Gearhart and H.A. Pangburn, "*In silico* identification of protein targets for chemical neurotoxins using ToxCast *in vitro* data and read-across within the QSAR toolbox", Toxicol. Res., 2018, 7, 423–431.

REFERENCES

Ahmed I., R. Tamouza, M. Delord, R. Krishnamoorthy, C. Tzourio, C. Mulot, M. Nacfer, J. C. Lambert, P. Beaune, P. Laurent-Puig, M. A. Loriot, D. Charron and A. Elbaz, Association between Parkinson's disease and the HLA-DRB1 locus, *Mov. Disord.*, 2012, **27**, 1104–1110.

Bal-Price A., K. M. Crofton, M. Sachana, T. J. Shafer, M. Behl, A. Forsby, A. Hargreaves, B. Landesmann, P. J. Lein, J. Louisse, F. Monnet-Tschudi, A. Paini, A. Rolaki, A. Schrattenholz, C. Suñol, C. van Thriel, M. Whelan and E. Fritsche, Putative adverse outcome pathways relevant to neurotoxicity, *Crit. Rev. Toxicol.*, 2015, **45**, 83–91.

Bertram L., M. B. McQueen, K. Mullin, D. Blacker and R. E. Tanzi, Systematic meta-analyses of Alzheimer disease genetic association studies: the AlzGene database, *Nat. Genet.*, 2007, **39**, 17–23.

Bose S. and J. Cho, Role of chemokine CCL2 and its receptor CCR2 in neurodegenerative diseases, *Arch. Pharm. Res.*, 2013, **36**, 1039–1050.

Chai N.C., B. L. Peterlin and A. H. Calhoun, Migraine and estrogen, *Curr. Opin. Neurol.*, 2014, **27**, 315–324.

Chakrabarti M., A. Haque, N. L. Banik, P. Nagarkatti, M. Nagarkatti and S. K. Ray, Estrogen receptor agonists for attenuation of neuroinflammation and neuro-degeneration, *Brain Res. Bull.*, 2014, **109**, 22–31.

Conductier G., N. Blondeau, A. Guyon, J. L. Nahon and C. Rovère, The role of mono-cyte chemoattractant protein MCP1/CCL2 in neuroinflammatory diseases, *J. Neuroimmunol.*, 2010, **224**, 93–100.

European Chemicals Agency, Guidance on information requirements and chemical safety assessment, Chapter R.6: QSARs and grouping of chemicals, https://echa.europa.eu/guidance-documents/guidance-on-information-requirements-and-chemical-safety-assessment (accessed January 2016).

Dimitrov S. D., R. Diderich, T. Sobanski, T. S. Pavlov, G. V. Chankov, A. S. Chapkanov, Y. H. Karakolev, S. G. Temelkov, R. A. Vasilev, K. D. Gerova, C. D. Kuseva, N. D. Todorova, A. M. Mehmed, M. Rasenberg, O. G. Mekenyan, QSAR Toolbox – workflow and major functionalities, *SAR QSAR Environ. Res.*, 2016, **27**, 203–219.

Dix D. J., K. A. Houck, M. T. Martin, A. M. Richard, R. W. Setzer and R. J. Kavlock, The ToxCast program for prioritizing toxicity testing of environmental chemicals, *Toxicol. Sci.*, 2007, **95**, 5–12.

Gallegos-Saliner A., A. Poater, N. Jeliazkova, G. Patlewicz and A. P. Worth, Toxmatch – a chemical classification and activity prediction tool based on similarity measures, *Regul. Toxicol. Pharmacol.*, 2008, **52**, 77–84.

Gini G., A. M. Franchi, A. Manganaro, A. Golbamaki and E. Benfenati, ToxRead: a tool to assist in read across and its use to assess mutagenicity of chemicals, *SAR QSAR Environ. Res.*, 2014, **25**, 999–1011.

International Multiple Sclerosis Genetics Consortium, D. A. Hafler, A. Compston, S. Sawcer, E. S. Lander, M. J. Daly, P. L. De Jager, P. I. de Bakker, S. B. Gabriel, D. B. Mirel, A. J. Ivinson, M. A. Pericak-Vance, S. G. Gregory, J. D. Rioux, J. L. McCauley, J. L. Haines, L. F. Barcellos, B. Cree, J. R. Oksenberg and S. L. Hauser, Risk alleles for multiple sclerosis identified by a genomewide study, *N. Engl. J. Med.*, 2007, **357**, 851–862.

Krishnan B. M. and B. M. Prakhya, In vitro evaluation of pyrethroid-mediated changes on neuronal burst parameters using microelectrode arrays, *Neurotoxicology*, 2016, **57**, 270–281.

Liu J., K. Mansouri, R. S. Judson, M. T. Martin, H. Hong, M. Chen, X. Xu, R. S. Thomas and I. Shah, Predicting hepatotoxicity using ToxCast *in vitro* bioactivity and chemical structure, *Chem. Res. Toxicol.*, 2015, **28**, 738–751.

Mansouri K., A. Abdelaziz, A. Rybacka, A. Roncaglioni, A. Tropsha, A. Varnek, A. Zakharov, A. Worth, A. M. Richard, C. M. Grulke, D. Trisciuzzi, D. Fourches, D. Horvath, E. Benfenati, E. Muratov, E. B. Wedebye, F. Grisoni, G. F. Mangiatordi, G. M. Incisivo, H. Hong, H. W. Ng, I. V. Tetko, I. Balabin, J. Kancherla, J. Shen, J. Burton, M. Nicklaus, M. Cassotti, N. G. Nikolov, O. Nicolotti, P. L. Andersson, Q. Zang, R. Politi, R. D. Beger, R. Todeschini, R. Huang, S. Farag, S. A. Rosenberg, S. Slavov, X. Hu and R. S. Judson, CERAPP: Collaborative Estrogen Receptor Activity Prediction Project, *Environ. Health Perspect.*, 2016, **124**, 1023–1033.

Mansouri K. and R. S. Judson, In Silico Study of In Vitro GPCR Assays by QSAR Modeling, in *In Silico Methods for Predicting Drug Toxicity*, ed. E. Benfenati, Springer, New York, 2016, chapter 16, 361–381.

Ng H.W., R. Perkins, W. Tong and H. Hong, Versatility or promiscuity: the estrogen receptors, control of ligand selectivity and an update on subtype selective ligands, *Int. J. Environ. Res. Public Health*, 2014, **11**, 8709–8742.

Novotarskyi S., A. Abdelaziz, Y. Sushko, R. Körner, J. Vogt and I. V. Tetko, ToxCast EPA *in vitro* to *in vivo* challenge: insight into the Rank-I model, *Chem. Res. Toxicol.*, 2016, **29**, 768–775.

Organization for Economic Co-operation and Development, *Guidance on Grouping of Chemicals*, Organization for Economic Co-operation and Development, Paris, 2nd edition, 2014, OECD Environment, Health and Safety Publications Series on Testing and Assessment No. 194, ENV/JM/MONO(2014)4.

Patlewicz G. and J. M. Fitzpatrick, Current and future perspectives on the development, evaluation, and application of *in silico* approaches for predicting toxicity, *Chem. Res. Toxicol.*, 2016, **29**, 438–451.

Roth B.L., E. Lopez, S. Patel and W. K. Kroeze, The multiplicity of serotonin receptors: uselessly diverse molecules or an embarrassment of riches? *The Neuroscientist*, 2000, **6**, 252–262.

Shah I., J. Liu, R. S. Judson, R. S. Thomas and G. Patlewicz, Systematically evaluating read-across prediction and performance using a local validity approach characterized by chemical structure and bioactivity information, *Regul. Toxicol. Pharmacol.*, 2016, **79**, 12–24.

Sipes N. S., M. T. Martin, P. Kothiya, D. M. Reif, R. S. Judson, A. M. Richard, K. A. Houck, D. J. Dix, R. J. Kavlock and T. B. Knudsen, Profiling 976 ToxCast chemicals across 331 enzymatic and receptor signalling assays, *Chem. Res. Toxicol.*, 2013, **26**, 878–895.

Thomas R. S., M. B. Black, L. Li, E. Healy, T. M. Chu, W. Bao, M. E. Andersen and R. D. Wolfinger, A comprehensive statistical analysis of predicting *in vivo* hazard using high-throughput *in vitro* screening, *Toxicol. Sci.*, 2012, **128**, 398–417.

Tice R. R., C. P. Austin, R. J. Kavlock and J. R. Bucher, Improving the human hazard characterization of chemicals: a Tox21 update, *Environ. Health Perspect.*, 2013, **121**, 756–765.

US Environmental Protection Agency, Toxicity ForeCaster (ToxCast™) data, ToxCast & Tox21 data spreadsheet from invitrodb_v2, http://www2.epa.gov/chemical-research/toxicity-forecaster-toxcasttm-data (accessed January 2016).

Valdivia P., M. Martin, W. R. LeFew, J. Ross, K. A. Houck and T. J. Shafer. Multi-well microelectrode array recordings detect neuroactivity of ToxCast compounds, *Neurotoxicology*, 2014, **44**, 204–217.

Vijverberg H. P. and J. van den Bercken, Neurotoxicological effects and the mode of action of pyrethroid insecticides, *Crit. Rev. Toxicol.*, 1990, **21**, 105–126.

Vinken M., The adverse outcome pathway concept: a pragmatic tool in toxicology, *Toxicology*, 2013, **312**, 158–165.

Wishart D. S., C. Knox, A. C. Guo, D. Cheng, S. Shrivastava, D. Tzur, B. Gautam and M. Hassanali, DrugBank: a knowledgebase for drugs, drug actions and drug targets, *Nucleic Acids Res.*, 2008, **36**, D901–D906.

8 "Omics"
An Introduction

Roland Saldanha
Wright-Patterson Air Force Base

CONTENTS

8.1 INTRODUCTION

The maximum period of time one is at optimum health ("healthspan") results from the interaction of our genetic fate encoded by our unique individual genomes with the complex set of exposures we experience from conception to death. In contrast to infectious disease where onset can be traced to a single cause, "health" is a cumulative result of multiple intrinsic and extrinsic exposures accumulated over a lifetime, each of which may be neither necessary nor sufficient in isolation to evoke a disease state (Vineis 2018). The Total Exposure Health (TEH) model recognizes this and seeks to integrate and model the interactions of an individual's genetic propensities with the totality of occupational, lifestyle and environmental exposures

DOI: 10.1201/9780429263286-10

to enable optimal choices to maximize health in an individually tailored manner enabling "high definition medicine" (Torkamani et al. 2017). Omics encompasses the superset of technologies and data streams that inform on the molecular determinants and dynamic connections that encompass a living system's intrinsic properties and interactions with the extrinsic environment. Omics provides insight into our genetic fate as encoded in our genes ("Genomics"), the playback of this information ("Transcriptomics"), the major structural and catalytic and regulatory effectors of this information ("Proteomics") and the collection of endogenous and exogenous chemical molecules whose flux are the currency of biological systems ("Metabolomics"). Emerging omic technologies include "Microbiomics" capturing the diverse microflora that interact with the host and their influences, "Epigenomics" reflecting a series of molecular marks that influence the playback of genetic information and "Connectomics" reflecting the complex web of cellular or molecular interactions that occur in systems such as neurons and are at the heart of emergent behaviors like "consciousness". This short review will highlight the information to be gleaned from each of the major "omic" study areas, an introduction to the methodology and highlight a few examples of how the broad vision of TEH can be informed by their deployment.

8.2 GENOMICS

The whole human genome is distributed over 23 pairs of chromosomes and extra-chromosomal maternally inherited mitochondrial deoxyribonucleic acid (DNA) with the haploid genome size of ~3.2 billion nucleotides. A large public and private effort spanning ~11 years and at cost of ~$3 billion created the first draft of the Human Genome Project (Lander et al. 2001). It should be noted that difficulties with spanning disease-causing long repetitive elements, extreme GC content regions, etc. have precluded obtaining a complete reference genome in the absolute sense.

A mosaic of several individuals is represented in the Genome Reference Consortium's (GRC) human reference genome version GRCh38. Several large genome sequencing projects have captured a large amount of the variability, and GRCH38 has 261 alternate scaffolds to account for the "benign" variability in ethnically diverse populations. It is estimated that unrelated individuals would differ at ~15 million positions and carry as many as 2,000 structural variations like copy number variations (duplications and deletions) and genome rearrangements like inversions and translocations. Based on a genome size of 3.2 billion nucleotides, it can be expected that each human may have ~3 million nucleotide differences from the reference genome (1 every 300 base pair (bp)). Thus, variants (alleles) have to be contextualized and could be benign or associated with a phenotype or disease or yet to be determined significance (Jackson et al. 2018). Allelic variants are referred as single nucleotide variants (SNVs), and when present in >1% of the population are called polymorphisms (SNP). About 11 million SNPs in the human genome have been cataloged with any one individual carrying about 3 million of them (Chong et al. 2015). Currently, about 4,100 mutations linked to a phenotype have been documented; their current count and statistical breakdown of the spectrum of phenotypes associated with the genes can be found at (https://www.omim.org/statistics/geneMap).

8.2.1 SEQUENCING TECHNOLOGIES

Contemporary sequencing technologies fall into either short (<600 bp) or long (>10 Kb) reads, and their evolution has been well traced (Levy and Myers 2016, Goldfeder et al. 2017, Shendure et al. 2017). A good example of the current short-read platform is Illumina's family of products which capture adapter-tagged libraries of nucleic acids on a flow cell with short complimentary oligonucleotides. These oligonucleotides are clonally amplified to form millions of "clusters" that form the substrate on which sequencing chemistry is performed. Each cluster is a subset of the nucleic acid being sequenced, and they are "read" through iterative rounds of synthesis using specially designed fluorescently labeled nucleotides. The labeled nucleotides have a cleavable terminator which restricts polymerization to a single nucleotide at each cluster whose identities are recorded in parallel using charge-coupled device (CCD) technology. The terminator is then cleaved, and a fresh round of reagents flood the flow cell for the cycle to repeat.

Long-read technologies, on the other hand, use direct single-molecule reading technologies obviating the need for amplification. Their lengths help in *de novo* assembly, read through of repetitive regions, assigning variants to the paternal or maternal chromosome (phasing) and detecting complex splicing isoforms in ribo-nucleic acid (RNA). In addition, they can permit readout of epigenetic modifications on DNA as well as direct readout of RNA without reverse transcription (Rhoads and Au 2015, Jain et al. 2018). In the approach adopted by Oxford Nanopore, an electrical field is applied across a lipid membrane in which nanopores are embedded. Adapter-linked nucleic acids are directed through these pores, and minute changes in electrical current are sensed to read out the sequence. PacBio platforms use a zero-mode waveguide within which a polymerase is immobilized creating a zeptoliter-sized observation chamber enabling detection of single fluorescent nucleotides.

8.2.2 UTILITY OF WHOLE-GENOME SEQUENCE IN TOTAL EXPOSURE HEALTH

For many modern diseases, it has been stated that genetics loads the gun, lifestyle pulls the trigger and the complex interplay of intrinsic and extrinsic factors determines our health span (McHale et al. 2018). The interaction of lifestyle and disease is seen in examples such as coronary artery disease (Said et al. 2019), type 2 diabetes (Franks and Merino 2018), cancer (Simonds et al. 2016) and actionable pharmacogenetic variants (Chanfreau-Coffinier et al. 2019) among many other model examples (Ritz et al. 2017). Genomic information can also inform precision medicine decisions within the TEH framework. For example, *CHRNA5* and *CYP2A6* are strongly implicated in nicotine dependence (a major driver of preventable death), and cessation strategies can be built around genomic data (Chen et al. 2018, Saccone et al. 2018).

8.3 TRANSCRIPTOMICS

The translation of genetic information from DNA to RNA is the first step in expressing genetic information and opens a window into the dynamic processes that occur under normal physiological conditions or in response to changing environments

(Mele et al. 2015). The human transcriptome consists of ~111,451 messenger RNA (mRNA), ~89,981 long non-coding RNA (ncRNA) and ~11,366 small ncRNA (Pertea 2012). Changing cellular, physiological or environmental conditions are quantitatively reflected in changes in gene expression and changes in transcript stability or qualitatively by RNA editing or utilization of alternate splicing sites to create different combinations of exons leading to different protein isoforms (McHale et al. 2013).

8.3.1 ANALYTIC METHODS FOR TRANSCRIPTOMICS

Array-based detection schemes dominated early studies with their results frequently validated by quantitative polymerase chain reaction (qPCR) (Brazma et al. 2001, Bustin et al. 2009). Since this technique is based on hybridization, it limits detection to the targets placed on the array and suffers from a limited dynamic range of detection. In the long-read technologies, RNA can be directly sequenced which permits accurate assemblies of complex isoforms and references-free transcriptome analysis (Hardwick et al. 2019). With the drop in next-generation sequencing (NGS) costs, contemporary studies are dominated by short-read RNA sequencing, and rigorous validation highlights its advantages (Xu et al. 2016, Sa et al. 2018). In these methods, total RNA is often enriched for a desired fraction (multiple adenosine monophosphates (poly A), micro RNA (miRNA), etc.) or depleted of RNA that would dominate the read counts (ribosomal RNA, globin RNA, etc.). There are a large number of protocols that are tailored to the goals for transcriptomics studies (preserving strand specificity, differential gene expression, isoforms, etc.). They generically involve fragmentation (chemical, mechanical, enzymatic or tagmentation), conversion to complementary DNA (cDNA) and ligation to sequencing adapters before being subjected to iterative rounds of sequencing as described for DNA (Hrdlickova et al. 2017, Sa et al. 2018).

8.3.2 TRANSCRIPTOMICS ROLE IN TEH

The dynamic response to challenges like infection, chemicals, pollution and physical stress (heat, radiation, etc.) is reflected in the transcriptome, and these responses serve to mechanistically understand how their impacts on the organism are mitigated or neutralized (Barton et al. 2017, Richards et al. 2017, O'Beirne et al. 2018, Pai and Luca 2019). In addition, transcriptomics has been used to study the impact of phytonutrients and their interactions with genotypes to inform disease prevention through dietary factors (van Breda et al. 2015, Corella et al. 2018, Lin et al. 2019).

8.4 EPIGENOMICS

The epigenome broadly refers to molecular marks and mechanisms that control the structural organization of the genome and thus exert an influence on gene expression without changing the actual coding sequence (Rivera and Ren 2013). Epigenetic changes can act as an on/off switch to activate/inactivate large genomic areas (an example being X-chromosome inactivation) or as a "rheostat" finely tuning gene expression. The deposition of epigenetic marks (and thus gene expression levels) is a mechanism by which cell and tissue types are determined. Epigenetic control is achieved most commonly by modifications of DNA or histones or through regulatory RNA. Common epigenetic marks include methylation/demethylation at cytosine residues of cytosine-guanosine dinucleotides (CpG) or histone tails (which can also be modified by acetylation/deacetylation). The modifications at histones modulate chromatin structure and accessibility of transcription factors, while cytosine methylation/hydroxymethylation generally leads to gene silencing through recruitment of repressors like methyl-binding protein domain protein and histone deacetylases. CpG dinucleotides are overrepresented in promoters and regulatory regions and some repetitive DNA elements.

8.4.1 MEASURING EPIGENOMIC MARKS

Sun et al. (2015) and Dirks et al. (2016) have reviewed the status of genome-wide epigenetic profiling technologies. To probe the methylation status genome wide, methylated DNA is treated with sodium bisulfite which converts methylated cytosine to uracil (read as thymine when sequenced or probed by a methylation microarray such as the Illumina Methylation Epic BeadChip assay). For known human genes, the Illumina Methylation Epic BeadChip assay reports methylation status at ~853,307 CpG sites with coverage of >90% of ~26,000 CpG islands (regions of >200 bp with %GC >50%), North and South Shores of islands (2,000 bp regions upstream and downstream of CpG islands) and 80% coverage of North and South Shelves (regions between 2,000–4,000 bp upstream and downstream of CpG islands). A limitation of array-based technology is that it is difficult to incorporate single nucleotide polymorphism-type data that might be uncovered by bisulfite sequencing approaches. Whole-genome bisulfite sequencing offers the ability to probe all 28 million known CpG and correlate genotype and methylation patterns. Reduced representation bisulfite sequencing and variants offer coverage of 1.5–4 million unique CpG by using methylation-sensitive restriction digestion to enrich CpG-rich regions and sequence only these. The impact of histone modifications is frequently assayed by immunoprecipitation of chromatin using affinity tags directed against specific histone modifications followed by sequencing.

8.4.2 THE EPIGENOME IN TEH

Epigenetic marks are deposited in response to a wide range of environmental exposures from pre-conception and extending from gestation through life in response to numerous life experiences (Leenen et al. 2016). In a natural experiment of a cohort of births following a Dutch famine, the methylation state and spectrum of adult disease states varied depending on the trimester in which nutrient deprivation occurred (Tobi et al. 2014). Similarly, gestational high-fat diets influence the methylome and increase probability of metabolic syndrome obesity and diabetes (Lee 2015). Some infections leave both a pathogen-specific and generic epigenetic signature (Cizmeci et al. 2016). A wide range of epigenetic marks have been correlated with specific environmental chemical exposures (Hou et al. 2012). In a review of epigenome-wide association studies (EWAS), the methylation statuses of cg05575921 (AHRR), cg03636183 (F2RL3) and cg19859270 (GPR15) are strongly correlated with smoking, and smoking cessation is correlated with reversion of the methylation mark at the aryl hydrocarbon receptor AHRR and other loci (Philibert et al. 2016, McCartney et al. 2018). The impact of the environment on the epigenome and its consequence in health and disease is being incorporated into the Adverse Outcome Pathway framework (Angrish et al. 2018, Wang et al. 2018).

8.5   PROTEOME

The proteome reflects both structural and enzymatic effectors of genomics function. Because of the vast range of post-transcriptional and post-translational modifications, the number of proteoforms vastly outnumbers the estimated number of protein coding genes (~20,245) and could be in the millions (Aebersold et al. 2018). Proteins frequently assemble into higher order "molecular machines" and form signaling networks controlling cellular function in both spatial and temporal domains. Because of this complexity, changes in proteome mirror cellular activities more closely than changes in the transcriptome. Proteomics focuses on analyzing changes in proteins in response to a perturbation (lifestyle, exposure, developmental condition, etc.) and includes both qualitative and quantitative assessments. Qualitative metrics might include the presence/absence of a particular polypeptide, the composition of multi-subunit proteins complexes or cellular structures or the distribution of proteins within cellular compartments or tissues. Quantitative assessments could include accurate estimation of concentrations and dynamic changes in concentration in response to changing conditions, as well as enumeration of post-translational modifications like phosphorylation, acetylation, glycosylation, etc. that underlie regulatory control of the enzymatic or structural properties of proteins.

8.5.1   PROTEOMICS METHODS

Targeted assays use affinity reagents (antibodies, aptamers, etc.) to detect/quantify the protein analyte. Newer platforms like that from Luminex or SomaLogic allow highly multiplexed assays against targets spanning a vast abundance range (Smith and Gerszten 2017). Like all targeted assays, they are limited by the availability of an affinity reagent. Untargeted approaches survey the entire proteome largely enabled by advances in liquid chromatography and mass spectrometry (MS) (Hosp and Mann 2017, Mertins et al. 2018). Typically, an extract of interest is digested to peptides and separated using several high-resolution techniques (reverse phase, polarity based, etc.) and analyzed by high-resolution MS. Typically, peptides are scanned and peaks fragmented and resolved in a second MS, and peak and fragment libraries allow identification of proteins (Bakalarski and Kirkpatrick 2016).

8.5.2   PROTEOMICS UTILITY IN TEH

Current workflows in plasma proteomics can detect >40 clinically relevant markers that inform on health (Geyer et al. 2016). Proteins have a number of reactive amino acids and readily form adducts with both environmental chemicals and natural metabolites making them reporters of these exposures. For example, albumin readily reacts with numerous environmental chemicals (Preston and Phillips 2019), and hemoglobin readily reacts with glucose to form glycated hemoglobin (HbA1C) providing a 3-month window of circulating glucose levels enabling both diagnosis of metabolic disease and an assay for glucose control in diabetics. Also of note, benzene is known to cause cancer, and analysis of protein adducts have provided insight into mechanisms of increased leukemia risk (Grigoryan et al. 2018).

8.6 METABOLOME

The metabolome represents a vast array of small molecules spanning a 10^{11}-fold dynamic range of femtomolar (fM) to millimolar (mM) representing both endogenous and exogenous molecules like amino acids, metabolites, carbohydrates, lipids, and dietary and environmental chemicals. The human metabolite database (http://www.hmdb.ca/metabolites) catalogs ~114,156 metabolites as of October 2019, while METLIN has over 1 million (Guijas et al. 2018). Rattray et al. (2018) recently reviewed strategies for exploiting the metabolome for gene environment interaction epidemiological studies.

8.6.1 METABOLOME METHODS

Because the metabolome spans a vast chemical space differing in mass, charge, lipophilicity, etc., no single analytical step is capable of capturing the entire complexity and usually a mixture of high-resolution techniques is required to capture a representative sample or targeted approaches may be directed at a particular class of metabolites like lipids. Nuclear magnetic resonance (NMR) and MS-based techniques are the dominant analytical platforms for metabolomics (Amberg et al. 2017, Balashova et al. 2018, Jang et al. 2018). A recent study using US Department of Defense (DoD) biobanked serum samples compared varying chromatographic separation strategies, modes of ionization and high-resolution MS illustrated the chemical and metabolic pathway space that can be analytically captured (Liu et al. 2016).

8.6.2 METABOLOME IN TEH

Metabolomics on banked serum samples of military populations have been used to evaluate the impacts of military deployment operations (Walker et al. 2016). Furthermore, traffic-related air pollution from two sites with different geographic profiles (diesel or mixed urban) were followed using personal exposure monitors, and specific pollutants were found to be associated with metabolic products. Notably, NO_2 was associated with the acyl-carnitine pathway and was implicated in cardio-respiratory disease (van Veldhoven et al. 2019). In an analogous study, Liang et al. (2019) identified pollutants associated with inflammatory and redox pathways; the arginine levels in asthmatics decreased upon exposure to vanadium in contrast to individuals without asthma that showed the opposite response illustrating the individualized nature of inflammatory and oxidative stress response to common pollutants. Lead exposure in military populations was shown to be associated with high blood pressure and oxidative stress (Obeng-Gyasi and Obeng-Gyasi 2018). Rappaport et al. (2014) analyzed blood concentrations of 1,561 small molecules distributed over 100 chemical classes ranging from fM to mM of which 361 had at least one disease association. In a recent review, Rappaport (2018) highlighted small molecules in the metabolome associated with cardiovascular disease, diabetes and cancer. In addition, numerous dietary compounds are activated through bacterial or cellular metabolism to highly reactive forms which increase disease risk. The International Agency for Research on Cancer working group estimates that colon cancer risk increases 18% for every 50 grams of processed meat or 100 grams of red meat consumed relative to those who consumed the least amount of meat; Turesky (2018) reviewed the mechanistic routes through which reactive metabolites contribute to this.

8.7 MICROBIOME

Microbes are in close symbiosis with their human hosts and play a vital role in combating infection from pathogens, extracting or synthesizing nutrients (e.g., amino acids, vitamins and isoprenoids) and digesting complex fibers to short-chain fatty acids that are critical for intestinal health (Goodrich et al. 2017, Thomas et al. 2017). The microbiome is critical for educating the immune system and neurodevelopment (Pronovost and Hsiao 2019). Dysbiosis has been associated with a range of human diseases from obesity to gut-brain associated maladaptations (Gilbert et al. 2018). The cell count of the human microbiome at a minimum matches the number of human cells, but expressed as a gene count vastly outnumbers the human gene count and confers significant advantages to the host (Sender et al. 2016).

8.7.1 ENUMERATING THE MICROBIOME

Culture-based enumeration is often performed in clinical settings and remains relevant for diagnostics. The full range of omic technologies is readily applied to the microbiome and achieved at a lower cost because of their relatively compact size (Aguiar-Pulido et al. 2016). Historically, the diversity of the human microbiome was characterized using amplicon sequencing targeting the 16S ribosomal gene used for taxonomic classification (McDonald et al. 2018). The 16S ribosomal RNA has nine hypervariable regions targeted for taxonomic classification of the microbiome. In this approach, primers hybridize to conserved regions flanking one or more of the nine highly variable regions of the 16S ribosomal RNA (V1–V3, V3–V4, V3–V5, etc.), are used to amplify genomic DNA and then sequenced. The main advantage is relatively low-cost taxonomic classification of the bacterial communities and historical use in the human microbiome project. 16S amplicon sequencing has known limitations in terms of bacterial diversity captured by amplicon choice, inability to capture fungal and viral representation, inability to detect certain genera, inability to identify to species and sub-species levels, and most metabolic predictions are based on operational taxonomic units (OTUs) rather than direct identification of the genes. However, these limitations can be overcome by whole-genome shotgun metagenomics sequencing (Ranjan et al. 2016, Knight et al. 2018).

8.7.2 Microbiome Relevance in TEH

Recently, we have begun to recognize that the host microbiome may influence and modulate exposure risk, for example, by biotransforming chemicals and drugs (Klaassen and Cui 2015, Koppel et al. 2017, Vazquez-Baeza et al. 2018). Microbial composition and interaction with diet strongly influences many metabolic diseases like obesity and diabetes (Palau-Rodriguez et al. 2015). The promotion of arthrosclerosis by meat has been traced to microbes metabolizing dietary choline and carnithine to the proatherogenic metabolite Trimethylamine-N-Oxide (TMAO) in concert with host enzymes (Tang and Hazen 2017). Evidence for this comes from mice rendered free of microbes through antibiotic treatment or raised under germ-free conditions who fail to synthesize TMAO from choline/carnithine-rich diets (Koeth et al. 2013). Interestingly, an omnivore which was fed a steak (~180 mg carnithine) or isotopically labeled carnithine responds with an increase in TMAO. However, a vegetarian/vegan fed the same steak/isotopically labeled carnithine fails to produce TMAO since the resident gut microflora between carnivores and long-term vegans/vegetarians have different compositions. This observation vividly illustrates the interplay of exposure, host and microbiome (Koeth et al. 2013).

8.8 PAN-OMICS IN A TEH MODEL

The TEH Model seeks to integrate a lifetime of exposures from all sources (work, home, geo-location) with lifestyle and genomic information to present actionable information in a participatory health model (Dennis et al. 2016). The utility of this approach is beginning to emerge from several recent studies that range from extensive tracking of a single individual to small cohorts to multi-national proof of concept studies. Here we briefly consider these studies to illustrate the power of "omics" and the "exposome" in enabling personalized health decisions.

Undoubtedly the best longitudinally studied individual is Michael Snyder who pioneered deep longitudinal data collection on himself (omic and sensor based) which enabled detection of lyme disease based on the knowledge of being in a lyme endemic area, an atypical elevated body temperature and onset of type 2 diabetes subsequent to a respiratory syncytial virus infection (both clinically confirmed). Appropriate lifestyle changes enabled control of diabetes almost from the point of clinical detection, and subsequent studies on larger cohorts illustrated the complex dynamics between individuals, disparate pathogen challenges and the utility of panomics in teasing these out (Chen et al. 2012, Stanberry et al. 2013, Li et al. 2017, Schussler-Fiorenza Rose et al. 2019, Zhou et al. 2019). Several large European projects such as EXPOsOMICS and HELIX are attempting to integrate exposures to molecular and health outcomes covering diverse exposures such as environmental and chemical exposures from in-utero to death (Vineis et al. 2017, Tamayo-Uria et al. 2019). Furthermore, differences in exposures to traffic-related pollutants have impacted telomere length indicating an impact of a molecular marker of longevity (Clemente et al. 2019). Finally, "All of Us," a part of the Precision Medicine Initiative, seeks to enroll 1 million Americans in a program to integrate health data with omic, lifestyle and environmental information whose successful conclusion will contribute to realizing the goals of TEH (All of Us Research Program, Denny et al. 2019).

REFERENCES

Aebersold, R., J. N. Agar, I. J. Amster, M. S. Baker, C. R. Bertozzi, E. S. Boja, C. E. Costello, B. F. Cravatt, C. Fenselau, B. A. Garcia, Y. Ge, J. Gunawardena, R. C. Hendrickson, P. J. Hergenrother, C. G. Huber, A. R. Ivanov, O. N. Jensen, M. C. Jewett, N. L. Kelleher, L. L. Kiessling, N. J. Krogan, M. R. Larsen, J. A. Loo, R. R. Ogorzalek Loo, E. Lundberg, M. J. MacCoss, P. Mallick, V. K. Mootha, M. Mrksich, T. W. Muir, S. M. Patrie, J. J. Pesavento, S. J. Pitteri, H. Rodriguez, A. Saghatelian, W. Sandoval, H. Schluter, S. Sechi, S. A. Slavoff, L. M. Smith, M. P. Snyder, P. M. Thomas, M. Uhlen, J. E. Van Eyk, M. Vidal, D. R. Walt, F. M. White, E. R. Williams, T. Wohlschlager, V. H. Wysocki, N. A. Yates, N. L. Young and B. Zhang (2018). "How Many Human Proteoforms Are There?" *Nat Chem Biol* **14**(3): 206–214.

Aguiar-Pulido, V., W. Huang, V. Suarez-Ulloa, T. Cickovski, K. Mathee and G. Narasimhan (2016). "Metagenomics, Metatranscriptomics, and Metabolomics Approaches for Microbiome Analysis." *Evol Bioinform Online* **12**(Suppl 1): 5–16.

All of Us Research Program Investigators, J. C. Denny, J. L. Rutter, D. B. Goldstein, A. Philippakis, J. W. Smoller, G. Jenkins and E. Dishman (2019). "The "All of Us" Research Program." *N Engl J Med* **381**(7): 668–676.

Amberg, A., B. Riefke, G. Schlotterbeck, A. Ross, H. Senn, F. Dieterle and M. Keck (2017). "NMR and MS Methods for Metabolomics." *Methods Mol Biol* **1641**: 229–258.

Angrish, M. M., P. Allard, S. D. McCullough, I. L. Druwe, L. Helbling Chadwick, E. Hines and B. N. Chorley (2018). "Epigenetic Applications in Adverse Outcome Pathways and Environmental Risk Evaluation." *Environ Health Perspect* **126**(4): 045001.

Bakalarski, C. E. and D. S. Kirkpatrick (2016). "A Biologist's Field Guide to Multiplexed Quantitative Proteomics." *Mol Cell Proteomics* **15**(5): 1489–1497.

Balashova, E. E., D. L. Maslov and P. G. Lokhov (2018). "A Metabolomics Approach to Pharmacotherapy Personalization." *J Pers Med* **8**(3): 1–15 doi:10.3390/jpm8030028.

Barton, A. J., J. Hill, A. J. Pollard and C. J. Blohmke (2017). "Transcriptomics in Human Challenge Models." *Front Immunol* **8**: 1839.

Brazma, A., P. Hingamp, J. Quackenbush, G. Sherlock, P. Spellman, C. Stoeckert, J. Aach, W. Ansorge, C. A. Ball, H. C. Causton, T. Gaasterland, P. Glenisson, F. C. Holstege, I. F. Kim, V. Markowitz, J. C. Matese, H. Parkinson, A. Robinson, U. Sarkans, S. Schulze-Kremer, J. Stewart, R. Taylor, J. Vilo and M. Vingron (2001). "Minimum Information about a Microarray Experiment (MIAME)-Toward Standards for Microarray Data." *Nat Genet* **29**(4): 365–371.

Bustin, S. A., V. Benes, J. A. Garson, J. Hellemans, J. Huggett, M. Kubista, R. Mueller, T. Nolan, M. W. Pfaffl, G. L. Shipley, J. Vandesompele and C. T. Wittwer (2009). "The MIQE Guidelines: Minimum Information for Publication of Quantitative Real-Time PCR Experiments." *Clin Chem* **55**(4): 611–622.

Chanfreau-Coffinier, C., L. E. Hull, J. A. Lynch, S. L. DuVall, S. M. Damrauer, F. E. Cunningham, B. F. Voight, M. E. Matheny, D. W. Oslin, M. S. Icardi and S. Tuteja (2019). "Projected Prevalence of Actionable Pharmacogenetic Variants and Level a Drugs Prescribed among US Veterans Health Administration Pharmacy Users." *JAMA Netw Open* **2**(6): e195345.

Chen, L. S., L. Zawertailo, T. M. Piasecki, J. Kaprio, M. Foreman, H. R. Elliott, S. P. David, A. W. Bergen, J. W. Baurley, R. F. Tyndale, T. B. Baker, L. J. Bierut, N. L. Saccone, Genetics, N. Treatment Workgroup of the Society for Research on and Tobacco (2018). "Leveraging Genomic Data in Smoking Cessation Trials in the Era of Precision Medicine: Why and How." *Nicotine Tob Res* **20**(4): 414–424.

Chen, R., G. I. Mias, J. Li-Pook-Than, L. Jiang, H. Y. Lam, R. Chen, E. Miriami, K. J. Karczewski, M. Hariharan, F. E. Dewey, Y. Cheng, M. J. Clark, H. Im, L. Habegger, S. Balasubramanian, M. O'Huallachain, J. T. Dudley, S. Hillenmeyer, R. Haraksingh, D. Sharon, G. Euskirchen, P. Lacroute, K. Bettinger, A. P. Boyle, M. Kasowski, F. Grubert, S. Seki, M. Garcia, M. Whirl-Carrillo, M. Gallardo, M. A. Blasco, P. L. Greenberg, P. Snyder, T. E. Klein, R. B. Altman, A. J. Butte, E. A. Ashley, M. Gerstein, K. C. Nadeau, H. Tang and M. Snyder (2012). "Personal Omics Profiling Reveals Dynamic Molecular and Medical Phenotypes." *Cell* **148**(6): 1293–1307.

Chong, J. X., K. J. Buckingham, S. N. Jhangiani, C. Boehm, N. Sobreira, J. D. Smith, T. M. Harrell, M. J. McMillin, W. Wiszniewski, T. Gambin, Z. H. Coban Akdemir, K. Doheny, A. F. Scott, D. Avramopoulos, A. Chakravarti, J. Hoover-Fong, D. Mathews, P. D. Witmer, H. Ling, K. Hetrick, L. Watkins, K. E. Patterson, F. Reinier, E. Blue, D. Muzny, M. Kircher, K. Bilguvar, F. Lopez-Giraldez, V. R. Sutton, H. K. Tabor, S. M. Leal, M. Gunel, S. Mane, R. A. Gibbs, E. Boerwinkle, A. Hamosh, J. Shendure, J. R. Lupski, R. P. Lifton, D. Valle, D. A. Nickerson, G. Centers for Mendelian and M. J. Bamshad (2015). "The Genetic Basis of Mendelian Phenotypes: Discoveries, Challenges, and Opportunities." *Am J Hum Genet* **97**(2): 199–215.

Cizmeci, D., E. L. Dempster, O. L. Champion, S. Wagley, O. E. Akman, J. L. Prior, O. S. Soyer, J. Mill and R. W. Titball (2016). "Mapping Epigenetic Changes to the Host Cell Genome Induced by Burkholderia Pseudomallei Reveals Pathogen-Specific and Pathogen-Generic Signatures of Infection." *Sci Rep* **6**: 30861.

Clemente, D. B. P., M. Vrijheid, D. S. Martens, M. Bustamante, L. Chatzi, A. Danileviciute, M. de Castro, R. Grazuleviciene, K. B. Gutzkow, J. Lepeule, L. Maitre, R. R. C. McEachan, O. Robinson, P. E. Schwarze, I. Tamayo, M. Vafeiadi, J. Wright, R. Slama, M. Nieuwenhuijsen and T. S. Nawrot (2019). "Prenatal and Childhood Traffic-Related Air Pollution Exposure and Telomere Length in European Children: The HELIX Project." *Environ Health Perspect* **127**(8): 87001.

Corella, D., O. Coltell, F. Macian and J. M. Ordovas (2018). "Advances in Understanding the Molecular Basis of the Mediterranean Diet Effect." *Annu Rev Food Sci Technol* **9**: 227–249.

Dennis, K. K., S. S. Auerbach, D. M. Balshaw, Y. Cui, M. D. Fallin, M. T. Smith, A. Spira, S. Sumner and G. W. Miller (2016). "The Importance of the Biological Impact of Exposure to the Concept of the Exposome." *Environ Health Perspect* **124**(10): 1504–1510.

Dirks, R. A., H. G. Stunnenberg and H. Marks (2016). "Genome-Wide Epigenomic Profiling for Biomarker Discovery." *Clin Epigenetics* **8**: 122.

Franks, P. W. and J. Merino (2018). "Gene-Lifestyle Interplay in Type 2 Diabetes." *Curr Opin Genet Dev* **50**: 35–40.

Geyer, P. E., N. A. Kulak, G. Pichler, L. M. Holdt, D. Teupser and M. Mann (2016). "Plasma Proteome Profiling to Assess Human Health and Disease." *Cell Syst* **2**(3): 185–195.

Gilbert, J. A., M. J. Blaser, J. G. Caporaso, J. K. Jansson, S. V. Lynch and R. Knight (2018). "Current Understanding of the Human Microbiome." *Nat Med* **24**(4): 392–400.

Goldfeder, R. L., D. P. Wall, M. J. Khoury, J. P. A. Ioannidis and E. A. Ashley (2017). "Human Genome Sequencing at the Population Scale: A Primer on High-throughput DNA Sequencing and Analysis." *Am J Epidemiol* **186**(8): 1000–1009.

Goodrich, J. K., E. R. Davenport, A. G. Clark and R. E. Ley (2017). "The Relationship between the Human Genome and Microbiome Comes into View." *Annu Rev Genet* **51**: 413–433.

Grigoryan, H., W. M. B. Edmands, Q. Lan, H. Carlsson, R. Vermeulen, L. Zhang, S. N. Yin, G. L. Li, M. T. Smith, N. Rothman and S. M. Rappaport (2018). "Adductomic Signatures of Benzene Exposure Provide Insights into Cancer Induction." *Carcinogenesis* **39**(5): 661–668.

Guijas, C., J. R. Montenegro-Burke, X. Domingo-Almenara, A. Palermo, B. Warth, G. Hermann, G. Koellensperger, T. Huan, W. Uritboonthai, A. E. Aisporna, D. W. Wolan, M. E. Spilker, H. P. Benton and G. Siuzdak (2018). "METLIN: A Technology Platform for Identifying Knowns and Unknowns." *Anal Chem* **90**(5): 3156–3164.

Hardwick, S. A., A. Joglekar, P. Flicek, A. Frankish and H. U. Tilgner (2019). "Getting the Entire Message: Progress in Isoform Sequencing." *Front Genet* **10**: 709.

Hosp, F. and M. Mann (2017). "A Primer on Concepts and Applications of Proteomics in Neuroscience." *Neuron* **96**(3): 558–571.

Hou, L., X. Zhang, D. Wang and A. Baccarelli (2012). "Environmental Chemical Exposures and Human Epigenetics." *Int J Epidemiol* **41**(1): 79–105.

Hrdlickova, R., M. Toloue and B. Tian (2017). "RNA-Seq Methods for Transcriptome Analysis." *Wiley Interdiscip Rev RNA* **8**(1): 1–24.

Jackson, M., L. Marks, G. H. W. May and J. B. Wilson (2018). "The Genetic Basis of Disease." *Essays Biochem* **62**(5): 643–723.

Jain, M., S. Koren, K. H. Miga, J. Quick, A. C. Rand, T. A. Sasani, J. R. Tyson, A. D. Beggs, A. T. Dilthey, I. T. Fiddes, S. Malla, H. Marriott, T. Nieto, J. O'Grady, H. E. Olsen, B. S. Pedersen, A. Rhie, H. Richardson, A. R. Quinlan, T. P. Snutch, L. Tee, B. Paten, A. M. Phillippy, J. T. Simpson, N. J. Loman and M. Loose (2018). "Nanopore Sequencing and Assembly of a Human Genome with Ultra-Long Reads." *Nat Biotechnol* **36**(4): 338–345.

Jang, C., L. Chen and J. D. Rabinowitz (2018). "Metabolomics and Isotope Tracing." *Cell* **173**(4): 822–837.

Klaassen, C. D. and J. Y. Cui (2015). "Review: Mechanisms of How the Intestinal Microbiota Alters the Effects of Drugs and Bile Acids." *Drug Metab Dispos* **43**(10): 1505–1521.

Knight, R., A. Vrbanac, B. C. Taylor, A. Aksenov, C. Callewaert, J. Debelius, A. Gonzalez, T. Kosciolek, L. I. McCall, D. McDonald, A. V. Melnik, J. T. Morton, J. Navas, R. A. Quinn, J. G. Sanders, A. D. Swafford, L. R. Thompson, A. Tripathi, Z. Z. Xu, J. R. Zaneveld, Q. Zhu, J. G. Caporaso and P. C. Dorrestein (2018). "Best Practices for Analysing Microbiomes." *Nat Rev Microbiol* **16**(7): 410–422.

Koeth, R. A., Z. Wang, B. S. Levison, J. A. Buffa, E. Org, B. T. Sheehy, E. B. Britt, X. Fu, Y. Wu, L. Li, J. D. Smith, J. A. DiDonato, J. Chen, H. Li, G. D. Wu, J. D. Lewis, M. Warrier, J. M. Brown, R. M. Krauss, W. H. Tang, F. D. Bushman, A. J. Lusis and S. L. Hazen (2013). "Intestinal Microbiota Metabolism of L-Carnitine, a Nutrient in Red Meat, Promotes Atherosclerosis." *Nat Med* **19**(5): 576–585.

Koppel, N., V. Maini Rekdal and E. P. Balskus (2017). "Chemical Transformation of Xenobiotics by the Human Gut Microbiota." *Science* **356**(6344), doi:10.1126/science.aag2770.

Lander, E. S., L. M. Linton, B. Birren, C. Nusbaum, M. C. Zody, J. Baldwin, K. Devon, K. Dewar, M. Doyle, W. FitzHugh, R. Funke, D. Gage, K. Harris, A. Heaford, J. Howland, L. Kann, J. Lehoczky, R. LeVine, P. McEwan, K. McKernan, J. Meldrim, J. P. Mesirov, C. Miranda, W. Morris, J. Naylor, C. Raymond, M. Rosetti, R. Santos, A. Sheridan, C. Sougnez, Y. Stange-Thomann, N. Stojanovic, A. Subramanian, D. Wyman, J. Rogers, J. Sulston, R. Ainscough, S. Beck, D. Bentley, J. Burton, C. Clee, N. Carter, A. Coulson, R. Deadman, P. Deloukas, A. Dunham, I. Dunham, R. Durbin, L. French, D. Grafham, S. Gregory, T. Hubbard, S. Humphray, A. Hunt, M. Jones, C. Lloyd, A. McMurray, L. Matthews, S. Mercer, S. Milne, J. C. Mullikin, A. Mungall, R. Plumb, M. Ross, R. Shownkeen, S. Sims, R. H. Waterston, R. K. Wilson, L. W. Hillier, J. D. McPherson,

M. A. Marra, E. R. Mardis, L. A. Fulton, A. T. Chinwalla, K. H. Pepin, W. R. Gish, S. L. Chissoe, M. C. Wendl, K. D. Delehaunty, T. L. Miner, A. Delehaunty, J. B. Kramer, L. L. Cook, R. S. Fulton, D. L. Johnson, P. J. Minx, S. W. Clifton, T. Hawkins, E. Branscomb, P. Predki, P. Richardson, S. Wenning, T. Slezak, N. Doggett, J. F. Cheng, A. Olsen, S. Lucas, C. Elkin, E. Uberbacher, M. Frazier, R. A. Gibbs, D. M. Muzny, S. E. Scherer, J. B. Bouck, E. J. Sodergren, K. C. Worley, C. M. Rives, J. H. Gorrell, M. L. Metzker, S. L. Naylor, R. S. Kucherlapati, D. L. Nelson, G. M. Weinstock, Y. Sakaki, A. Fujiyama, M. Hattori, T. Yada, A. Toyoda, T. Itoh, C. Kawagoe, H. Watanabe, Y. Totoki, T. Taylor, J. Weissenbach, R. Heilig, W. Saurin, F. Artiguenave, P. Brottier, T. Bruls, E. Pelletier, C. Robert, P. Wincker, D. R. Smith, L. Doucette-Stamm, M. Rubenfield, K. Weinstock, H. M. Lee, J. Dubois, A. Rosenthal, M. Platzer, G. Nyakatura, S. Taudien, A. Rump, H. Yang, J. Yu, J. Wang, G. Huang, J. Gu, L. Hood, L. Rowen, A. Madan, S. Qin, R. W. Davis, N. A. Federspiel, A. P. Abola, M. J. Proctor, R. M. Myers, J. Schmutz, M. Dickson, J. Grimwood, D. R. Cox, M. V. Olson, R. Kaul, C. Raymond, N. Shimizu, K. Kawasaki, S. Minoshima, G. A. Evans, M. Athanasiou, R. Schultz, B. A. Roe, F. Chen, H. Pan, J. Ramser, H. Lehrach, R. Reinhardt, W. R. McCombie, M. de la Bastide, N. Dedhia, H. Blocker, K. Hornischer, G. Nordsiek, R. Agarwala, L. Aravind, J. A. Bailey, A. Bateman, S. Batzoglou, E. Birney, P. Bork, D. G. Brown, C. B. Burge, L. Cerutti, H. C. Chen, D. Church, M. Clamp, R. R. Copley, T. Doerks, S. R. Eddy, E. E. Eichler, T. S. Furey, J. Galagan, J. G. Gilbert, C. Harmon, Y. Hayashizaki, D. Haussler, H. Hermjakob, K. Hokamp, W. Jang, L. S. Johnson, T. A. Jones, S. Kasif, A. Kaspryzk, S. Kennedy, W. J. Kent, P. Kitts, E. V. Koonin, I. Korf, D. Kulp, D. Lancet, T. M. Lowe, A. McLysaght, T. Mikkelsen, J. V. Moran, N. Mulder, V. J. Pollara, C. P. Ponting, G. Schuler, J. Schultz, G. Slater, A. F. Smit, E. Stupka, J. Szustakowski, D. Thierry-Mieg, J. Thierry-Mieg, L. Wagner, J. Wallis, R. Wheeler, A. Williams, Y. I. Wolf, K. H. Wolfe, S. P. Yang, R. F. Yeh, F. Collins, M. S. Guyer, J. Peterson, A. Felsenfeld, K. A. Wetterstrand, A. Patrinos, M. J. Morgan, P. de Jong, J. J. Catanese, K. Osoegawa, H. Shizuya, S. Choi, Y. J. Chen, J. Szustakowki and C. International Human Genome Sequencing (2001). "Initial Sequencing and Analysis of the Human Genome." *Nature* **409**(6822): 860–921.

Lee, H. S. (2015). "Impact of Maternal Diet on the Epigenome during in Utero Life and the Developmental Programming of Diseases in Childhood and Adulthood." *Nutrients* **7**(11): 9492–9507.

Leenen, F. A., C. P. Muller and J. D. Turner (2016). "DNA Methylation: Conducting the Orchestra from Exposure to Phenotype?" *Clin Epigenetics* **8**: 92.

Levy, S. E. and R. M. Myers (2016). "Advancements in Next-Generation Sequencing." *Annu Rev Genomics Hum Genet* **17**: 95–115.

Li, X., J. Dunn, D. Salins, G. Zhou, W. Zhou, S. M. Schussler-Fiorenza Rose, D. Perelman, E. Colbert, R. Runge, S. Rego, R. Sonecha, S. Datta, T. McLaughlin and M. P. Snyder (2017). "Digital Health: Tracking Physiomes and Activity using Wearable Biosensors Reveals Useful Health-Related Information." *PLoS Biol* **15**(1): e2001402.

Liang, D., C. N. Ladva, R. Golan, T. Yu, D. I. Walker, S. E. Sarnat, R. Greenwald, K. Uppal, V. Tran, D. P. Jones, A. G. Russell and J. A. Sarnat (2019). "Perturbations of the Arginine Metabolome Following Exposures to Traffic-Related Air Pollution in a Panel of Commuters with and without Asthma." *Environ Int* **127**: 503–513.

Lin, H., G. T. Rogers, K. L. Lunetta, D. Levy, X. Miao, L. M. Troy, P. F. Jacques and J. M. Murabito (2019). "Healthy Diet Is Associated with Gene Expression in Blood: The Framingham Heart Study." *Am J Clin Nutr* **110**(3): 742–749.

Liu, K. H., D. I. Walker, K. Uppal, V. Tran, P. Rohrbeck, T. M. Mallon and D. P. Jones (2016). "High-Resolution Metabolomics Assessment of Military Personnel: Evaluating Analytical Strategies for Chemical Detection." *J Occup Environ Med* **58**(8 Suppl 1): S53–S61.

McCartney, D. L., A. J. Stevenson, R. F. Hillary, R. M. Walker, M. L. Bermingham, S. W. Morris, T. K. Clarke, A. Campbell, A. D. Murray, H. C. Whalley, D. J. Porteous, P. M. Visscher, A. M. McIntosh, K. L. Evans, I. J. Deary and R. E. Marioni (2018). "Epigenetic Signatures of Starting and Stopping Smoking." *EBioMedicine* **37**: 214–220.

McDonald, D., E. Hyde, J. W. Debelius, J. T. Morton, A. Gonzalez, G. Ackermann, A. A. Aksenov, B. Behsaz, C. Brennan, Y. Chen, L. DeRight Goldasich, P. C. Dorrestein, R. R. Dunn, A. K. Fahimipour, J. Gaffney, J. A. Gilbert, G. Gogul, J. L. Green, P. Hugenholtz, G. Humphrey, C. Huttenhower, M. A. Jackson, S. Janssen, D. V. Jeste, L. Jiang, S. T. Kelley, D. Knights, T. Kosciolek, J. Ladau, J. Leach, C. Marotz, D. Meleshko, A. V. Melnik, J. L. Metcalf, H. Mohimani, E. Montassier, J. Navas-Molina, T. T. Nguyen, S. Peddada, P. Pevzner, K. S. Pollard, G. Rahnavard, A. Robbins-Pianka, N. Sangwan, J. Shorenstein, L. Smarr, S. J. Song, T. Spector, A. D. Swafford, V. G. Thackray, L. R. Thompson, A. Tripathi, Y. Vazquez-Baeza, A. Vrbanac, P. Wischmeyer, E. Wolfe, Q. Zhu, C. American Gut and R. Knight (2018). "American Gut: An Open Platform for Citizen Science Microbiome Research." *mSystems* **3**(3), doi:10.1128/mSystems.00031-18.

McHale, C. M., G. Osborne, R. Morello-Frosch, A. G. Salmon, M. S. Sandy, G. Solomon, L. Zhang, M. T. Smith and L. Zeise (2018). "Assessing Health Risks from Multiple Environmental Stressors: Moving from GxE to IxE." *Mutat Res* **775**: 11–20.

McHale, C. M., L. Zhang, R. Thomas and M. T. Smith (2013). "Analysis of the Transcriptome in Molecular Epidemiology Studies." *Environ Mol Mutagen* **54**(7): 500–517.

Mele, M., P. G. Ferreira, F. Reverter, D. S. DeLuca, J. Monlong, M. Sammeth, T. R. Young, J. M. Goldmann, D. D. Pervouchine, T. J. Sullivan, R. Johnson, A. V. Segre, S. Djebali, A. Niarchou, G. T. Consortium, F. A. Wright, T. Lappalainen, M. Calvo, G. Getz, E. T. Dermitzakis, K. G. Ardlie and R. Guigo (2015). "Human Genomics. The Human Transcriptome across Tissues and Individuals." *Science* **348**(6235): 660–665.

Mertins, P., L. C. Tang, K. Krug, D. J. Clark, M. A. Gritsenko, L. Chen, K. R. Clauser, T. R. Clauss, P. Shah, M. A. Gillette, V. A. Petyuk, S. N. Thomas, D. R. Mani, F. Mundt, R. J. Moore, Y. Hu, R. Zhao, M. Schnaubelt, H. Keshishian, M. E. Monroe, Z. Zhang, N. D. Udeshi, D. Mani, S. R. Davies, R. R. Townsend, D. W. Chan, R. D. Smith, H. Zhang, T. Liu and S. A. Carr (2018). "Reproducible Workflow for Multiplexed Deep-Scale Proteome and Phosphoproteome Analysis of Tumor Tissues by Liquid Chromatography-Mass Spectrometry." *Nat Protoc* **13**(7): 1632–1661.

O'Beirne, S. L., S. A. Shenoy, J. Salit, Y. Strulovici-Barel, R. J. Kaner, S. Visvanathan, J. S. Fine, J. G. Mezey and R. G. Crystal (2018). "Ambient Pollution-Related Reprogramming of the Human Small Airway Epithelial Transcriptome." *Am J Respir Crit Care Med* **198**(11): 1413–1422.

Obeng-Gyasi, E. and B. Obeng-Gyasi (2018). "Blood Pressure and Oxidative Stress among U.S. Adults Exposed to Lead in Military Environments–A Preliminary Study." *Diseases* **6**(4), doi:10.3390/diseases6040097.

Pai, A. A. and F. Luca (2019). "Environmental Influences on RNA Processing: Biochemical, Molecular and Genetic Regulators of Cellular Response." *Wiley Interdiscip Rev RNA* **10**(1): e1503.

Palau-Rodriguez, M., S. Tulipani, M. Isabel Queipo-Ortuno, M. Urpi-Sarda, F. J. Tinahones and C. Andres-Lacueva (2015). "Metabolomic Insights into the Intricate Gut Microbial-Host Interaction in the Development of Obesity and Type 2 Diabetes." *Front Microbiol* **6**: 1151.

Pertea, M. (2012). "The Human Transcriptome: An Unfinished Story." *Genes (Basel)* **3**(3): 344–360.

Philibert, R., N. Hollenbeck, E. Andersen, S. McElroy, S. Wilson, K. Vercande, S. R. Beach, T. Osborn, M. Gerrard, F. X. Gibbons and K. Wang (2016). "Reversion of AHRR Demethylation Is a Quantitative Biomarker of Smoking Cessation." *Front Psychiatry* **7**: 55.

Preston, G. W. and D. H. Phillips (2019). "Protein Adductomics: Analytical Developments and Applications in Human Biomonitoring." *Toxics* **7**(2).

Pronovost, G. N. and E. Y. Hsiao (2019). "Perinatal Interactions between the Microbiome, Immunity, and Neurodevelopment." *Immunity* **50**(1): 18–36.

Ranjan, R., A. Rani, A. Metwally, H. S. McGee and D. L. Perkins (2016). "Analysis of the Microbiome: Advantages of Whole Genome Shotgun versus 16S Amplicon Sequencing." *Biochem Biophys Res Commun* **469**(4): 967–977.

Rappaport, S. M. (2018). "Redefining Environmental Exposure for Disease Etiology." *NPJ Syst Biol Appl* **4**: 30.

Rappaport, S. M., D. K. Barupal, D. Wishart, P. Vineis and A. Scalbert (2014). "The Blood Exposome and Its Role in Discovering Causes of Disease." *Environ Health Perspect* **122**(8): 769–774.

Rattray, N. J. W., N. C. Deziel, J. D. Wallach, S. A. Khan, V. Vasiliou, J. P. A. Ioannidis and C. H. Johnson (2018). "Beyond Genomics: Understanding Exposotypes through Metabolomics." *Hum Genomics* **12**(1): 4.

Rhoads, A. and K. F. Au (2015). "PacBio Sequencing and Its Applications." *Genomics Proteomics Bioinformatics* **13**(5): 278–289.

Richards, A. L., D. Watza, A. Findley, A. Alazizi, X. Wen, A. A. Pai, R. Pique-Regi and F. Luca (2017). "Environmental Perturbations Lead to Extensive Directional Shifts in RNA Processing." *PLoS Genet* **13**(10): e1006995.

Ritz, B. R., N. Chatterjee, M. Garcia-Closas, W. J. Gauderman, B. L. Pierce, P. Kraft, C. M. Tanner, L. E. Mechanic and K. McAllister (2017). "Lessons Learned from Past Gene-Environment Interaction Successes." *Am J Epidemiol* **186**(7): 778–786.

Rivera, C. M. and B. Ren (2013). "Mapping Human Epigenomes." *Cell* **155**(1): 39–55.

Sa, A. C. C., W. Sadee and J. A. Johnson (2018). "Whole Transcriptome Profiling: An RNA-Seq Primer and Implications for Pharmacogenomics Research." *Clin Transl Sci* **11**(2): 153–161.

Saccone, N. L., J. W. Baurley, A. W. Bergen, S. P. David, H. R. Elliott, M. G. Foreman, J. Kaprio, T. M. Piasecki, C. L. Relton, L. Zawertailo, L. J. Bierut, R. F. Tyndale, L. S. Chen, Genetics, N. Treatment Networks of the Society for Research on and Tobacco (2018). "The Value of Biosamples in Smoking Cessation Trials: A Review of Genetic, Metabolomic, and Epigenetic Findings." *Nicotine Tob Res* **20**(4): 403–413.

Said, M. A., Y. J. van de Vegte, M. M. Zafar, M. Y. van der Ende, G. K. Raja, N. Verweij and P. van der Harst (2019). "Contributions of Interactions between Lifestyle and Genetics on Coronary Artery Disease Risk." *Curr Cardiol Rep* **21**(9): 89.

Schussler-Fiorenza Rose, S. M., K. Contrepois, K. J. Moneghetti, W. Zhou, T. Mishra, S. Mataraso, O. Dagan-Rosenfeld, A. B. Ganz, J. Dunn, D. Hornburg, S. Rego, D. Perelman, S. Ahadi, M. R. Sailani, Y. Zhou, S. R. Leopold, J. Chen, M. Ashland, J. W. Christle, M. Avina, P. Limcaoco, C. Ruiz, M. Tan, A. J. Butte, G. M. Weinstock, G. M. Slavich, E. Sodergren, T. L. McLaughlin, F. Haddad and M. P. Snyder (2019). "A Longitudinal Big Data Approach for Precision Health." *Nat Med* **25**(5): 792–804.

Sender, R., Fuchs, S. and Milo, R. (2016). "Revised Estimates for the Number of Human and Bacteria Cells in the Body." *PLoS Biology* **14**(8): e1002533.

Shendure, J., S. Balasubramanian, G. M. Church, W. Gilbert, J. Rogers, J. A. Schloss and R. H. Waterston (2017). "DNA Sequencing at 40: Past, Present and Future." *Nature* **550**(7676): 345–353.

Simonds, N. I., A. A. Ghazarian, C. B. Pimentel, S. D. Schully, G. L. Ellison, E. M. Gillanders and L. E. Mechanic (2016). "Review of the Gene-Environment Interaction Literature in Cancer: What Do We Know?" *Genet Epidemiol* **40**(5): 356–365.

Smith, J. G. and R. E. Gerszten (2017). "Emerging Affinity-based Proteomic Technologies for Large-Scale Plasma Profiling in Cardiovascular Disease." *Circulation* **135**(17): 1651–1664.

Stanberry, L., G. I. Mias, W. Haynes, R. Higdon, M. Snyder and E. Kolker (2013). "Integrative Analysis of Longitudinal Metabolomics Data from a Personal Multi-Omics Profile." *Metabolites* **3**(3): 741–760.

Sun, Z., J. Cunningham, S. Slager and J. P. Kocher (2015). "Base Resolution Methylome Profiling: Considerations in Platform Selection, Data Preprocessing and Analysis." *Epigenomics* **7**(5): 813–828.

Tamayo-Uria, I., L. Maitre, C. Thomsen, M. J. Nieuwenhuijsen, L. Chatzi, V. Siroux, G. M. Aasvang, L. Agier, S. Andrusaityte, M. Casas, M. de Castro, A. Dedele, L. S. Haug, B. Heude, R. Grazuleviciene, K. B. Gutzkow, N. H. Krog, D. Mason, R. R. C. McEachan, H. M. Meltzer, I. Petraviciene, O. Robinson, T. Roumeliotaki, A. K. Sakhi, J. Urquiza, M. Vafeiadi, D. Waiblinger, C. Warembourg, J. Wright, R. Slama, M. Vrijheid and X. Basagana (2019). "The Early-Life Exposome: Description and Patterns in Six European Countries." *Environ Int* **123**: 189–200.

Tang, W. H. and S. L. Hazen (2017). "Microbiome, Trimethylamine N-oxide, and Cardiometabolic Disease." *Transl Res* **179**: 108–115.

Thomas, S., J. Izard, E. Walsh, K. Batich, P. Chongsathidkiet, G. Clarke, D. A. Sela, A. J. Muller, J. M. Mullin, K. Albert, J. P. Gilligan, K. DiGuilio, R. Dilbarova, W. Alexander and G. C. Prendergast (2017). "The Host Microbiome Regulates and Maintains Human Health: A Primer and Perspective for Non-Microbiologists." *Cancer Res* **77**(8): 1783–1812.

Tobi, E. W., J. J. Goeman, R. Monajemi, H. Gu, H. Putter, Y. Zhang, R. C. Slieker, A. P. Stok, P. E. Thijssen, F. Muller, E. W. van Zwet, C. Bock, A. Meissner, L. H. Lumey, P. Eline Slagboom and B. T. Heijmans (2014). "DNA Methylation Signatures Link Prenatal Famine Exposure to Growth and Metabolism." *Nat Commun* **5**: 5592.

Torkamani, A., K. G. Andersen, S. R. Steinhubl and E. J. Topol (2017). "High-Definition Medicine." *Cell* **170**(5): 828–843.

Turesky, R. J. (2018). "Mechanistic Evidence for Red Meat and Processed Meat Intake and Cancer Risk: A Follow-up on the International Agency for Research on Cancer Evaluation of 2015." *Chimia (Aarau)* **72**(10): 718–724.

van Breda, S. G., L. C. Wilms, S. Gaj, D. G. Jennen, J. J. Briede, J. C. Kleinjans and T. M. de Kok (2015). "The Exposome Concept in a Human Nutrigenomics Study: Evaluating the Impact of Exposure to a Complex Mixture of Phytochemicals using Transcriptomics Signatures." *Mutagenesis* **30**(6): 723–731.

van Veldhoven, K., A. Kiss, P. Keski-Rahkonen, N. Robinot, A. Scalbert, P. Cullinan, K. F. Chung, P. Collins, R. Sinharay, B. M. Barratt, M. Nieuwenhuijsen, A. A. Rodoreda, G. Carrasco-Turigas, J. Vlaanderen, R. Vermeulen, L. Portengen, S. A. Kyrtopoulos, E. Ponzi, M. Chadeau-Hyam and P. Vineis (2019). "Impact of Short-Term Traffic-Related Air Pollution on the Metabolome - Results from Two Metabolome-Wide Experimental Studies." *Environ Int* **123**: 124–131.

Vazquez-Baeza, Y., C. Callewaert, J. Debelius, E. Hyde, C. Marotz, J. T. Morton, A. Swafford, A. Vrbanac, P. C. Dorrestein and R. Knight (2018). "Impacts of the Human Gut Microbiome on Therapeutics." *Annu Rev Pharmacol Toxicol* **58**: 253–270.

Vineis, P. (2018). "From John Snow to Omics: The Long Journey of Environmental Epidemiology." *Eur J Epidemiol* **33**(4): 355–363.

Vineis, P., M. Chadeau-Hyam, H. Gmuender, J. Gulliver, Z. Herceg, J. Kleinjans, M. Kogevinas, S. Kyrtopoulos, M. Nieuwenhuijsen, D. H. Phillips, N. Probst-Hensch, A. Scalbert, R. Vermeulen, C. P. Wild and E. X. Consortium (2017). "The Exposome in Practice: Design of the EXPOsOMICS Project." *Int J Hyg Environ Health* **220**(2 Pt A): 142–151.

Walker, D. I., C. T. Mallon, P. K. Hopke, K. Uppal, Y. M. Go, P. Rohrbeck, K. D. Pennell and D. P. Jones (2016). "Deployment-Associated Exposure Surveillance with High-Resolution Metabolomics." *J Occup Environ Med* **58**(8 Suppl 1): S12–S21.

Wang, T., E. C. Pehrsson, D. Purushotham, D. Li, X. Zhuo, B. Zhang, H. A. Lawson, M. A. Province, C. Krapp, Y. Lan, C. Coarfa, T. A. Katz, W. Y. Tang, Z. Wang, S. Biswal, S. Rajagopalan, J. A. Colacino, Z. T. Tsai, M. A. Sartor, K. Neier, D. C. Dolinoy, J. Pinto, R. B. Hamanaka, G. M. Mutlu, H. B. Patisaul, D. L. Aylor, G. E. Crawford, T. Wiltshire, L. H. Chadwick, C. G. Duncan, A. E. Garton, K. A. McAllister, R. I. I. C. Ta, M. S. Bartolomei, C. L. Walker and F. L. Tyson (2018). "The NIEHS TaRGET II Consortium and Environmental Epigenomics." *Nat Biotechnol* **36**(3): 225–227.

Xu, J., B. Gong, L. Wu, S. Thakkar, H. Hong and W. Tong (2016). "Comprehensive Assessments of RNA-seq by the SEQC Consortium: FDA-Led Efforts Advance Precision Medicine." *Pharmaceutics* **8**(1), doi:10.3390/pharmaceutics8010008.

Zhou, W., M. R. Sailani, K. Contrepois, Y. Zhou, S. Ahadi, S. R. Leopold, M. J. Zhang, V. Rao, M. Avina, T. Mishra, J. Johnson, B. Lee-McMullen, S. Chen, A. A. Metwally, T. D. B. Tran, H. Nguyen, X. Zhou, B. Albright, B. Y. Hong, L. Petersen, E. Bautista, B. Hanson, L. Chen, D. Spakowicz, A. Bahmani, D. Salins, B. Leopold, M. Ashland, O. Dagan-Rosenfeld, S. Rego, P. Limcaoco, E. Colbert, C. Allister, D. Perelman, C. Craig, E. Wei, H. Chaib, D. Hornburg, J. Dunn, L. Liang, S. M. S. Rose, K. Kukurba, B. Piening, H. Rost, D. Tse, T. McLaughlin, E. Sodergren, G. M. Weinstock and M. Snyder (2019). "Longitudinal Multi-Omics of Host-Microbe Dynamics in Prediabetes." *Nature* **569**(7758): 663–671.

9 Silicone Wristbands and Wearables to Assess Chemical Exposures

Holly M. Dixon, Carolyn M. Poutasse,
and Kim A. Anderson
Oregon State University

CONTENTS

DOI: 10.1201/9780429263286-11

9.1 PERSONAL CHEMICAL EXPOSURES

Chemicals in our everyday environment may have unintended effects on human and environmental health. Increasing evidence indicates that environmental exposures impact the risk of disease (Advancing Science, Improving Health 2018), but researchers and community members often lack knowledge about the frequency and magnitude of personal exposures to many chemicals. In order to monitor such exposures, low-cost and easy-to-use technologies are critical tools that inform cutting-edge research in toxicology and environmental epidemiology. These exposure assessment tools will further complement recent research initiatives, such as understanding total exposures throughout a person's lifespan ("exposome") and pairing personal exposure data with genetic information ("total exposure health" and "precision medicine").

9.2 PASSIVE SAMPLING

9.2.1 PASSIVE SAMPLING BACKGROUND

Passive sampling devices (PSDs) for organic chemicals are lipophilic polymers that mimic biological cellular membranes (Figure 9.1) (Huckins et al. 2006, Anderson et al. 2008). Via simple diffusion, unbound chemicals in environmental media (e.g. air, sediment, soil, and water) are sequestered into PSD polymers (Anderson et al. 2008, O'Connell et al. 2014a). Researchers can then extract and quantify the chemicals in the polymer. PSDs do not sequester all chemicals in the environment, but rather the fraction biologically available to transport across cellular membranes (Forsberg et al. 2011, Booij et al. 2016, Paulik et al. 2016). A chemical's bioavailability is not an inherent property. Rather, bioavailability is dependent upon

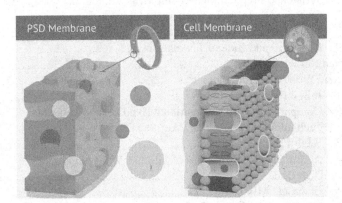

FIGURE 9.1 Simplified representation of a passive sampling device (PSD) membrane and biological cell membrane, illustrating functional similarities. Both membranes are lipophilic and have similar pore sizes (estimated 10 Å for PSD membrane and 9.5 Å for cell membrane) (Anderson et al. 2008). Chemicals are represented by spheres, with some chemicals able to cross the membranes (bioavailable fraction) and some chemicals unable to cross the membranes. (Adapted from Anderson and Hillwalker 2008.).

physiological uptake processes and physical–chemical properties (Bioavailability of Contaminants 2003, Anderson et al. 2008). When examining the relationship between chemical exposures and health effects, it is important to characterize the bioavailable fraction of chemicals.

Over 16,700 scientific publications have mentioned passive sampling since 1980, and over 45 percent of those papers were published between 2014 and 2018 (Google Scholar search; accessed January 4, 2019). Growing interest in passive sampling is partly attributed to low cost, ease of deployment, high sensitivity to low chemical concentrations, and ability to sequester a wide range of bioavailable chemicals (Bohlin et al. 2007, Lohmann 2011). In addition, PSD chemical concentrations represent an average chemical concentration over the study period (i.e. time-weighted average) (Bohlin et al. 2007, Booij et al. 2016, Bergmann et al. 2017b). A time-weighted average can be a benefit in comparison to conventional chemical assessment methods, such as taking water or soil grab samples. Grab samples, which represent a snapshot of chemicals at one time point, require repeated sampling campaigns to characterize long-term exposures, resulting in comparatively high costs (Anderson et al. 2008). For chemical monitoring programs, passive sampling is an effective long-term solution compared to grab sampling (O'Connell et al. 2014b).

9.2.2 SILICONE WRISTBANDS

Many different types of polymers, including silicone, have been optimized for use as PSDs. A novel application of PSDs are silicone wristbands, first described by O'Connell et al. in 2014. Wristbands are used to characterize personal exposure to organic chemicals. As of March 2019, wristband results have been included in 23 peer-reviewed manuscripts and have been worn by several thousand volunteers on six continents. To date, several different chemical classes including flame retardants, pesticides, polycyclic aromatic hydrocarbons (PAHs), phthalates, and consumer product-related chemicals, have been detected and quantified in silicone wristbands. The ability to concurrently monitor all these different chemical classes offers a unique opportunity to assess the effect of chemical mixtures on human health.

9.3 SILICONE WRISTBAND CHARACTERIZATION

9.3.1 WRISTBAND ADVANTAGES

Silicone wristbands are a robust, simple technology used to characterize an individual's chemical exposures from dermal, inhalation, and limited ingestion exposure pathways. Due to their small size and mass (less than five grams), wristbands are comfortable, rugged, and do not interfere with daily activities (Figure 9.2). Wristbands also do not require a battery or maintenance, allowing an individual to continuously wear the sampler. Finally, as a noninvasive chemical monitor, wristbands studies have high volunteer compliance (Donald et al. 2016, Kile et al. 2016, Bergmann et al. 2017a, Vidi et al. 2017, Harley et al. 2019).

Silicone wristbands sequester a wide range of chemicals, including volatile organic chemicals (VOCs) and semi-volatile organic chemicals (SVOCs). Depending

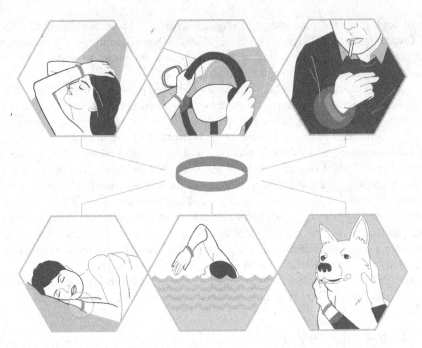

FIGURE 9.2 Silicone wristbands can be worn during normal daily activities, such as showering, driving, smoking, sleeping, swimming, and interacting with animals.

on physical–chemical properties, different chemicals will sequester at different rates into the wristband, which can be characterized by chemical partition coefficients (e.g. octanol-air partition coefficient, log K_{oa}) (Anderson et al. 2017, Bergmann et al. 2018, Hammel et al. 2018). Wristbands can sample chemicals that span over twelve orders of magnitude for octanol-air partition coefficients, with log K_{oa} ranging from 3.3 to 16 (toluene to di(2-ethylhexyl)tetrabromophthalate) (Bergmann et al. 2018). As an analogy for several orders of magnitude, the temperature of water freezing at 0°C (log 0) and the temperature at the sun center is 15,000,000°C (log 7). This wide range enables the PSD to function as a broad, nonspecific organic chemical sampler.

9.3.2   CHEMICAL UPTAKE

Uptake into the silicone wristband, or other silicone wearable, is unique to each chemical based on its physical–chemical properties, environmental concentrations, and exposure time. The uptake of organic chemicals into the wristband over time includes linear, curvilinear, and equilibrium phases (Figure 9.3) (Shoeib and Harner 2002, Huckins et al. 2006, Bohlin et al. 2007). In the linear phase, a chemical's concentration in the wristband is lower than in the environment and the uptake rate is constant. In the curvilinear phase, a chemical's concentration in the wristband increases and the uptake rate is reduced. In the next phase, the wristband is in equilibrium with the surrounding environment; the chemical concentration in the wristband becomes constant if the environmental concentration is not changing.

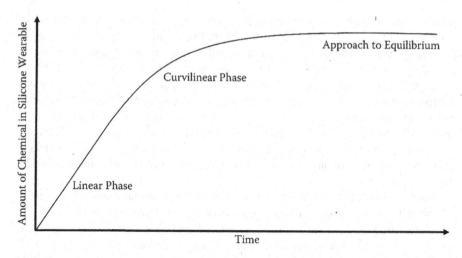

FIGURE 9.3 Theoretical chemical uptake curve for silicone wearables over time. Each chemical will have a different uptake curve.

Regardless of whether a chemical is in the linear, curvilinear, or equilibrium phase, chemical uptake is dynamic and chemicals are actively moving in and out of the silicone wristband during the entire sampling period.

Some chemicals will reach equilibrium between the wristband and the environment, representing the estimated average concentration of the chemical over the time worn. This is the case for small, volatile chemicals (e.g. naphthalene). Saturation of the wristbands is not a concern at equilibrium; the wristbands have been tested in highly contaminated environments for long deployment times with no evidence of saturation. At equilibrium, wristbands can detect changes in a chemical's concentration and will accurately reflect the average concentrations over the period worn. The chemicals are sequestered within the silicone polymer via simple diffusion (Figure 9.1), but the polymer pores do not behave like enzymatic binding sites (e.g. lock-and-key mechanism). Wristbands do not fill up nor stop sequestering chemicals during uptake; rather, chemicals can move freely between the environment and silicone wristband, resulting in relevant chemical concentrations.

Although the process of chemical uptake depends on several factors, researchers have tools to determine chemical uptake rates in wristbands. Performance reference compounds (PRCs) can be added to wristbands prior to deployment and they allow researchers to calculate a chemical's uptake rate and phase specific to each sampler's environment (Booij et al. 2002). There is significant precedence for using PRCs with PSDs (Shoeib and Harner 2002, Bohlin et al. 2007, Lohmann 2011, Anderson et al. 2017).

9.3.3 WRISTBAND DATA APPLICATIONS

Understanding the process of chemical uptake is essential when making conclusions about chemical exposure. Wristband results are often used to make comparisons between different groups of study volunteers. For exposure comparisons, chemical concentrations can be reported as ng/wristband, ng/g wristband, or pmol/g wristband (Donald et al. 2016, Poutasse et al. 2019). Even if specific uptake rates are not known, the uptake rate of a given chemical will be approximately equivalent for all samplers, enabling comparisons of the given chemical between samplers. Because different chemicals have unique uptake curves, researchers have to be cautious when making comparisons between different chemicals (e.g. toluene compared to benzo[a]pyrene), either within a wristband or between different wristbands (Donald et al. 2016). Screening for the presence and absence of a large number of chemicals can also be an efficient way to make comparisons between groups of volunteers and inform future toxicology and exposure science studies (Bergmann et al. 2017a, Dixon et al. 2019).

Current research is addressing how environmental concentrations can be calculated from silicone wristbands via partition coefficients (Anderson et al. 2017). For PAHs, partition coefficients between wristbands and air have been reported from two paired studies: one using wristbands and active air samplers (Anderson et al. 2017) and one using wristbands and low-density polyethylene, another common PSD (Donald et al. 2019).

Another application of wristband data sets is to predict chemical concentrations in biological matrices. This is similar to other research that has used PSD data to predict chemical concentrations in organisms such as crayfish, clams, mussels, and aquatic worms (Muijs et al. 2012, Fernandez et al. 2015, Joyce et al. 2015, Paulik et al. 2016). Data from Dixon et al. (2018) was used to generate a linear regression model of phenanthrene in wristbands and associated metabolites in urine from participants in an urban environment (Figure 9.4). When looking at the sum of

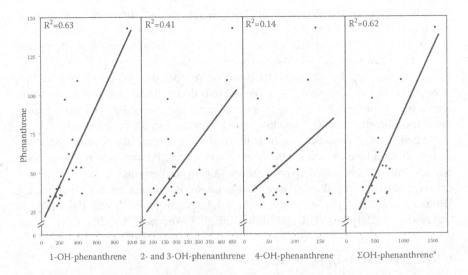

FIGURE 9.4   Linear regression model of phenanthrene in wristbands and associated phenanthrene metabolites in urine from data in Dixon et al. (2018). ([a]Sum of 1-OH-phenanthrene, 2-OH- and 3-OH-phenanthrene, 4-OH-phenanthrene concentrations.)

phenanthrene urinary metabolites, the associated R-squared value for the line of best fit was 0.62 (Figure 9.4). This type of approach could be used with other chemicals and types of biological matrices (e.g. blood and breast milk) to predict internal biomarker concentrations.

9.3.4 Silicone Wristband Limitations and Additional Considerations

While wristbands and other silicone wearables offer many opportunities to examine personal chemical exposures, wristbands are not real-time samplers (e.g. do not change color nor notify the wearer when chemical exposure occurs). A sampler must be sent back to a laboratory for chemical analysis. Wristband extracts from either liquid extraction or thermal desorption methods can be stored and reanalyzed later with other analytical methods after sampling has occurred.

Additionally, when worn on the wrist, chemical concentrations in wristbands represent a combination of several exposure routes (e.g. dermal and inhalation) (Weschler et al. 2012, Aerts et al. 2018, Dixon et al. 2019). Although determining the contribution from specific exposure routes may be difficult, it can be advantageous to evaluate chemical exposures from multiple routes to address human health questions.

There are other types of methodologies beyond silicone wristbands that are currently available to monitor personal organic chemical exposures (O'Connell 2017). Stakeholders (e.g. researchers, communities, non-government organizations) need to consider which method aligns best with their objectives. For example, biomonitoring samples are traditionally analyzed to monitor chemical exposures (Ospina et al. 2018). However, biomarker concentrations can vary due to several factors, such as individual variability in metabolism, gender, age, and health status (Aylward et al. 2014, Koch et al. 2014). Additionally, some chemicals remain in the body for a long time or lack a clear link to an internal biomarker (Forsberg et al. 2011). These factors complicate efforts to evaluate chemical exposures, assess intervention strategies, and set regulatory limits via biomonitoring samples. The characteristics of any chemical exposure assessment method must be fit-for-purpose to best address stakeholder questions.

9.4 LABORATORY PRACTICES

9.4.1 Wristband Preparation and Shipment

Silicone wristband stock material is low cost and commercially available. Yet, the stock material must be properly prepared in order to remove chemicals that can adversely impact analysis and chemicals that are in the desired analytical method. To minimize solvent use, wristband preparation can occur via vacuum oven conditioning when prepared according to Anderson et al. (2017). Alternatively, wristband preparation can also occur using Soxhlet extraction (Hammel et al. 2016, Hammel et al. 2018, Romanak et al. 2018). Following the preparation processes, wristbands can be analyzed using chromatography and spectrometry to ensure removal of chemicals (Anderson et al. 2017).

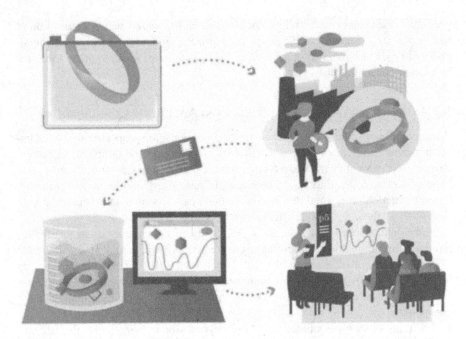

FIGURE 9.5 Silicone wristbands can promote collaborations between diverse stakeholders. Process steps to assess personal chemical exposures can include preparation in the laboratory, study volunteer participation, sampler transport, chemical extraction and analysis, and community engagement.

Silicone wristbands can be individually transported to study locations in airtight, impermeable containers, such as airtight polytetrafluoroethylene (PTFE) bags (Figure 9.5) (Anderson et al. 2017). Each PTFE bag can be labeled with necessary study information, such as sample identification number and the sampler on and off dates and times. Wristbands can be transported to each study location at ambient temperature through standard mail services (Figure 9.5).

9.4.2 CHEMICAL STABILITY IN WRISTBANDS

When stored in PTFE bags, both VOCs and SVOCs have been demonstrated to be stable in the wristbands for extended periods of time (Anderson et al. 2017). Under simulated transport conditions (30°C), 17 VOCs were stable in the wristbands for 7 days and 131 SVOCs for up to 1 month (Anderson et al. 2017). Because there was no chemical loss in wristbands stored in PTFE bags at elevated temperatures, wristbands and other wristbands can be shipped long distances at ambient temperature, reducing transportation costs. Similarly, during long-term storage at −20°C, all chemical levels were stable for up to 3 months for VOCs and 6 months for SVOCs (Anderson et al. 2017), and this dataset has since been extended to 21 months. The transport and storage stability of organic chemicals provides time and cost advantages over other exposure assessment methods. By comparison, the US EPA SVOC method 8270 for water samples maintains that extractions be completed in 14 days. Storage stability of chemicals in wristbands allows greater flexibility for stakeholders.

9.4.3 Chemical Extraction

The extraction of chemicals from wristbands can vary depending upon study design and analytes of interest. The majority of literature on wristbands include a post-deployment cleaning step to remove surface particulates (O'Connell et al. 2014a, Donald et al. 2016, Kile et al. 2016, Anderson et al. 2017, Bergmann et al. 2017a, Vidi et al. 2017, Dixon et al. 2018, Paulik et al. 2018, Dixon et al. 2019, Harley et al. 2019). Particle-bound contaminants, which are generally not bioavailable for dermal exposure, can be removed by washing the wristbands (Anderson et al. 2008, Anderson et al. 2017). Following post-deployment cleaning, wristbands are amenable to a wide variety of chemical extraction procedures. Solvent extractions are currently the most common method (Anderson et al. 2017). For example, wristbands can be extracted with ethyl acetate (O'Connell et al. 2014a, Anderson et al. 2017, Aerts et al. 2018). Alternatively, thermal desorption onto sorbent tubes is another option which can significantly decrease extraction time compared to solvent extractions.

For any extraction method, researchers must consider the number and amount of chemicals that are removed by the silicone preparation step compared to the extraction steps after use. If the silicone preparation process removes fewer interference chemicals than the post-use extraction process, researchers are potentially analyzing chemicals left over from the original silicone manufacturing process. In practice, the silicone preparation steps should be more rigorous (e.g. higher temperature) than the post-use solvent extraction.

9.4.4 Chemical and Biological Analysis

Solvent extracts from wristbands can be analyzed for chemicals on a wide variety of different analytical methods, using both gas and liquid chromatography. One analytical method is a quantitative screen for 1530 target organic chemicals with only 50 minutes of instrument time per sample (Bergmann et al. 2018). Experienced chemists spend under 20 minutes per sample reviewing the chromatographic results. The target analytes include pesticides, PAHs, polychlorinated biphenyls (PCBs), polybrominated diphenyl ethers (PBDEs), phthalates, and fragrances, which can all contribute to chemical mixtures. Although this method is a targeted screen, there is interest in applying non-targeted chemical analysis to extracts from wristbands as demonstrated by Manzano et al. (2019) and Ulrich et al. (2019).

For biological analysis, extracts can be applied to bioassays and investigated using an effects-directed analysis (Bergmann et al. 2017b, Geier et al. 2018). For instance, the developmental zebrafish model has allowed researchers to test multiple toxicity endpoints, such as physiological deformities and neurobehavioral changes, with chemical extracts from PSDs (Geier et al. 2018). The zebrafish developmental model, or other bioassays, paired with extracts from wristbands offers countless opportunities for chemical risk assessment.

9.5   HUMAN RESEARCH ETHICS

Silicone wristbands can be easily integrated into studies requiring Institutional Review Board (IRB) approval. At academic institutions, IRB approval is required for all studies involving human participants. This process ensures volunteers understand the risks, benefits, and expectations of participating in a research study. As determined by Oregon State University's IRB on silicone wristband research, "The probability and magnitude of harm or discomfort anticipated in the research are not greater in and of themselves than those ordinarily encountered in daily life." For other stakeholders interested in using silicone wristbands outside of a research study, IRB approval might not be required.

In several studies from Oregon State University, volunteers are given the option to have their wristband chemical results returned to them. Returning chemical results gives volunteers opportunities to learn more about scientific studies, reduce their chemical exposures, and engage in public discourse (Brody et al. 2007, Brody et al. 2014, Ohayon et al. 2017). Even if chemical exposure limits and potential health effects of exposure are not known, previous research has demonstrated that participants report benefits from receiving their chemical results (Morello-Frosch et al. 2009, Adams et al. 2011, Ohayon et al. 2017, Dixon et al. 2019). For example, members of the Swinomish Indian Tribal Community received their wristband results and volunteers reported that this information helped them become more aware of potential PAH sources in their community (Rohlman et al. 2019b). Several volunteers also reported changing their behaviors to try to reduce their exposure to PAHs (Rohlman et al. 2019b).

9.6   SILICONE WRISTBAND APPLICATIONS

Since 2014, researchers have demonstrated the applicability of wristbands, compared wristbands with other conventional exposure assessment methodologies, and investigated associations between wristband results and health effects (Table 9.1).

9.6.1   INITIAL FIELD APPLICATIONS

In two occupational settings with hot asphalt applications in O'Connell et al. (2014a), silicone wristbands were worn by roofers at an outdoor and indoor training facility and analyzed for PAHs and oxygenated-PAHs. Average PAH concentrations were three times higher at the indoor worksite compared to the outdoor worksite (O'Connell et al. 2014a). This initial wristband publication garnered significant interest in applications in areas of exposure science, occupational health, and epidemiology.

Paulik et al. (2018) focused on personal PAH exposures in non-occupational settings ($n = 19$) of rural Ohio, using both silicone wristbands and stationary air PSDs nearby. With the expansion of natural gas extraction (NGE) in the United States, this was one of few studies documenting personal PAH exposures with NGE occurring nearby. Wristbands from participants with active NGE wells on their properties had a significantly higher sum of 62 PAHs than participants without (Wilcoxon ranked sum, $p < 0.005$) (Paulik et al. 2018). Furthermore, PAH concentrations in wristbands were positively correlated with PAH concentrations sampled in air near participants' homes (simple linear regression, $p < 0.0001$). This linear relationship underestimated

TABLE 9.1

Silicone Wearable References as of March 2019, Organized by Chemical Class

	Chemical Class	Analytical Instrument	References
Targeted Chemical Analysis	Polycyclic aromatic hydrocarbons (PAHs)	GC-MS[a]	(O'Connell et al. 2014a, Donald et al. 2016, Bergmann et al. 2017a, Bergmann et al. 2018, Romanak et al. 2018, Dixon et al. 2019)
		GC-MS/MS	(Anderson et al. 2017, Paulik et al. 2018, Dixon et al. 2019, Rohlman et al. 2019a, Rohlman et al. 2019b)
		GCxGC/ToF-MS[b]	(Manzano et al. 2018)
	Polychlorinated biphenyls (PCBs)	GC-MS	(O'Connell et al. 2014a, Anderson et al. 2017, Bergmann et al. 2017a, Bergmann et al. 2018, Dixon et al. 2019)
	Flame Retardants	GC-MS	(O'Connell et al. 2014a, Hammel et al. 2016, Kile et al. 2016, Anderson et al. 2017, Bergmann et al. 2017a, Lipscomb et al. 2017, Bergmann et al. 2018, Hammel et al. 2018, Romanak et al. 2018, Dixon et al. 2019, Donald et al. 2019)
	• Polybrominated diphenyl ethers (PBDEs)		
	• Novel brominated flame retardants (BFRs)		
	• Organophosphate esters (OPEs)		
	Pesticides	GC-MS	(O'Connell et al. 2014a, Bergmann et al. 2017a, Bergmann et al. 2018, Dixon et al. 2019, Donald et al. 2019, Harley et al. 2019)
	• Organochlorines		
	• Organophosphates	GC-ECD[c]	(O'Connell et al. 2014a, Donald et al. 2016, Bergmann et al. 2017a, Vidi et al. 2017, Bergmann et al. 2018, Harley et al. 2019)
	• Neonicotinoids		
	• Pyrethroids	UHPLC-MS/MS[d]	(Aerts et al. 2018)
	• Amides		
	• Pyrazoles		
	• Other		

(Continued)

TABLE 9.1 (*Continued*)
Silicone Wearable References as of March 2019, Organized by Chemical Class

	Chemical Class	Analytical Instrument	References
	Phthalates	GC-MS	(O'Connell et al. 2014a, Bergmann et al. 2017a, Bergmann et al. 2018, Dixon et al. 2019)
		GCxGC/ToF-MS	(Manzano et al. 2018)
	Consumer product-related chemicals	GC-MS	(O'Connell et al. 2014a, Bergmann et al. 2017a, Bergmann et al. 2018, Dixon et al. 2019, Donald et al. 2019)
		LC-MS/MS	(Quintana et al. 2019)
	Industrial-related chemicals	GC-MS	(O'Connell et al. 2014a, Bergmann et al. 2017a, Bergmann et al. 2018, Dixon et al. 2019, Donald et al. 2019)
		GCxGC/ToF-MS	(Manzano et al. 2018)
	Volatile organic compounds (VOCs)	GC-MS	Anderson 2017, Donald 2019 (Anderson et al. 2017, Donald et al. 2019)
	Dioxins and Furans	GC-MS	(Bergmann et al. 2017a, Bergmann et al. 2018, Dixon et al. 2019)
		GCxGC/ToF-MS	(Manzano et al. 2018)
Nontargeted Chemical Analysis		Assorted LC analyses (interlaboratory comparison study)	(Ulrich et al. 2019)

a Gas chromatography (GC)-mass spectrometry (MS).
b GCxGC-time of flight (ToF)-MS.
c GC-electron capture detector (ECD).
d Ultra-high performance liquid chromatography (UHPLC)-MS/MS.

and overestimated some personal PAH exposures based on stationary air monitors, indicating the importance of personal wristband data.

In Aerts et al. (2018), volunteers (n = 30) in Leuven, Belgium, wore silicone wristbands to assess non-occupational pesticide exposures in an urban setting, while a second wristband was placed near each volunteer's home (Aerts et al. 2018). Researchers analyzed wristband extracts for 200 polar pesticides. Thirty-one pesticides were detected, with 48% of those pesticides being detected only in the wristbands worn by volunteers and not detected in the wristbands placed outside. Volunteers with diets featuring increased vegetable consumption were associated with increased pesticide detections, demonstrating that wristbands capture ingestion and dermal exposures. Aside from five wristbands with only *N,N*-diethyl-meta-toluamide (DEET) detected, all other wristbands had a unique profile of pesticide detections, revealing how highly individualized chemical exposures can be and the importance of personal monitoring (Aerts et al. 2018).

As further evidence of individualized exposures, Donald et al. (2016) found that no two wristbands worn by different volunteers (n = 35) had the exact same pesticides detected. In this study, volunteers from rural farming families in Diender, Senegal, wore wristbands in the first assessment of personal occupational pesticide exposures in West Africa (Donald et al. 2016). Each volunteer wore a wristband for two separate periods, for a total of 70 wristbands in the study (100% compliance). Although inter-individual differences were large between different volunteers for the 63 pesticides in the analysis, the pairs of wristbands worn by the same individuals revealed that intra-individual differences were small. Within each individual's paired wristbands neither the number of detections nor concentrations were significantly different (Wilcoxon signed-rank, p < 0.003). These results may be attributable to consistent behaviors and activities of individuals from week to week, whereas behaviors can vary widely between different people. Researchers can use wristbands to detect inter- and intra-individual chemical exposure patterns.

In the remote region of Alto Mayo, Peru, volunteers (n = 68) from rural and urban communities wore wristbands, as described in Bergmann et al. (2017). Wristbands were screened for the presence of 1,397 chemicals, and chemical patterns based on demographics were identified (Bergmann et al. 2017a). For example, wristbands from rural communities had a higher number of pesticide and PAH detections than urban communities, and wristbands from urban communities had higher personal care product chemical detections than rural communities (chi-square likelihood ratio test, p < 0.05). Together, these studies demonstrated silicone wristband applications across diverse communities.

9.6.2 COMPARISONS WITH CONVENTIONAL EXPOSURE ASSESSMENT TECHNOLOGIES

Concentrations in silicone wearables (i.e. wristband) have been directly compared to concentrations in paired conventional exposure assessment technologies, including hand wipes, active air samplers, serum, and urine. These studies all demonstrated strong correlations between wristband chemical concentrations and paired biological metabolite concentrations, providing further evidence that wristbands sequester the bioavailable fraction.

In Hammel et al. (2016), adults from Durham, North Carolina, wore wristbands and provided one hand wipe and three spot urine samples. Pooled urine was analyzed for metabolites of four organophosphate flame retardants (OPFRs): tris(1,3-dichloroisopropyl)phosphate (TDCIPP), tris(1,3-dichloro-2-propyl)phosphate (TCIPP), triphenyl phosphate (TPHP), and monosubstitued isopropylated triaryl phosphate (mono-ITP). Concentrations of TDCIPP and TCIPP in the wristbands strongly correlated with the associated urinary metabolites (r_s = 0.5–0.65, p < 0.001), suggesting wristbands predict internal exposure to OPFRs (Hammel et al. 2016). Wristbands may be an improved OPFR exposure assessment tool compared to hand wipes.

In follow-up to Hammel et al. (2016), Hammel et al. (2018) continued the validation study by examining wristbands for PBDE exposures. PBDEs, which also act as household flame retardants, biomagnify and have longer half-lives in the body compared to OPFRs. Participants (n = 30) provided serum samples to correlate PBDE biomarkers with wristband data (Hammel et al. 2018). Between wristbands and serum biomarkers, BDE-47, -99, -100, and -153 were positively correlated (r_s = 0.39–0.57, p < 0.05), demonstrating that silicone wristbands can quantify personal PBDE exposures, as wells as OPFR exposures.

In Dixon et al. (2018), pregnant women (n = 22) in a birth cohort in New York City wore a wristband, provided a urine sample, and wore an active air sampler (i.e. polyurethane foam (PUF) and filter housed in a personal backpack). Researchers compared concentrations of PAHs and PAH metabolites between wristbands, PUFs, filters, and urine. Researchers found three times more positive, significant correlations between PAH and PAH metabolite pairs in wristbands and urine samples than between PUF-filters and urine samples (Dixon et al. 2018). Specifically, concentrations of six PAHs in the wristbands strongly correlated with concentrations of the associated urinary metabolites (r_s = 0.44–0.76, p = 0.04 to <0.001), indicating that wristband PAH exposures are predictive of internal biomarkers.

In Quintana et al. (2019), children in California (n = 31) wore silicone wristbands and provided a urine sample to investigate nicotine exposures between smoking and nonsmoking homes. Similar to Hammel et al. (2016, 2018) and Dixon et al. (2018), Quintana et al. reported strong significant correlations between concentrations in the wristbands and in the urine (r^2 = 0.85, p < 0.001), further demonstrating that wristbands are reflecting the bioavailable chemical fraction and body burden (Quintana et al. 2019).

9.6.3   Health Effects

Several studies have begun to examine chemical concentrations from wristbands in association with adverse health effects. In Kile et al. (2016) and Lipscomb et al. (2017), wristbands quantified preschool-aged children's flame retardant exposures (n = 72) and examined exposures in the context of emotional and social behaviors. Children from Corvallis and Eugene, Oregon, enjoyed wearing the wristbands, with one child referring to it as "their own personal science bracelet" (Kile et al. 2016). Flame retardant concentrations and sociodemographic data were correlated for multiple variables, such as house age and vacuuming frequency. In the companion article, social behaviors were measured using the Social Skills Improvement Rating Scale as rated by a child's teacher (Lipscomb et al. 2017). Higher flame retardant exposures were associated with less responsible behavior and increased external-izing behavior problems (Lipscomb et al. 2017). This study suggested that the cor-relation of higher flame retardant exposures with poorer social skills may impact a child's ability to succeed academically and socially.

Vidi et al. (2018) also characterized children's chemical exposures, but focused on para-occupational pesticide exposures and DNA damage in hair follicles. The long-term effects of pesticide exposures on health and development are poorly under-stood, but indirect exposures (e.g. shared housing with an agricultural worker) may lead to adverse health effects (Vidi et al. 2017). Latino children (n = 10) from farmworker households in rural North Carolina were recruited as part of a community-based par-ticipatory research project. Each child wore a wristband to quantify pesticide exposures and provided plucked hair follicle samples to quantify DNA damage. An increasing number of pesticide detections was significantly associated with DNA damage in the papilla region of the hairs, indicative of DNA damage to epithelial cells.

Rohlman et al. (2019a) developed the novel Exposure, Location and lung Function (ELF) tool to concurrently collect daily individualized chemical exposure (silicone wristbands), location (cell phone), and respiratory health outcomes (spirometer and questionnaires) (Rohlman et al. 2019a). An ELF phone app collected questionnaire data about personal behavior, potential exposure sources, and respiratory health symptoms. Volunteers also used a handheld, Bluetooth-linked spirometer to assess lung function throughout the study. In an initial pilot study using this ELF tech-nology in Eugene, Oregon, volunteers used the ELF with high compliance (>90%) (Rohlman et al. 2019a).

9.6.4 ADDITIONAL CONFIGURATIONS OF SILICONE WRISTBANDS

Since the first report of silicone wristbands in 2014, new configurations of silicone PSDs have also been developed. Multiple pilot studies have demonstrated the use of novel silicone PSDs that are not worn on the wrist (e.g. wearables).

To characterize chemical exposures in animal health studies, horses have worn silicone wearables on their halters, and cats have worn silicone pet tags. The horse cohort study evaluated broodmare PAH exposures in New York and Pennsylvania in relationship to the incidence of foal dysphagia (Rivera et al. In Preparation). A sili-cone wearable was secured to the horses' halter (Figure 9.6a). A cat case-control study evaluated flame retardant exposures using pet tags (Figure 9.6b) worn by geriatric cats diagnosed with feline hyperthyroidism. Community cat owners vol-unteered their cats (n = 78) to wear the tag. With extremely positive feedback from the owners (e.g. "The tag didn't bother her/him at all!"), the results indicated that elevated exposures to tris(1,3,-dichloro-2-isopropyl) phosphate were correlated with feline hyperthyroidism (Poutasse et al. 2019). These two examples demonstrate the widespread applicability of silicone wearables to answer chemical exposure ques-tions for animals, as well as humans.

Additional configurations for human volunteers include lapels and military-style dog tags. A lapel configuration on top of clothing (Figure 9.6c) selectively samples

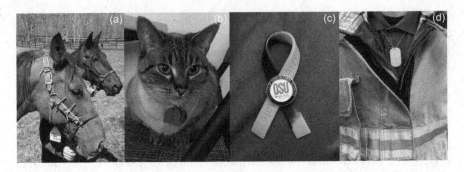

FIGURE 9.6 Silicone wearable options: (a) horse halter, (b) pet tag, (c) lapel, and (d) military-style dog tag.

inhalation exposures, as demonstrated in O'Connell et al. (2014a). By altering where and how the silicone sampler is worn, the lapel minimizes dermal uptake. Similarly, a military-style dog tag (Figure 9.6d) can be worn around the neck to assess firefighter chemical exposures. The exposure study was driven by firefighter concern over high incidences of cancer diagnoses (Daniels et al. 2014), and firefighter participants had significant input in developing the dog tag sampler. Dog tags can be worn under or over clothing to address different chemical exposure questions. Examining occupational chemical exposure mixtures provides unique opportunities for assessing behavioral health interventions.

9.7 FUTURE DIRECTIONS

9.7.1 CHEMICAL MIXTURES

The ability to analyze personal chemical samplers for many chemical classes at one time allows for efficient and realistic chemical mixture analysis on a global scale. With more research studies including silicone wristbands, researchers can use PSDs as population screening tools as demonstrated in Dixon et al. (2019). The presence of 1,530 chemical detections was reported for 262 wristbands worn on three continents (Dixon et al. 2019). Common chemical mixtures were identified, and the characterization of such chemical mixtures offers significant advances for toxicological testing. When certain chemicals co-occur, there can be synergistic, antagonistic, or additive effects (Carpenter et al. 2002), and wristbands allow for the identification of realistic chemical mixtures.

9.7.2 DISASTER-RELATED EXPOSURES

Wristbands can be worn in disaster situations to characterize chemical exposures because they do not interfere with important activities, such as response and recovery to a flood or fire (Figure 9.7). After Hurricane Harvey made landfall in Texas in 2017, over a dozen federal Superfund sites were flooded and/or experienced possible storm damage (Status of Superfund Sites 2017, Griggs et al. 2017). Communities were concerned about chemicals in the floodwater (Wristbands Given Out... 2017).

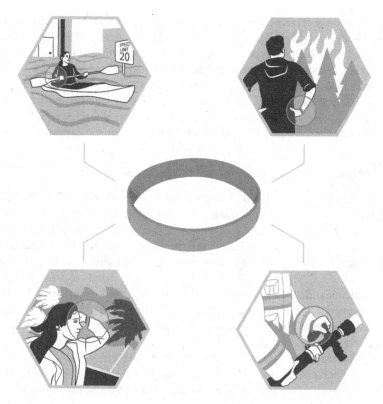

FIGURE 9.7 Silicone wristbands can be used to assess personal chemical exposure in several disaster scenarios, including flooding, hurricanes, and fires.

People involved in the hurricane recovery process wore wristbands within four weeks post-Hurricane Harvey. Even in the aftermath of Harvey, wristband compliance was 85%, illustrating the approachability of this technology. Although only a small, non-random sample of wristbands was analyzed, wristbands worn after Harvey had a higher mean number of chemical detections compared to several other geographic regions unaffected by recent disasters (Dixon et al. 2019). In the future, wristbands can be worn by people impacted by other disasters, such as people in close proximity to wildfire smoke.

9.7.3 Behavioral Health Interventions

Identifying risk factors associated with elevated chemical exposures provides insight into how exposures can be mitigated in the future via behavioral interventions. Harley et al. (2019) used silicone wristbands to characterize pesticide exposures among 14- to 16-year-old girls (n = 97) living in the Salinas Valley, California. California's Salinas Valley (Monterey County) is an extremely productive agricultural region, but some pesticide exposures are associated with various adverse health effects (e.g. disruption of hormonal function). In this study, the majority of detected pesticides were used only for residential pest control, suggesting that this community experiences pesticides exposures beyond agriculture (Harley et al. 2019). Higher odds of detecting select pesticides were associated with living within 100 m of agricultural fields, having carpet in the home, and having an exterminator treating the home within the past 6 months. The study volunteers reported these major findings to the larger agricultural community and recommended lifestyle changes for reducing pesticide exposures (Harley et al. 2019). In the future, wristband studies could assess the impact of behavioral health interventions on personal chemical exposure.

9.7.4 Precision Health and Precision Prevention

Individualized chemical exposure data obtained from silicone wristbands can be paired with personalized genomic data. A combination of chemical exposure and genetic data is necessary to understand human health. The cost to sequence an individual's genome has decreased dramatically in the past decade (The Cost of Sequencing a Human Genome 2016), and the cost to assess personal chemical exposures is dropping with the development of silicone wristbands. Wristbands can fulfill the need for large chemical dataset generation in the emerging field of precision health and precision prevention (Gillman et al. 2016). The power of large-scale chemical datasets enables researchers to improve overall understanding of exposures, to improve health through reducing certain chemical exposures, and to answer health-related questions previously unable to be addressed with genetic information alone. Silicone wristbands can be an integral piece of the collaborative strategy that shifts the current healthcare paradigm from retroactively curing disease to proactively preventing disease.

ACKNOWLEDGMENTS

The authors give thanks to all past and current members of the Food Safety and Environmental Stewardship Laboratory at Oregon State University. Our special thanks go to Dr. Carey Donald, Dr. Julie Herbstman, Dr. Sara Jahnke, Sean Carver, Kyla Tom, and Jacob Del Savio.

CONFLICT OF INTEREST

Kim A. Anderson, author of this research, discloses a financial interest in MyExposome, Inc., which is marketing products related to the research being reported. The terms of this arrangement have been reviewed and approved by Oregon State University in accordance with its policy on research conflicts of interest. The authors have no other disclosures.

REFERENCES

Adams, C., Brown, P., Morello-Frosch, R., Brody, J. G., Rudel, R., Zota, A., Dunagan, S., Tovar, J., and Patton, S. 2011. "Disentangling the Exposure Experience: The Roles of Community Context and Report-Back of Environmental Exposure Data." *J Health Soc Behav* 52 (2):180–196. doi: 10.1177/0022146510395593.

Advancing Science, Improving Health: A Plan for Environmental Health Research. 2018. National Institute of Health Publication 18-ES–7935.

Aerts, R., Joly, L., Szternfeld, P., Tsilikas, K., De Cremer, K., Castelain, P., Aerts, J. M., Van Orshoven, J., Somers, B., Hendrickx, M., Andjelkovic, M., and Van Nieuwenhuyse, A. 2018. "Silicone Wristband Passive Samplers Yield Highly Individualized Pesticide Residue Exposure Profiles." *Environ Sci Technol* 52 (1):298–307. doi: 10.1021/acs. est.7b05039.

Anderson, K., and Hillwalker, W. 2008. "Bioavailability." In *Ecotoxicology*, edited by Sven Erik Jorgensen and Brian D. Fath, 348–357. Oxford: Elsevier.

Anderson, K. A., Points III, G. L., Donald, C. E., Dixon, H. M., Scott, R. P., Wilson, G., Tidwell, L. G., Hoffman, P. D., Herbstman, J. B., and O'Connell, S. G. 2017. "Preparation and Performance Features of Wristband Samplers and Considerations for Chemical Exposure Assessment." *J Expo Sci Environ Epidemiol* 27 (6):551.

Aylward, L. L., Hays, S. M., Smolders, R., Koch, H. M., Cocker, J., Jones, K., Warren, N., Levy, L., and Bevan, R. 2014. "Sources of Variability in Biomarker Concentrations." *J Toxicol Env Heal B* 17 (1):45–61. doi: 10.1080/10937404.2013.864250.

Bergmann, A. J., North, P. E., Vasquez, L., Bello, H., Ruiz, M. d. C. G., and Anderson, K. A. 2017a. "Multi-Class Chemical Exposure in Rural Peru Using Silicone Wristbands." *J Expo Sci Environ Epidemiol* 27 (6):560.

Bergmann, A. J., Points, G. L., Scott, R. P., Wilson, G., and Anderson, K. A. 2018. "Development of Quantitative Screen for 1550 Chemicals with GC-MS." *Anal Bioanal Chem* 410 (13):3101–3110. doi: 10.1007/s00216-018-0997-7.

Bergmann, A. J., Tanguay, R. L., and Anderson, K. A. 2017b. "Using Passive Sampling and Zebrafish to Identify Developmental Toxicants in Complex Mixtures." *Environ Toxicol Chem* 36 (9):2290–2298. doi: 10.1002/etc.3802.

Bioavailability of Contaminants in Soils and Sediments: Processes, Tools, and Applications. 2003. National Research Council: National Academies Press.

Bohlin, P., Jones, K. C., and Strandberg, B. 2007. "Occupational and Indoor Air Exposure to Persistent Organic Pollutants: A Review of Passive Sampling Techniques and Needs." *J Environ Monit* 9 (6):501–509. doi: 10.1039/b700627f.

Booij, K., Robinson, C. D., Burgess, R. M., Mayer, P., Roberts, C. A., Ahrens, L., Allan, I. J., Brant, J., Jones, L., Kraus, U. R., Larsen, M. M., Lepom, P., Petersen, J., Profrock, D., Roose, P., Schafer, S., Smedes, F., Tixier, C., Vorkamp, K., and Whitehouse, P. 2016. "Passive Sampling in Regulatory Chemical Monitoring of Nonpolar Organic Compounds in the Aquatic Environment." *Environ Sci Technol* 50 (1):3–17. doi: 10.1021/acs.est.5b04050.

Booij, K., Smedes, F., and Van Weerlee, E. M. 2002. "Spiking of Performance Reference Compounds in Low Density Polyethylene and Silicone Passive Water Samplers." *Chemosphere* 46 (8):1157–1161.

Brody, J. G., Dunagan, S. C., Morello-Frosch, R., Brown, P., Patton, S., and Rudel, R. A. 2014. "Reporting Individual Results for Biomonitoring and Environmental Exposures: Lessons Learned from Environmental Communication Case Studies." *Environ Health* 13:8. doi: 10.1186/1476-069x-13–40.

Brody, J. G., Morello-Frosch, R., Brown, P., Rudel, R. A., Altman, R. G., Frye, M., Osimo, C. A., Perez, C., and Seryak, L. M. 2007. "Improving Disclosure and Consent: "Is It Safe?": New Ethics for Reporting Personal Exposures to Environmental Chemicals." *Am J Public Health* 97 (9):1547–1554.

Carpenter, D. O., Arcaro, K., and Spink, D. C. 2002. "Understanding the Human Health Effects of Chemical Mixtures." *Environ Health Perspect* 110 (Suppl 1):25.

The Cost of Sequencing a Human Genome. 2016. National Institute of Health: National Human Genome Research Institute.

Daniels, R. D., Kubale, T. L., Yiin, J. H., Dahm, M. M., Hales, T. R., Baris, D., Zahm, S. H., Beaumont, J. J., Waters, K. M., and Pinkerton, L. E. 2014. "Mortality and Cancer Incidence in a Pooled Cohort of US Firefighters from San Francisco, Chicago and Philadelphia (1950–2009)." *Occup Environ Med* 71 (6):388–397. doi: 10.1136/oemed–2013–101662.

Dixon, H. M., Armstrong, G., Barton, M., Bergmann, A. J., Bondy, M., Halbleib, M. L., Hamilton, W., Haynes, E., Herbstman, J., Hoffman, P., Jepson, P., Kile, M. L., Kincl, L., Laurienti, P. J., North, P., Paulik, L. B., Petrosino, J., Points, G. L., Poutasse, C. M., Rohlman, D., Scott, R. P., Smith, B., Tidwell, L. G., Walker, C., Waters, K. M., and Anderson, K. A. 2019. "Discovery of Common Chemical Exposures across Three Continents Using Silicone Wristbands." *R Soc Open Sci* 6 (2). doi: 10.1098/rsos.181836.

Dixon, H. M., Scott, R. P., Holmes, D., Calero, L., Kincl, L. D., Waters, K. M., Camann, D. E., Calafat, A. M., Herbstman, J. B., and Anderson, K. A. 2018. "Silicone Wristbands Compared with Traditional Polycyclic Aromatic Hydrocarbon Exposure Assessment Methods." *Anal Bioanal Chem* 410 (13):3059–3071. doi: 10.1007/s00216-018-0992-z.

Donald, C. E., Scott, R. P., Blaustein, K. L., Halbleib, M. L., Sarr, M., Jepson, P. C., and Anderson, K. A. 2016. "Silicone Wristbands Detect Individuals' Pesticide Exposures in West Africa." *R Soc Open Sci* 3 (8):13. doi: 10.1098/rsos.160433.

Donald, C. E., Scott, R. P., Wilson, G., Hoffman, P. D., and Anderson, K. A. 2019. "Artificial Turf: Chemical Flux and Development of Silicone Wristband Partitioning Coefficients." *Air Quality, Atmos Health*. doi: 10.1007/s11869-019-00680-1.

Fernandez, L. A., and Gschwend, P. M. 2015. "Predicting Bioaccumulation of Polycyclic Aromatic Hydrocarbons in Soft-Shelled Clams (*Mya Arenaria*) Using Field Deployments of Polyethylene Passive Samplers." *Environ Toxicol Chem* 34 (5):993–1000. doi: 10.1002/etc.2892.

Forsberg, N. D., Rodriguez-Proteau, R., Ma, L., Morre, J., Christensen, J. M., Maier, C. S., Jenkins, J. J., and Anderson, K. A. 2011. "Organophosphorus Pesticide Degradation Product in Vitro Metabolic Stability and Time-Course Uptake and Elimination in Rats Following Oral and Intravenous Dosing." *Xenobiotica* 41 (5):422–429. doi: 10.3109/00498254.2010.550656.

Geier, M. C., James Minick, D., Truong, L., Tilton, S., Pande, P., Anderson, K. A., Teeguardan, J., and Tanguay, R. L. 2018. "Systematic Developmental Neurotoxicity Assessment of a Representative PAH Superfund Mixture Using Zebrafish." *Toxicol Appl Pharmacol*. doi: 10.1016/j.taap.2018.03.029.

Gillman, M. W., and Hammond, R. A. 2016. "Precision Treatment and Precision Prevention: Integrating "Below and Above the Skin"." *JAMA Pediatr* 170 (1):9–10. doi: 10.1001/jamapediatrics.2015.2786.

Griggs, T., Lehren, A. W., Popovich, N., Singhvi, A., and Tabuchi, H. 2017. "More Than 40 Sites Released Hazardous Pollutants Because of Hurricane Harvey." *New York Times*, 09/08/2017. https://www.nytimes.com/interactive/2017/09/08/us/houston-hurricane-harvey-harzardous-chemicals.html.

Hammel, S. C., Hoffman, K., Webster, T. F., Anderson, K. A., and Stapleton, H. M. 2016. "Measuring Personal Exposure to Organophosphate Flame Retardants Using Silicone Wristbands and Hand Wipes." *Environ Sci Technol* 50 (8):4483–4491. doi: 10.1021/acs.est.6b00030.

Hammel, S. C., Phillips, A. L., Hoffman, K., and Stapleton, H. M. 2018. "Evaluating the Use of Silicone Wristbands to Measure Personal Exposure to Brominated Flame Retardants." *Environ Sci Technol* 52 (20):11875–11885. doi: 10.1021/acs.est.8b03755.

Harley, K. G., Parra, K. L., Camacho, J., Bradman, A., Nolan, J. E., Lessard, C., Anderson, K. A., Poutasse, C. M., Scott, R. P., and Lazaro, G. 2019. "Determinants of Pesticide Concentrations in Silicone Wristbands Worn by Latina Adolescent Girls in a California Farmworker Community: The COSECHA Youth Participatory Action Study." *Sci Total Environ* 652:1022–1029.

Huckins, J. N., Petty, J. D., and Booij, K. 2006. *Monitors of Organic Chemicals in the Environment: Semipermeable Membrane Devices.* Springer Science & Business Media, New York.

Joyce, A. S., Pirogovsky, M. S., Adams, R. G., Lao, W., Tsukada, D., Cash, C. L., Haw, J. F., and Maruya, K. A. 2015. "Using Performance Reference Compound-Corrected Polyethylene Passive Samplers and Caged Bivalves to Measure Hydrophobic Contaminants of Concern in Urban Coastal Seawaters." *Chemosphere* 127:10–17. doi: 10.1016/j.chemosphere.2014.12.067.

Kile, M. L., Scott, R. P., O'Connell, S. G., Lipscomb, S., MacDonald, M., McClelland, M., and Anderson, K. A. 2016. "Using Silicone Wristbands to Evaluate Preschool Children's Exposure to Flame Retardants." *Environ Res* 147:365–372 doi: 10.1016/j.envres.2016.02.034.

Koch, H. M., Aylward, L. L., Hays, S. M., Smolders, R., Moos, R. K., Cocker, J., Jones, K., Warren, N., Levy, L., and Bevan, R. 2014. "Inter- and Intra-Individual Variation in Urinary Biomarker Concentrations over a 6-Day Sampling Period. Part 2: Personal Care Product Ingredients." *Toxicol Lett* 231 (2):261–269. doi: 10.1016/j.toxlet.2014.06.023.

Lipscomb, S. T., McClelland, M. M., MacDonald, M., Cardenas, A., Anderson, K. A., and Kile, M. L. 2017. "Cross-Sectional Study of Social Behaviors in Preschool Children and Exposure to Flame Retardants." *Environ Health* 16:10. doi: 10.1186/s12940-017-0224-6.

Lohmann, R. 2011. "Critical Review of Low-Density Polyethylene's Partitioning and Diffusion Coefficients for Trace Organic Contaminants and Implications for Its Use as a Passive Sampler." *Environ Sci Technol* 46 (2):606–618.

Manzano, C. A., Dodder, N. G., Hoh, E., and Morales, R. G. E. 2018. "Patterns of Personal Exposure to Urban Pollutants Using Personal Passive Samplers and GCxGC/ToF-MS." *Environ Sci Technol.* doi: 10.1021/acs.est.8b06220.

Morello-Frosch, R., Brody, J. G., Brown, P., Altman, R. G., Rudel, R. A., and Pérez, C. 2009. "Toxic Ignorance and Right-to-Know in Biomonitoring Results Communication: A Survey of Scientists and Study Participants." *Environ Health* 8 (1):6.

Muijs, B., and Jonker, M. T. 2012. "Does Equilibrium Passive Sampling Reflect Actual in Situ Bioaccumulation of PAHs and Petroleum Hydrocarbon Mixtures in Aquatic Worms?" *Environ Sci Technol* 46 (2):937–944. doi: 10.1021/es202951w.

O'Connell, S. G. 2017. Commercially Available Personal Passive Organic Chemical Montiors. *International Society of Exposure Science Newsletter.*

O'Connell, S. G., Kincl, L. D., and Anderson, K. A. 2014a. "Silicone Wristbands as Personal Passive Samplers." *Environ Sci Technol* 48 (6):3327–3335. doi: 10.1021/es405022f.

O'Connell, S. G., McCartney, M. A., Paulik, L. B., Allan, S. E., Tidwell, L. G., Wilson, G., and Anderson, K. A. 2014b. "Improvements in Pollutant Monitoring: Optimizing Silicone for Co-Deployment with Polyethylene Passive Sampling Devices." *Environ Pollut* 193:71–78. doi: 10.1016/j.envpol.2014.06.019.

Ohayon, J. L., Cousins, E., Brown, P., Morello-Frosch, R., and Brody, J. G. 2017. "Researcher and Institutional Review Board Perspectives on the Benefits and Challenges of Reporting Back Biomonitoring and Environmental Exposure Results." *Environ Res* 153:140–149. doi: 10.1016/j.envres.2016.12.003.

Ospina, M., Jayatilaka, N. K., Wong, L. Y., Restrepo, P., and Calafat, A. M. 2018. "Exposure to Organophosphate Flame Retardant Chemicals in the U.S. General Population: Data from the 2013–2014 National Health and Nutrition Examination Survey." *Environ Int* 110:32–41. doi: 10.1016/j.envint.2017.10.001.

Paulik, L. B., Hobbie, K. A., Rohlman, D., Smith, B. W., Scott, R. P., Kincl, L., Haynes, E. N., and Anderson, K. A. 2018. "Environmental and Individual PAH Exposures near Rural Natural Gas Extraction." *Environ Pollut* 241:397–405. doi: 10.1016/j.envpol.2018.05.010.

Paulik, L. B., Smith, B., Bergmann, A. J., Sower, G. J., Forsberg, N. D., Teeguarden, J. G., and Anderson, K. A. 2016. "Passive Samplers Accurately Predict PAH Levels in Resident Crayfish." *Sci Total Environ* 544:782–791. doi: 10.1016/j.scitotenv.2015.11.142.

Poutasse, C. M., Herbstman, J. B., Peterson, M. E., Gordon, J. M., Soboroff, P. H., Holmes, D., Gonzalez, D., Tidwell, L. G., and Anderson, K. A. 2019. "Silicone Pet Tags Associate Tris(1,3-Dichloro-2-Isopropyl) Phosphate Exposures with Feline Hyperthyroidism." *Environ Sci Technol* 53(15):9201–9213. doi: 10.1021/acs.est.9b02226.

Quintana, P. J. E., Hoh, E., Dodder, N. G., Matt, G. E., Zakarian, J. M., Anderson, K. A., Akins, B., Chu, L., and Hovell, M. F. 2019. "Nicotine Levels in Silicone Wristband Samplers Worn by Children Exposed to Secondhand Smoke and Electronic Cigarette Vapor Are Highly Correlated with Child's Urinary Cotinine." *J Exposure Sci Environ Epidemiol.* doi: 10.1038/s41370-019-0116-7.

Rivera, B., Mullen, K. M., Tidwell, L. G., Ainsworth, D. M., and Anderson, K. A. In Preparation. "Silicone Passive Sampling Devices Measure Exposures to Unconventional Natural Gas Extraction in Sentinel Farm Animals."

Rohlman, D., Dixon, H. M., Kincl, L., Larkin, A., Evoy, R., Barton, M., Phillips, A. L., Peterson, E., Scaffidi, C., Herbstman, J. B., Waters, K. M., and Anderson, K. A. 2019a. "Development of an Environmental Health Tool Linking Chemical Exposures, Physical Location and Lung Function." *BMC Public Health* 19(1):854. doi: 10.1186/s12889-019-7217-z.

Rohlman, D., Donatuto, J., Heidt, M., Barton, M., Campbell, L., Anderson, K. A., and Kile, M. L. 2019b. "A Case Study Describing a Community-Engaged Approach for Evaluating Polycyclic Aromatic Hydrocarbon Exposure in a Native American Community." *Int J Env Res Public Health* 16 (3). doi: 10.3390/ijerph16030327.

Romanak, K. A., Wang, S., Stubbings, W. A., Hendryx, M., Venier, M., and Salamova, A. 2018. "Analysis of Brominated and Chlorinated Flame Retardants, Organophosphate Esters, and Polycyclic Aromatic Hydrocarbons in Silicone Wristbands Used as Personal Passive Samplers." *J Chromatogr A.* doi: 10.1016/j.chroma.2018.12.041.

Shoeib, M., and Harner, T. 2002. "Characterization and Comparison of Three Passive Air Samplers for Persistent Organic Pollutants." *J Toxicol Env Heal B* 36 (19):4142–4151.

Status of Superfund Sites in Areas Affected by Harvey. 2017. United States Environmental Protection Agency.

Ulrich, E. M., Sobus, J. R., Grulke, C. M., Richard, A. M., Newton, S. R., Strynar, M. J., Mansouri, K., and Williams, A. J. 2019. "EPA's Non-Targeted Analysis Collaborative Trial (Entact): Genesis, Design, and Initial Findings." *Anal Bioanal Chem* 411 (4):853–866. doi: 10.1007/s00216-018-1435-6.

Vidi, P. A., Anderson, K. A., Chen, H. Y., Anderson, R., Salvador-Moreno, N., Mora, D. C., Poutasse, C., Laurienti, P. J., Daniel, S. S., and Arcury, T. A. 2017. "Personal Samplers of Bioavailable Pesticides Integrated with a Hair Follicle Assay of DNA Damage to Assess Environmental Exposures and Their Associated Risks in Children." *Mutat Res* 822:27–33. doi: 10.1016/j.mrgentox.2017.07.003.

Weschler, C. J., and Nazaroff, W. W. 2012. "SVOC Exposure Indoors: Fresh Look at Dermal Pathways." *Indoor Air* 22 (5):356–377. doi: 10.1111/j.1600–0668.2012.00772.x.

Wristbands Given Out… 2017. In *Wristbands Given Out to Test for Chemical Exposure from Harvey Floodwaters*, edited by Grace White: KHOU 11.

10 Total Exposure Hearing Health Preservation

Jeremy Slagley
Wright-Patterson Air Force Base

CONTENTS

10.1 INTRODUCTION

Total exposure health (TEH) incorporates occupational and non-occupational (environmental and recreational) exposures, as well as individual genetic makeup and health habits, to assess possible risk of negative health outcomes. The long-used paradigm of assessing occupational risk by individual chemical, physical, and biological agents may have worked well in years past. Preventive medicine practitioners would assess worker exposure to a single chemical agent and estimate risk levels. Then we could consider similar target organs among several chemical exposures and combine estimated exposures. While this is a simplistic view of possible chemical interactions within the human receiver, it would be difficult to produce appropriate toxicological and epidemiological studies on the near infinite possible multiple chemical interaction scenarios in industry to address the possible risk levels. Implicit in these risk assessments is also the underlying bias of epidemiological studies and exposure levels drawn largely from American industry, with some limits on work cycles, some controls on worker exposure, and a worker population of a particular genetic background generally receiving healthcare, clean water and sufficient nutrition for vigorous life. As scientific research probes further into the varied exposures which may impact an organ system or the entire human person, we find more links

DOI: 10.1201/9780429263286-12

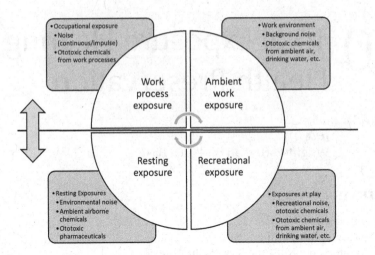

FIGURE 10.1 Total exposure health exposures that could affect hearing health.

between chemical, physical, and biological exposures, and more links between the exposure and the individual person's response to the exposure when considering that person's diet, health history, habits, and genetics. If we can estimate risk better, perhaps we can control risk better with better health outcomes for the individual as well as the herd.

Hearing health is especially well suited for TEH analysis as the hearing organ is sensitive to noise (continuous and impulse), other industrial chemicals (ototoxic lead, styrene, xylene, etc.), and pharmaceuticals (see Figure 10.1). These exposures can impact the person's body from the workplace, in recreation, at rest, via airborne, ingestion, and sometimes skin absorption, and make up the previously elucidated internal and external "exposome" from conception in the mother's womb until natural death (Wild 2012). There may also be individual genetic predisposition to hearing health damage. In 2018, Captain Bill Murphy of the National Institute for Occupational Safety and Health (NIOSH) presented these aspects and the many years of NIOSH research contribution to hearing health preservation, entitled *Total Hearing Health* (Murphy 2018).

10.2 OVERVIEW OF HEARING HEALTH

Human hearing health is a vital sensory function that affects quality of life and safety. Some practicing preventive medicine professionals accept a level of typical hearing loss in a population where they would become much more concerned with a different injury or illness, such as amputation or cancer. Noise exposure and hearing loss are so prevalent, almost ubiquitous, in our society, that we become accustomed to accepting a level of damage. Almost all Americans know someone or have a dear relative who suffers from hearing loss. There is a significant social isolation and emotional suffering component among victims of hearing loss since humans are designed as social creatures.

The scale of hearing loss makes it a very significant problem. The World Health Organization (WHO) estimates 466 million people (greater than 5% of the world's population) suffer from disabling hearing loss and estimates the financial loss at US $750 billion annually (WHO 2019). Within the United States (US), The National Institutes of Health, National Institute on Deafness and Other Communication Disorders (NIDCD) reports 15% (37.5 million) of American adults have some trouble hearing (NIDCD 2019). Hearing loss is associated with exposure to high levels of noise, some infectious diseases, exposure to ototoxic chemicals in the workplace, ambient environment, and some pharmaceuticals (Sliwinska-Kowalska et al. 2003, Sliwinska-Kowalska and Davis 2012). Noise exposure may also affect developing humans in their mother's womb (Selander et al. 2019, ACGIH 2019). Noise-induced hearing loss may also be affected by genetic factors (Konings et al. 2009, Sliwinska-Kowalska and Pawelczyk 2013). Hearing loss is the most common occupational illness in the US with some 22 million workers exposed to high noise (Masterson et al. 2016). Within the US Department of Defense (USDOD), auditory illness is the second most prevalent disability, accounting for 13.4% of veterans' disability claims – 3.3 million of a total 25 million disabilities (Department of Veterans Affairs 2019). This is an enormous problem affecting health, stress, social interaction, and quality of life. To reduce the global burden of hearing loss, we must understand all the exposure and individual genetic factors that affect human hearing. Then we must develop measures to estimate risk from the factors and develop methods to control those risks to acceptable levels. Individuals do not always adhere to control measures, so we must also understand and account for factors that affect individuals' risk control behaviors. Many researchers have dedicated their careers to improving and protecting hearing health. Recent review articles are excellent summaries of published work (Lie et al. 2016, Kerr et al. 2017, Suter 2017, Murphy 2018).

10.3   AUDITORY AND NON-AUDITORY HEALTH EFFECTS

As noted previously, noise exposure can result in both auditory and non-auditory health effects. Noise-induced hearing loss (NIHL) and tinnitus are auditory effects associated with excessive exposure to noise. NIHL presents as a loss of hearing acuity as well as a loss of speech perception with background noise. At this point, it is permanent and not ameliorated by medical treatment. Tinnitus is a subjective report of "ringing in the ears," not directly detectable by the clinician, but still maddening and permanent for the suffering patient. The effects of hearing loss and tinnitus for those continuing to work may also result in unsafe acts when workers do not detect warning signals or cross-traffic from forklifts, for example.

Non-auditory effects include social isolation, withdrawal, depression, hypertension, heart disease, and others. When considering impacts to a baby *in utero*, excessive noise exposure to expectant mothers has been associated with low birth weights (Belojevic et al. 2008, Berglund et al. 1999, Stansfield and Matheson 2003). Risk estimates should include all effects on hearing health, as well as other non-auditory effects from noise.

10.4   EXPOSURE LIFETIME

TEH should also consider the exposure lifetime. Hearing health begins at conception and ends with (hopefully natural) death. Studies have shown that noise passes through the abdominal wall, reaching the developing fetal hearing organs, primarily in the lower frequencies (Abrams and Gerhardt 2000). We also know that the hearing organ changes during gestation so that low-frequency damage in the first trimester may result in higher-frequency hearing loss at birth (Harris and Dallos 1984, Müller 1996). There are standards limiting fetal exposure to noise, but some have argued for a specific frequency weighting curve for fetal exposures (Eninger and Slagley 2017). Ambient noise exposures are termed "environmental noise," and US Environmental Protection Agency (USEPA) and WHO guidelines exist to limit those exposures from aircraft, traffic noise, and the general environment (USEPA 1974, Berglund et al. 1999). Both ambient and industrial noise exposures contain an important risk consideration. It is assumed that the receiver is not voluntarily accepting the excess risk, and therefore the entity creating the noise risk is responsible to mitigate the risk or compensate the victim. However, children can voluntarily receive important noise exposures in school, musical bands, sporting events, and recreationally. Generations have had the opportunity for almost constant noise input from voluntary music-listening with headphones and ear buds. All of these other exposures may still affect the same ears which employers have a responsibility to protect.

10.5   NOISE TYPE: CONTINUOUS AND IMPULSE

Another important distinction emerges when considering the type of noise exposure. Gaussian, or continuous, noise has been shown to acceptably follow an equal energy exchange damage risk. The well-known 3-dB exchange rate works acceptably well to predict hearing loss of a cohort of workers. An average working lifetime of exposure kept below 85 A-weighted decibels (dBA) would result in an average of 5-dB NIHL for the group according to the International Organization for Standardization (ISO 2013). Non-Gaussian, or impulse noise, consists of a rapid, often transient, rise in pressure. Note that practitioners often differentiate impulse from impact noise based on the causative agent. Impulse noise arises from the rapid release of pressure into the fluid medium. Impact noise arises from striking two solids and often has an accompanying "ringing." Peak levels can be very high in level, far exceeding the equal energy assumption limits. Current research is inconclusive on the appropriate levels of risk from impulse noise, and even how to best measure the risk. Measurement of noise signal kurtosis, or "peakiness," shows some promise (Fuente et al. 2018) but is beyond the capabilities of most practicing occupational hygienists. Some have been working on better noise dose measurement systems (Kardous and Willson 2004, Kardous et al. 2005, Davis et al. 2019). Researchers active in the field of impulse noise suggest that the potential damage from impulse noise may be worse than current risk models indicate (Chan et al. 2016, Suter 2017). This is even more important for TEH when considering the popularity of recreational impulse noise exposures from firearms, fireworks, and other sources (Meinke et al. 2017).

10.6 NON-NOISE EXPOSURES

Two important non-noise exposures affecting hearing health are ototoxic chemicals and pharmaceuticals. They could be considered different ends of the same spectrum. Any chemical agent in the body, which affects the nervous system, may have some effect on the auditory nerve. Several solvents and heavy metals have substantial evidence in toxicological and epidemiological studies that they have an ototoxic property. Pharmaceutical preparations such as aminoglycosidic antibiotics, loop diuretics, certain analgesics, antipyretics, and antineoplastic agents also have warnings that they may induce hearing loss (NIOSH and OSHA 2018). A worker co-exposed to noise and ototoxic chemicals should be considered as "hypersensitive" for NIHL. Also, some agencies, such as the US Army, advise that airborne exposure to ototoxins above 50% of the occupational exposure limit requires workers to receive annual audiograms as a measure of possible ototoxic health effects (US Army 2015). Further, the combination of impulse noise and ototoxins may be more injurious than either alone or the assumed additive effects (Pons et al. 2017).

10.7 GENETICS

For TEH, the exposome is only one side of the equation of worker health. The other very important component is the individual person. There has already been published toxicological and epidemiological work looking for genetic markers of predisposition toward hearing loss. Many toxicological studies suggested specific genes, but some epidemiological studies failed to produce the same results. A review in 2013 recommended that toxicology studies should be confirmed with a relevant epidemiological finding before confirming the genetic hearing loss link in a specific gene (Sliwinksa-Kowalska and Pawelczyk 2013). Regardless, precision preventive medicine may have to include genetics along with the exposure to help manage individual hearing health risk.

10.8 HOW DO I MEASURE RISK?

Risk from continuous noise has traditionally been estimated by estimating noise dose. The dose definition includes the sound energy and the time exposure, with an exchange rate. The most common acceptable level of occupational NIHL risk, echoed by the American Conference of Governmental Industrial Hygienists (ACGIH), is a 100% dose limit of 85 dBA equivalent continuous level (ECL, effectively a time-weighted average) over 8 hours with a 3-dB exchange rate. The 3-dB exchange rate is considered the "equal energy" exchange, so that an increase in level by 3 dB would halve the allowed time of exposure for the same percent dose. Impulse noise is limited to a peak of 140 C-weighted decibels (dBC) (ACGIH 2019) or 140 dB (unweighted)

(OSHA 1974). ACGIH also recommends limiting exposures to the abdomen of pregnant mothers beyond the fifth month of gestation to an 8-hour time-weighted average of 115 dBC and 155-dBC peak (ACGIH 2019).

The relationship between high noise exposure and hearing loss has long been established (Mirza et al. 2018). It has also been shown in toxicological and epidemiological studies that impulse noise is associated with hearing loss, but at a different rate of loss than continuous noise (Suter 2017). The USDOD suggests several methods to estimate impulse noise risk via military acquisition standard 1474E (USDOD 2015). The instrumentation and the measurement standard for impulse noise risk are still in development. Researchers at NIOSH (Kardous and Willson 2004, Kardous et al. 2005) and the Massachusetts Institute of Technology (Smalt et al. 2017) have been developing instruments for characterizing impulse noise. Others have been exploring hearing loss associations to impulse noise by such novel measurements as kurtosis (Fuente et al. 2018), or an interim A-weighted equivalent level (Zagadou et al. 2016), the equal energy of the impulse over 100 milliseconds of the peak ($L_{IAeq100ms}$), Auditory Risk Units, or others (USDOD 2015).

Adding off-duty noise exposure is of particular importance when workers have high noise exposures outside of work, as the assumption of noise-free recovery period for an acceptable exposure level is violated (Schaal et al. 2019a, 2019b). ACGIH notes that the level of residual risk for 85 dBA, 8-hour ECL dose of 100% also assumes a rest period away from noise (<70 dBA). If workers are exposed occupationally for 24 hours, the average should be limited to 80 dBA (ACGIH 2019). This also demonstrates the importance of including ambient environmental and recreational noise in the risk estimate.

Environmental noise limits are set primarily to avoid disturbing sleep and preventing annoyance. The WHO recommends sleeping area indoor noise levels be kept below 30 dBA averaged over 8 hours of night (L_{Aeq}) with a continuous maximum level (L_{Amax}) limited to 45 dBA for a single noise event. Daytime indoor noise levels should be kept below an L_{Aeq} of 35 dBA, and outdoor daytime levels below 55 dBA for serious annoyance. Outdoor daytime levels 50–55 dBA might excite moderate annoyance. These daytime ambient noise levels are averaged over 16 hours of daytime and evening (Berglund et al. 1999). The USEPA once had an Office of Noise Abatement and Control (ONAC) and regulated ambient noise under the 1972 Noise Control Act, the 1978 Quiet Communities Act, and Title IV of the Clean Air Act (Noise Pollution) (USEPA 2019). The ONAC was closed in 1982; however, the USEPA still recommends that the 24-hour equivalent level ($L_{eq(24)}$) should be below 70 dBA to prevent hearing loss, and a day-night level (L_{dn}) should be kept below 55 dBA for outdoor activity or less than 45 dBA for indoor residential areas (USEPA 1974). Day-night levels are 24-hour equivalent levels with a 10 dB penalty added to those nighttime sound levels between 2200 hours (10:00 pm) and 0700 hours (7:00 am).

Further, other exposures, particularly ototoxic chemicals such as styrene (Sliwinska-Kowalska et al. 2003), solvents (Sliwinska-Kowalska et al. 2001, Vyskocil et al. 2008, Metwally et al. 2012, Behar 2018, Lewkowski et al. 2019, Staudt et al. 2019), solvents and heavy metals (Schaal et al. 2017, Schaal et al. 2018), lead (Carlson and Neitzel 2019), and pharmaceuticals add to the risk of hearing health impairment

(Watts 2019). Most airborne exposure limits are not set with ototoxicity as the toxicological endpoint. Exposures below a limit may not be protective for hearing.

10.9   HOW DO I CONTROL RISK?

The traditional hierarchy of controls paradigm can also be employed for hearing health. Removing the noise source, whether at work or not, reduces risk. Engineered controls for noise are well-understood, and many acoustics companies specialize in noise control. From a consumer product perspective, market forces can drive manufacturers to control noise in their products. NIOSH has worked on its "Buy Quiet" program for many years, to include developing standards for product noise (Beamer et al. 2016, Camargo et al. 2017). From the acquisition standpoint, the USDOD specifies noise standards for new systems in MIL-STD-1474E. After a noise source is present in the environment, effective passive controls can be devised and constructed sometimes for little capital investment (Sweeney et al. 2010). The field of active noise control (ANC), sampling noise and then adding an out-of-phase noise to effectively decouple the acoustic energy from the medium it travels through, can also reduce noise. ANC application works best in a volume-constrained problem and best for lower frequency noise (<500 Hz) (Hansen 1999). While practicing occupational hygienists can implement ANC controls, they tend to be expensive and specific to the particular noise situation (Slagley and Guffey 2006, 2007a, 2007b). As further evidence that markets drive innovation, ANC earmuffs have found a comfortable niche among consumers.

Administrative controls include an effective Hearing Conservation Program (HCP) besides auditory risk zones, where non-noise workers are excluded. Effective HCPs include noise surveys and data analysis, education and motivation, noise control, hearing protection devices (HPDs), and audiometric monitoring (Stewart 2000). Most audiograms use pure tone audiometry (PTA). Much research has also suggested that PTA is insufficient to detect early hearing health effects (Vermiglio et al. 2012, Liberman et al. 2016). The data analysis should include characterizing similar exposure groups for later epidemiological surveillance (Soderlund et al. 2016).

The last level of risk control is personal protection in the form of HPDs. Smalt et al. (2017) described the process well. The goal of HPD control is to reduce the sound level at the eardrum. Occupational hygienists apply exposure assessment strategies to estimate noise dose through instantaneous task measurements and reported exposure durations, or through integrated dose measurements on a representative random sample of (willing) workers. Guidance is to place the dosimeter microphone on the dominant shoulder as a surrogate for the sound level at the position of the center of the receiver's head if they were not there to disturb the sound field. The measured estimate of noise dose is used to select HPDs. HPD noise attenuation ratings come from a variety of standard methods. The only binding required method is the 1974 ANSI method noise reduction ratings of HPDs, so many manufacturers apply the minimum legal standard and ignore modern advances in HPD attenuation measurement. NIOSH recommends a model to conservatively reduce the effective attenuation (NIOSH 1998). The result is that we use inaccurate estimates of average exposure to a group and then apply a lower level estimate of HPD attenuation from an old standard method to come up with a less-than-ideal guess at the noise level impacting the receiver's eardrum. Then we train workers and expect them to use the HPD correctly every time.

Many occupational health practitioners are advocating for individual HPD fit-testing, similar to respiratory protection fit-testing (Murphy et al. 2016). This can be a more precise estimate of attenuation and also serves as a training opportunity and encouragement for workers to wear HPDs properly and consistently (Trompette et al. 2015).

Many researchers have examined worker self-protective behaviors for noise dose reduction. The microphone-in-real-ear (MIRE) technology used by some noise dosimeters allows immediate feedback to the worker on noise levels inside their ear canals. Researchers have shown a significant reduction in noise dose when workers receive the feedback (Rabinowitz et al. 2011, McTague et al. 2013, Trawick et al. 2019). This same idea of informed self-protective behavior is also seen as a key for off-work ambient and recreational exposure. The US Air Force has begun a study using 24-hour personal measurements of individual noise exposure. Awareness of noise levels and potential health risk may result in people avoiding noise or using HPDs off-duty (Yamamoto et al. 2019).

Finally, the ACGIH recommends audiograms when listed ototoxic substances are present in the workplace (carbon monoxide, hydrogen cyanide, lead, and solvent mixtures with noise, or ethylbenzene, styrene, toluene, and xylene without noise). ACGIH lists in their 2019 Notice of Intended Changes that they may add the "OTO" notation to styrene, as an ototoxicant. In 2018, NIOSH and OSHA released a Safety and Health Information Bulletin with a list of 21 chemical ototoxins and four groups of pharmaceutical ototoxins possibly present in the workplace, with an admonition to limit exposures and add audiometric monitoring, even if below the noise and airborne chemical limits (NIOSH and OSHA 2018). The reverse of this is found when researchers test substances that may be protective against NIHL (Crowson et al. 2017).

10.10   CONCLUSION

In effect, hearing health risk management and control follows Figure 10.2. We must measure continuous and impulse noise at work and at home, consider individual genetics and pharmaceuticals, then select effective controls using the hierarchy of controls. If substitution and engineered solutions from the hierarchy of controls leave some residual risk, then administrative controls (hearing conservation program with audiograms) and personal protective equipment (HPDs) should be considered. Audiograms using pure tones may not be sensitive enough to detect early illness. HPDs require motivation and consistent use. Innovations like HPD fit-testing and MIRE HPDs may assist with proper use. Preventive medicine practitioners then monitor individual hearing health and continue the cycle of work to prevent excess impairment. Hearing health is a serious issue. NIHL and tinnitus have consequences beyond simple difficulty in hearing. The number of people suffering hearing health impairment is staggering, and the economic impact of disability and loss of productivity is enormous. Lastly, it is not a new problem. The TEH approach is best-suited to make progress to protect hearing.

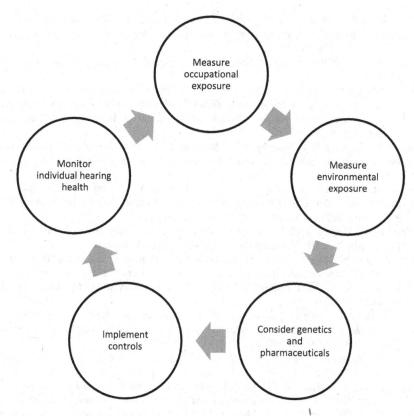

FIGURE 10.2 Total exposure health cycle for hearing health protection.

REFERENCES

Abrams, R. M., & Gerhardt, K. J. (2000). The acoustic environment and physiological responses of the fetus. *Journal of Perinatology, 20*(S1), S31.

American Conference of Governmental Industrial Hygienists (ACGIH). (2019). *Threshold Limit Values for Chemical Substances and Physical Agents & Biological Exposure Indices*. ACGIH Press, Cincinnati, OH.

Beamer, B., McCleery, T., & Hayden, C. (2016). Buy Quiet Initiative in the USA. *Acoustics Australia, 44*(1), 51–54.

Behar, A. (2018). Ototoxicity and Noise. *Journal of Otorhinolaryngology, Hearing and Balance Medicine, 1*(2), 10.

Belojević, G. A., Jakovljević, B. D., Stojanov, V. J., Slepcević, V. Z., & Paunović, K. Z. (2008). Nighttime road-traffic noise and arterial hypertension in an urban population. *Hypertension Research : Official Journal of the Japanese Society of Hypertension, 31*(4), 775–781. doi:10.1291/hypres.31.775

Berglund, B., Lindvall, T., & Schwela, D. (1999). *Guideline for Community Noise*. Geneva. Accessed September 17, 2019. https://apps.who.int/iris/handle/10665/66217

Camargo, H. E., Thompson, J. K., & Azman, A. (2017, December). The development of buy quiet options for the mining equipment industry. In *INTER-NOISE and NOISE-CON Congress and Conference Proceedings* (Vol. 255, No. 7, pp. 364–369). Institute of Noise Control Engineering, Hong Kong, China.

Carlson, K., & Neitzel, R. L. (2018). Hearing loss, lead (Pb) exposure, and noise: A sound approach to ototoxicity exploration. *Journal of Toxicology and Environmental Health, Part B, 21*(5), 335–355.

Chan, P., Ho, K., & Ryan, A. F. (2016). Impulse noise injury model. *Military Medicine, 181*(suppl_5), 59–69.

Crowson, M. G., Hertzano, R., & Tucci, D. (2017). Emerging therapies for sensorineural hearing loss. *Otology & Neurotology: Official Publication of the American Otological Society, American Neurotology Society [and] European Academy of Otology and Neurotology, 38*(6), 792.

Davis, S. K., Calamia, P. T., Murphy, W. J., & Smalt, C. J. (2019). In-ear and on-body measurements of impulse-noise exposure. *International Journal of Audiology, 58*(suppl_1), S49–S57.

Department of Veterans Affairs. (2019). Veterans Benefits Administration Annual Benefits Report Fiscal Year 2018-Compensation. Accessed August 26, 2019. https://www.benefits.va.gov/REPORTS/abr/docs/2018-compensation.pdf

Eninger, R., & Slagley, J. (2017). *Proposed New Noise Weighting for Pregnant Workers.* Presentation at AIHCE, Seattle, WA, 5–8 Jun 2017, podium session.

Fuente, A., Qiu, W., Zhang, M., Xie, H., Kardous, C. A., Campo, P., & Morata, T. C. (2018). Use of the kurtosis statistic in an evaluation of the effects of noise and solvent exposures on the hearing thresholds of workers: An exploratory study. *The Journal of the Acoustical Society of America, 143*(3), 1704–1710.

Hansen, C. H. (1999). *Understanding Active Noise Cancellation.* CRC Press, New York.

Harris, D. M., & Dallos, P. (1984). Ontogenetic changes in frequency mapping of a mammalian ear. *Science, 225*(4663), 741–743.

ISO. (2013). *Acoustics – Estimation of Noise-Induced Hearing Loss, ISO 1999:2013.* Geneva.

Kardous, C. A., & Willson, R. D. (2004). Limitations of using dosimeters in impulse noise environments. *Journal of Occupational and Environmental Hygiene, 1*(7), 456–462.

Kardous, C. A., Willson, R. D., & Murphy, W. J. (2005). Noise dosimeter for monitoring exposure to impulse noise. *Applied Acoustics, 66*(8), 974–985.

Kerr, M. J., Neitzel, R. L., Hong, O., & Sataloff, R. T. (2017). Historical review of efforts to reduce noise-induced hearing loss in the United States. *American Journal of Industrial Medicine, 60*(6), 569–577.

Konings, A., Van Laer, L., Michel, S., Pawelczyk, M., Carlsson, P. I., Bondeson, M. L., ... Huyghe, J. (2009). Variations in HSP70 genes associated with noise-induced hearing loss in two independent populations. *European Journal of Human Genetics, 17*(3), 329.

Lewkowski, K., Heyworth, J. S., Li, I. W., Williams, W., McCausland, K., Gray, C., ... Florath, I. (2019). Exposure to noise and ototoxic chemicals in the Australian workforce. *Occupational Environmental Medicine, 76*(5), 341–348.

Liberman, M. C., Epstein, M. J., Cleveland, S. S., Wang, H., & Maison, S. F. (2016). Toward a differential diagnosis of hidden hearing loss in humans. *PloS one, 11*(9), e0162726.

Lie, A., Skogstad, M., Johannessen, H. A., Tynes, T., Mehlum, I. S., Nordby, K. C., ... Tambs, K. (2016). Occupational noise exposure and hearing: a systematic review. *International Archives of Occupational and Environmental Health, 89*(3), 351–372.

Masterson, E. A., Bushnell, P. T., Themann, C. L., & Morata, T. C. (2016). Hearing impairment among noise-exposed workers — United States, 2003–2012. *MMWR Morbidity Mortality Weekly Report, 65*, 389–394. doi 10.15585/mmwr.mm6515a2

McTague, M. F., Galusha, D., Dixon-Ernst, C., Kirsche, S. R., Slade, M. D., Cullen, M. R., & Rabinowitz, P. M. (2013). Impact of daily noise exposure monitoring on occupational noise exposures in manufacturing workers. *International Journal of Audiology, 52*(supp_1), S3–S8.

Meinke, D. K., Finan, D. S., Flamme, G. A., Murphy, W. J., Stewart, M., Lankford, J. E., & Tasko, S. (2017, November). Prevention of noise-induced hearing loss from recreational firearms. *Seminars in Hearing 38*(04), 267–281.

Metwally, F. M., Aziz, H. M., Mahdy-Abdallah, H., ElGelil, K. S. A., & El-Tahlawy, E. M. (2012). Effect of combined occupational exposure to noise and organic solvents on hearing. *Toxicology and Industrial Health, 28*(10), 901–907.

Mirza, R., Kirchner, D. B., Dobie, R. A., & Crawford, J. (2018). Occupational noise-induced hearing loss. *Journal of Occupational and Environmental Medicine, 60*(9), e498–e501.

Müller, M. (1996). The cochlear place-frequency map of the adult and developing Mongolian gerbil. *Hearing Research, 94*(1–2), 148–156.

Murphy, W. J., Themann, C. L., & Murata, T. K. (2016). Hearing protector fit testing with offshore oil-rig inspectors in Louisiana and Texas. *International Journal of Audiology, 55*(11), 688–698.

Murphy, W. J. (2018). Total hearing health for preventing occupational hearing loss. *The Journal of the Acoustical Society of America, 143*(3), 1909–1909.

National Institute on Deafness and Other Communication Disorders (NIDCD). (2019). Quick Statistics about Hearing. Accessed August 26, 2019. https://www.nidcd.nih.gov/health/statistics/quick-statistics-hearing

NIOSH. (1998). Criteria for a Recommended Standard: Occupational Noise Exposure, Revised Criteria 1998, DHHS (NIOSH) Publication No. 98-126.

NIOSH and OSHA. (2018). Preventing Hearing Loss Caused by Chemical (Ototoxicity) and Noise Exposure. DHHS (NIOSH) Publication No. 2018-124, SHIB 03-08-2018. Accessed September 17, 2019. https://www.osha.gov/dts/shib/shib030818.html

Occupational Safety and Health Administration (OSHA). (1974). 29 CFR 1910.95-Occupational Noise Exposure. Accessed September 17, 2019. https://www.osha.gov/laws-regs/regulations/standardnumber/1910/1910.95

Pons, M. C., Chalansonnet, M., Venet, T., Thomas, A., Nunge, H., Merlen, L., ... Campo, P. (2017). Carbon disulfide potentiates the effects of impulse noise on the organ of Corti. *Neurotoxicology, 59*, 79–87.

Rabinowitz, P. M., Galusha, D., Kirsche, S. R., Cullen, M. R., Slade, M. D., & Dixon-Ernst, C. (2011). Effect of daily noise exposure monitoring on annual rates of hearing loss in industrial workers. *Occupational and Environmental Medicine, 68*(6), 414–418.

Schaal, N. C., Salaam, R. A., Stevens, M. E., & Stubner, A. H. (2019a). Living at work: 24-hour noise exposure aboard US Navy aircraft carriers. *Annals of Work Exposures and Health, 63*(3), 316–327.

Schaal, N. C., Salaam, R. A., Stevens, M., & Stubner, A. H. (2019b). Noise characterization of "effective quiet" areas on a US Navy aircraft carrier. *Journal of Occupational and Environmental Hygiene, 16*(5), 329–335.

Schaal, N. C., Slagley, J., Richburg, C., Zreiqat, M., & Paschold, H. (2018). Chemical induced hearing loss in shipyard workers. *Journal of Occupational and Environmental Medicine, 60*(1), e55–e62.

Schaal, N. C., Slagley, J., Zreiqat, M., & Paschold, H. (2017). Effects of combined exposure to metals, solvents, and noise on permanent threshold shifts. *American Journal of Industrial Medicine, 60*(3), 227–238. doi:10.1002/ajim.22690

Selander, J., Rylander, L., Albin, M., Rosenhall, U., Lewné, M., & Gustavsson, P. (2019). Full-time exposure to occupational noise during pregnancy was associated with reduced birth weight in a nationwide cohort study of Swedish women. *Science of the Total Environment, 651*, 1137–1143.

Slagley, J. M., & Guffey, S. E. (2006). Active noise control of stageloader noise in longwall mining. 2005 Transactions of the Society for Mining, Metallurgy, and Exploration, Inc., 318, 154–160.

Slagley, J. M., & Guffey, S. E. (2007a). Effects of cross-sectional partitioning on active noise control in round ducts. *Journal of Occupational and Environmental Hygiene, 4*(10), 751–761.

Slagley, J.M., & Guffey, S. E. (2007b). Effects of diameter on active noise control in rectangular and round ducts. *Journal of Occupational and Environmental Hygiene, 4*(7), 492–501.

Sliwinska-Kowalska, M., & Davis, A. (2012). Noise-Induced Hearing Loss. Noise Health [serial online] 2012 [cited August 26, 2019], *14*, 274–280. http://www.noiseandhealth.org/text.asp?2012/14/61/274/104893

Sliwinska-Kowalska, M., & Pawelczyk, M. (2013). Contribution of genetic factors to noise-induced hearing loss: A human studies review. *Mutation Research/Reviews in Mutation Research, 752*(1), 61–65.

Sliwinska-Kowalska, M., Zamyslowska-Szmytke, E., Szymczak, W., Kotylo, P., Fiszer, M., Dudarewicz, A., … Stolarek, R. (2001). Hearing loss among workers exposed to moderate concentrations of solvents. *Scandinavian Journal of Work, Environment & Health, 27*(5), 335–342.

Sliwinska-Kowalska, M., Zamyslowska-Szmytke, E., Szymczak, W., Kotylo, P., Fiszer, M., Wesolowski, W., & Pawlaczyk-Luszczynska, M. (2003). Ototoxic effects of occupational exposure to styrene and co-exposure to styrene and noise. *Journal of Occupational and Environmental Medicine, 45*(1), 15–24.

Smalt, C. J., Lacirignola, J., Davis, S. K., Calamia, P. T., & Collins, P. P. (2017). Noise dosimetry for tactical environments. *Hearing Research, 349*, 42–54.

Soderlund, L., McKenna, E. A., Tastad, K., & Paul, M. (2016). Prevalence of permanent threshold shifts in the United States Air Force hearing conservation program by career field, 2005–2011. *Journal of Occupational and Environmental Hygiene, 13*(5), 383–392.

Stansfeld, S. A., & Matheson, M. P. (2003). Noise pollution: Non-auditory effects on health. *British Medical Bulletin, 68*(1), 243–257. doi:10.1093/bmb/ldg033

Staudt, A. M., Whitworth, K. W., Chien, L. C., Whitehead, L. W., & de Porras, D. G. R. (2019). Association of organic solvents and occupational noise on hearing loss and tinnitus among adults in the US, 1999–2004. *International Archives of Occupational and Environmental Health, 92*(3), 403–413.

Stewart, A. P. *Program Overview and Administration.* Elliott H. Berger, L. H.

Royster, L. H., Royster, J. D., Driscoll, D. P., & Layne, M. (Eds.) (2000). The Noise Manual, 5th ed., chapter 6, pp. 149–164. American Industrial Hygiene Association, Indianapolis, IN.

Suter, A. H. (2017). Occupational hearing loss from Non-Gaussian noise. *Seminars in Hearing, 2017*(38), 225–262.

Sweeney, D. D., Slagley, J. M., & Smith, D. A. (2010). Insertion loss of noise barriers on an above ground full scale model longwall coal mining shearer. *Journal of Occupational and Environmental Hygiene, 7*(5), 272–279.

Trawick, J., Slagley, J., & Eninger, E. (2019). Occupational noise dose reduction via behavior modification using in-ear dosimetry among United States air force personnel exposed to continuous and impulse noise. *Open Journal of Safety Science and Technology, 9*(2), 61–81. doi:10.4236/ojsst.2019.92005

Trompette, N., Kusy, A., & Ducourneau, J. (2015). Suitability of commercial systems for earplug individual fit testing. *Applied Acoustics, 90*, 88–94.

United States Army. (2015, January 8). Army Hearing Program. DA Pamphlet 40-501. Washington, DC. Accessed September 23, 2019. https://armypubs.army.mil/epubs/DR_pubs/DR_a/pdf/web/p40_501.pdf

United States Department of Defense. (2015, April 15). Department of Defense Design Criteria Standard: Noise Limits. MIL-STD-1474E. Washington, DC. Accessed September 23, 2019. https://www.arl.army.mil/www/pages/343/MIL-STD-1474E-Final-15Apr2015.pdf

United States Environmental Protection Agency (USEPA). (2019). EPA History: Noise and the Noise Control Act. Accessed September 17, 2019. https://www.epa.gov/history/epa-history-noise-and-noise-control-act

United States Office of Noise Abatement. (1974). *Information on Levels of Environmental Noise Requisite to Protect Public Health and Welfare with an Adequate Margin of Safety* (Vol. 74, No. 4), https://www.nrc.gov/docs/ML1224/ML12241A393.pdf, accessed 20 March 2020.

Vermiglio, A. J., Soli, S. D., Freed, D. J., & Fisher, L. M. (2012). The relationship between high-frequency pure-tone hearing loss, hearing in noise test (HINT) thresholds, and the articulation index. *Journal American Academy of Audiology, 23*, 779–788.

Vyskocil, A., Leroux, T., Truchon, G., Gendron, M., El Majidi, N., & Viau, C. (2008). Occupational ototoxicity of n-hexane. *Human & Experimental Toxicology, 27*(6), 471–476.

Watts, K. L. (2019, May). Ototoxicity: visualized in concept maps. *Seminars in Hearing, 40*(02), 177–187.

Wild, C. P. (2012). The exposome: From concept to utility. *International Journal of Epidemiology, 41*(1), 24–32.

World Health Organization. (2019) Deafness and Hearing Loss. Accessed August 26, 2019. https://www.who.int/en/news-room/fact-sheets/detail/deafness-and-hearing-loss

Yamamoto, D. P., Kurzdorfer, J. W., & Fullerton, K. L. (2019). U.S. Air Force Noise Exposure Demonstration Project. *Air Force Research Laboratory,* Final Technical Report AFRL-SA-WP-TR-2019-0010.

Zagadou, B., Chan, P., & Ho, K. (2016). An interim LAeq8 criterion for impulse noise injury. *Military Medicine, 181*(suppl_5), 51–58.

11 The Role of Noise Exposure as an Element of Total Exposure Health
Determination of 24-Hour Noise Exposure Profiles on U.S. Navy Aircraft Carriers

N. Cody Schaal
Naval Medical Research Unit-Dayton
Uniformed Services University

CONTENTS

DOI: 10.1201/9780429263286-13

11.1   INTRODUCTION

Occupational and non-occupational noise exposure poses substantial public health challenges and has been linked to a variety of adverse health effects such as hearing loss, tinnitus, hypertension, ischemic heart disease, sleep disturbance, cognitive impairment, and annoyance (Basner et al. 2014; Babisch et al., 1999; Banerjee et al., 2014). It has been estimated that 22 million workers are exposed to potentially damaging noise at work each year (Tak et al., 2009).

The U.S. Department of Veterans Affairs (VA) reported 3.2 million veterans received disability compensation for hearing loss and tinnitus in FY18 (Department of Veteran's Affairs, 2019). Hearing loss and tinnitus were the two most prevalent service-connected disabilities representing 12.7% of all service-connected disabilities (Department of Veteran's Affairs, 2019). Adverse audiological outcomes have continued to grow over time with the VA reporting nearly 6% growth in new auditory related service-connected disabilities from 2014 to 2018 (Department of Veteran's Affairs, 2019).

A Total Exposure Health (TEH) approach may be used to quantify health risk associated with noise exposure both inside and outside the workplace. Occupational exposure limits (OELs) are typically designed to protect an occupational workforce for 8-hour exposure periods occurring within the workplace. Despite prolonged exposure to hazardous noise being associated with hearing impairment, there is little regulation governing environmental and recreational noise exposures (Berger et al., 2003). It is important to understand cumulative exposures both inside and outside the workplace to control exposures and prevent adverse health effects because in addition to on-duty periods (inside the workplace), noise exposures may continue during off-duty periods (outside the workplace). Activities occurring at home/outside the workplace, which may present additional noise exposure and hearing impairment risks to workers if not controlled include hobbies and second jobs. The challenge associated with controlling noise exposure both on-duty and off-duty is compounded within the military during operational deployments. Longer duration noise exposure via 12-hour on-duty and 12-hour off-duty shifts may result in both high-intensity noise exposure over a longer duration and reduced opportunity for auditory recovery in "effective quiet" areas thus increasing the risk of hearing impairment. Both of these situations may be found on a U.S. Navy aircraft carrier when at-sea.

11.2   NOISE EXPOSURE ON U.S. NAVY AIRCRAFT CARRIERS

Flight decks aboard aircraft carriers function as a forward operating airfield that allows for the launching and landing of fixed-wing and rotary-wing aircraft. Personnel assigned duty aboard aircraft carriers can be exposed to a wide variety of noise sources located in areas such as mechanical rooms, catapult spaces, engineering spaces, hotel service areas (galley, scullery, and laundry), maintenance areas, hangar bays, and the flight deck (Yankaskas and Shaw, 1999). Other noise sources that may affect personnel include noise emanating from the ship's propellers to adjacent spaces, noise radiating from the flight deck during launch and recovery operations directly to adjacent areas, and noise from operating heavy equipment in the hangar bays that expose passers-by. Flight deck operations involve a variety of noise-producing activities to include refueling, repairing, re-arming, launching, and recovery operations.

On an aircraft carrier, personnel working on the flight deck during flight operations (e.g., Air department), participating in aircraft maintenance activities (e.g., Aircraft Intermediate Maintenance department), or working in the engineering plants (e.g., Engineering department) are typically monitored in a Hearing Conservation Program (HCP) due to measured or anticipated exposures >85 dBA as an 8-hour time-weighted average (TWA). Aircraft carrier support personnel are also assigned to aircraft carriers to provide a variety of support services including professional/ administrative duties, anticipated to have low noise exposures (<85 dBA) based on their work tasks. These groups include Religious Ministries, Medical, Dental, Media, Navigation, and Operations departments, among others. During off-duty hours when an aircraft carrier is at-sea, personnel remain on the ship but are usually free to spend most of that time in their berthing (sleeping areas), or at mess decks (eating areas), libraries, classrooms, religious worship spaces, or spaces used for recreational physical training (on-board gyms). These leisure areas are commonly located adjacent to flight deck operations and machinery capable of producing noise levels >85 dBA. Total noise exposure on an aircraft carrier presents risk control challenges compared to traditional work situations that allow workers to leave industrial areas at the end of their daily work-shift and rest at home until the next duty day. On an operational aircraft carrier at-sea, noise exposure often does not cease during off-duty hours because noise sources associated with the flight deck and other shipboard activities are adjacent to off-duty locations. Noise transmission is compounded with aircraft carrier designs that feature hard surfaces. Walls, floors, and ceilings in most areas are bare, lacking carpet, draperies, and linen presenting an opportunity for sound reflection rather than absorption. Additionally, when at-sea, on-duty work shifts often are 12–14 hours in duration with the remaining time considered off-duty. If aircraft carrier personnel experience relatively high noise levels during on-duty and off-duty periods in leisure and sleeping areas rather than high noise levels on-duty and low noise levels during off-duty periods, personnel may be at higher risk to hearing loss than personnel that sleep in areas away from hazardous noise sources.

11.3   AUDITORY EFFECTS

Personnel working extended shifts may not have an opportunity to recover from Temporary Threshold Shifts (TTSs) incurred during their on-duty work-shift if noise exposures during off-duty periods are not sufficient to allow for auditory recovery. This is especially true with aircraft carriers since ships may remain at sea for weeks to months at a time. Because extended work-shifts, work-shifts >8 hours, are common on aircraft carriers, personnel are at risk of developing TTSs even when 8-hour TWAs are less than 85 dBA. Mills et al. studied personnel exposed to noise levels ranging 75–88 dB at 500–4,000 Hz for 16–24 hour durations and found threshold shifts increased 1.7 dB for every 1 dB increase in noise level beginning at 74 dB at 4,000 Hz, 78 dB at 2,000 Hz, and 82 dB at 1,000 and 500 Hz (Mills et al., 1979).

In addition to TTSs, cochlear synaptopathy has been identified as another adverse audiological effect where detriments in hearing acuity may not be detected in pure tone audiometry, but rather may contribute to other perceptual abnormalities such as difficulty understanding speech in noise and tinnitus (Liberman and Kujawa, 2017).

11.4 NON-AUDITORY EFFECTS

Non-auditory effects are also an important aspect of TEH and have been associated with noise exposure to include being unable to detect auditory cues, warnings, and signals as an element of situational awareness and being unable to detect and understand speech (Yankaskas, 2013). Some studies have estimated that 12.2% of accidents are attributable to workplace noise exposure and noise-induced hearing loss (Picard et al., 2008). Hansell et al. found a link between increased risk of stroke mortality, coronary heart disease, and cardiovascular disease and daytime aircraft noise exposure >63 dB and due to night-time aircraft noise exposure >55 dB (Hansell et al., 2013). Studies investigating sleep quality due to air, rail, and traffic noise found decreases in sleep quality and gradual increases in fatigue for noise levels reaching 74 dBA (Griefahn et al., 2006).

There may also be negative effects on readiness and safety as a result of poor sleep quality leading to fatigue and inadequate crew rest (Government Accountability Office, 2018). Noise's ability to interfere with sleep may be described by sleep deprivation such as lack of sufficient sleep, sleep disturbance/fragmentation, difficulty falling asleep, frequent awakenings, waking too early, and alternations in sleep stages and depth (Zaharna and Guilleminault, 2010). In 2017, the guided-missile destroyers USS Fitzgerald and USS John S. McCain were involved in two collisions resulting in 17 fatalities. Crew fatigue, high workload, and inadequate crew rest were cited as contributing factors of the accidents (Department of the Navy, 2017; Government Accountability Office, 2018).

11.5 REGULATION

The Occupational Safety and Health Administration (OSHA) regulates occupational noise exposures for 8-hour shifts rather than exposure durations that include situations where the employee rests/sleeps near their work space for longer than 8-hour durations. American Conference of Governmental Industrial Hygienist's (ACGIH's) 85 decibel "A"-weighted OEL is based on the assumption that an 8-hour TWA noise exposure will be balanced with 16 hours of auditory quiet to allow ears to rest. ACGIH further indicates when workers are restricted for periods >24 hours to employer-controlled areas that serve as both workplace and living quarters, the average noise exposure over a 24-hour period should not exceed 80 dBA (ACGIH, 2019). Threshold Limit Values (TLVs) such as 85 dBA for 8 hours, 82 dBA for 16 hours, and 80 dBA for 24-hours are based on daily exposures where there will be time away from work in effective quiet areas (i.e. <70 dBA) to rest and sleep after exposure and to allow recovery from any potential TTSs that may have developed (ACGIH, 2019). The Department of Defense (DoD) and U.S. Navy standards require personnel to be entered in an HCP when routine occupational noise exposure is equal to or greater than 85 dBA as an 8-hour TWA with a 3-dB exchange rate (ER) or 140-dB peak (Department of Defense, 2019; Department of the Navy, 2019).

In addition to OELs designed to prevent hearing loss, guidelines are also available to prevent adverse effects on sleep as a result of excessive noise exposure. World Health Organization (WHO) guidelines suggest noise levels less than 30 dBA for continuous background noise and 45 dBA for individual noise events are necessary to avoid negative effects on sleep (Berglund et al. 1999). WHO indicates sleep response to noise ranges from 32 to 42 dB (WHO, 2009). Noise levels necessary to induce awakenings begin at 35 dBA with a background noise level of 27 dBA (WHO, 2009).

The following sections summarize results of recent personal noise exposure and area noise measurement investigations on U.S. Navy aircraft carriers (Schaal et al., 2019a, 2019b, 2019c, 2019d).

11.6 24-HOUR NOISE EXPOSURE ABOARD U.S. NAVY AIRCRAFT CARRIERS (SCHAAL ET AL., 2019C)

Personnel noise exposure was investigated aboard a U.S. Navy Nimitz-class aircraft carrier during a routine at-sea period during flight operations. Fifty-nine study volunteers were divided into the following seven similar exposure groups (SEGs) using an observational approach considering departmental assignment, work location, and type/similarity of work performed.

- SEG 1: Flight Deck Controllers/Observers
- SEG 2: Launch and Recovery
- SEG 3: Damage Control Maintenance & Repair
- SEG 4: Hangar Bay Maintenance & Repair
- SEG 5: Supply
- SEG 6: Roving
- SEG 7: Administrative/Professional.

3M™ Quest Edge5, Edge4, and Quest NoisePro type II noise dosimeters (Quest Technologies, Oconomowoc, WI) were used to measure equivalent continuous noise levels (L_{eq}) in dBA by data logging at one-minute intervals during each 24-hour monitoring period. The sound pressure measurements were divided into on-duty and off-duty exposures for analysis and comparison. The data-logged measurements were logarithmically added then averaged to determine each worker's overall $L_{eq(24-hour)}$, $TWA_{(on-duty)}$, and $L_{eq(off-duty)}$ in dBA.

$L_{eq(24-hour)}$ and $TWA_{(on-duty)}$ ranged from 71 to 127 dBA. The 80 dBA ACGIH TLV for 24-hour noise exposure was exceeded by 93% of the study participants. The 85-dBA ACGIH TLV and DoD OEL for 8-hour noise exposures were exceeded by 68% of the population. $L_{eq(off-duty)}$ ranged from 38 to 102 dBA with 61% of the population exceeding the 70-dBA ACGIH TLV classified as effective quiet to allow for TTS recovery. SEG 2 Flight Deck Launch and Recovery had significantly higher 24-hour noise exposures, using a p of 0.05, than SEG 3 Damage Control Maintenance and Repair ($p = 0.01$), SEG 5 Supply ($p = 0.01$), and SEG 7 Administrative/Professional ($p = 0.009$). Similar results were found for $TWA_{(on-duty)}$ noise exposures. Median

$TWA_{(on-duty)}$ and $L_{eq(24-hour)}$ for SEG 2 were 16–21 dB higher than SEG 3, 5, and 7. There were no significant differences between $L_{eq(off-duty)}$ according to SEG. SEGs located on the flight deck (SEGs 1 and 2) and SEGs responsible for maintenance and repair activities (SEGs 3 and 4) supporting flight operations had the highest $TWA_{(on-duty)}$ and $L_{eq(24-hour)}$.

11.7 CHARACTERIZATION OF EXTENDED SHIFT NOISE EXPOSURES AMONG LOW NOISE HAZARD U.S. NAVY AIRCRAFT CARRIER SUPPORT PERSONNEL (SCHAAL ET AL., 2019A)

In another study of noise exposures among U.S. Navy aircraft carrier personnel, noise profiles were characterized for 12-hour on-duty ($L_{eq(on-duty)}$), 12-hour off-duty ($L_{eq(off-duty)}$), and 24-hour exposure periods ($L_{eq(24-hour)}$) in dBA among a relatively low noise hazard (<85 dBA) aircraft carrier support personnel population. Flight operations were the primary noise source during this at-sea period but other noise sources/evolutions included emergency response drills (General Quarters), Man Overboard Drills, and nightly propulsion-plant drills. Aircraft carrier support personnel assigned to departments not enrolled in the DoD HCP and with noise exposures <85 dBA were specifically invited to participate in the investigation. Personnel noise exposure was investigated aboard a U.S. Navy Nimitz-class aircraft carrier during a routine at-sea period during flight operations. Forty-seven study volunteers were divided into the following four similar exposure groups (SEGs) using an observational approach considering departmental assignment, work location, and type/similarity of work performed.

- SEG 1: Administration/Religious Ministries/Legal/Training
- SEG 2: Combat Systems/Operations
- SEG 3: Medical/Dental
- SEG 4: Supply.

3M™ Quest Technology NoisePro DLX (Oconomowoc, WI) and 3M™ Quest Technology Edge eg5 (Oconomowoc, WI) personal noise dosimeters were used to measure $L_{eq(on-duty)}$, $L_{eq(off-duty)}$, and $L_{eq(24-hour)}$. Dosimeters logged at one-minute intervals and were set to a 70-dBA threshold due to the anticipated noise exposures of the selected population. L_{eq} measurements were compared to TLVs and were compared to determine exposure differences between each group according to 12-hour on-duty, 12-hour off-duty, and 24-hour periods.

Mean $L_{eq(24-hour)}$ ranged from 69 to 88 dBA with 22% exceeding the 80-dBA TLV. $L_{eq(on-duty)}$ ranged from 71 to 90 dBA with 17% exceeding the 83-dBA 12-hour on-duty TLV. $L_{eq(off-duty)}$ ranged from 68 to 84 dBA with 95% exceeding the 70-dBA ACGIH TLV classified as effective quiet to allow for TTS recovery. SEG 2 Combat Systems/Operations had significantly higher 24-hour noise exposures, using a p of 0.05, than SEG 3 Medical/Dental ($p = 0.019$) and SEG 4 Supply ($p = 0.045$) by approximately 5 dBA. SEG 2 Combat Systems/Operations had significantly higher

12-hour on-duty noise exposure than SEG 3 Medical/Dental ($p = 0.030$) by nearly 5 dBA. There were no significant differences between $L_{eq(off-duty)}$ noise exposures according to SEG ($p = 0.096$).

11.8 NOISE CHARACTERIZATION OF "EFFECTIVE QUIET" AREAS ON A U.S. NAVY AIRCRAFT CARRIER (SCHAAL ET AL., 2019D)

Continued investigation to characterize noise levels on aircraft carriers was completed in spaces designated as "effective quiet" areas where personnel spend time off-duty. Area noise levels were measured with 3M™ Quest NoisePro type II noise dosimeters (Quest Technologies, Oconomowoc, WI) in 15 areas while at-sea during airwing carrier qualifications. Dosimeters were programmed to no threshold and to data log at one-minute intervals. Measurements during flight operations ($L_{eq\,(flt\,ops)}$), non-flight operations ($L_{eq\,(non-flt\,ops)}$), and over 24-hour periods ($L_{eq\,(24-hour)}$) were collected. These data were compared to the 70 dBA ACGIH TLV for "effective quiet" areas intended for TTS recovery when personnel live and work in a potentially noise hazardous environment for periods greater than 24 hours. The monitored areas were selected based on personnel occupancy/use during off-duty time periods. Areas were classified by:

- 1: leisure areas that included mess (eating areas), gyms, lounges, internet café, and fantail social area
- 2: berthing (sleeping) areas.

The berthing locations selected for 24-hour monitoring were located within two levels of the flight deck because these areas were expected to be most affected by flight operations. L_{eq} measurements in dBA were compared to determine significant differences between $L_{eq\,(flt\,ops)}$, $L_{eq\,(non-flt\,ops)}$, and $L_{eq\,(24-hour)}$ and were compared between leisure area and berthing area using an alpha level of 0.05.

While at-sea, personnel on aircraft carriers work in shifts, so segments of the population occupy "effective quiet" areas at different times throughout a 24-hour period. During this study, the majority of personnel on the aircraft carrier worked first shift (0,730–1,900 hours) and were off-duty for the remainder of the day in or near areas such as gyms, mess decks, lounges/social areas, and berthing, among other areas.

Measured noise levels according to time period ranged as follows: (1) $L_{eq\,(24-hour)}$: 70.8–105.4 dBA, (2) $L_{eq\,(flt\,ops)}$: 70–101.2 dBA, and (3) $L_{eq\,(non-flt\,ops)}$: 39.4–104.6 dBA. All area measurements over the 24-hour period and during flight operations and 46.7% of the areas during the non-flight operation time period exceeded the "effective quiet" 70-dBA ACGIH TLV. The highest $L_{eq\,(flt\,ops)}$, $L_{eq\,(non-flt\,ops)}$, and $L_{eq\,(24-hour)}$ were in the fantail social area ranging from 97.7 to 105.4 dBA. The two lowest $L_{eq\,(24-hour)}$ and $L_{eq\,(flt\,ops)}$ were in berthing (sleeping areas) ranging from 70.3 to 70.8 dBA. Similarly, the lowest $L_{eq\,(non-flt\,ops)}$ was predominantly in berthing ranging from 39.4 to 64.9 dBA. Noise levels decreased in all sleep areas, dining areas, and the internet café when flight operations ended each day.

The $L_{eq(24-hour)}$ of 83.2 dBA was not significantly different than the $L_{eq\,(flt\,ops)}$ of 82.2 dBA ($p = 0.065$). This small 1 dBA difference suggests $L_{eq\,(flt\,ops)}$ was the primary contributor to $L_{eq\,(24-hour)}$. Mean L_{eqs} were 15 dBA higher during flight operations compared to non-flight operations in "effective quiet" areas ($p = 0.001$). $L_{eq\,(24-hour)}$ and $L_{eq\,(flt\,ops)}$ in leisure areas were 5–6 dBA higher than in berthing areas; however, there were no significant differences between the "effective quiet" area types according to $L_{eq\,(24-hour)}$ ($p = 0.174$) and $L_{eq\,(flt\,ops)}$ ($p = 0.248$). The $L_{eq\,(non-flt\,ops)}$ in leisure areas was significantly higher than berthing areas by approximately 21 dBA ($p = 0.001$) during non-flight operation periods.

11.9   SOUND LEVEL MEASUREMENTS IN BERTHING AREAS OF AN AIRCRAFT CARRIER (SCHAAL ET AL., 2019B)

An investigation on a U.S. Navy Nimitz-class aircraft carrier during a routine at-sea training period was conducted to characterize L_{eq} and standardized octave band center frequency noise levels according to berthing (sleeping) area location during flight operation and non-flight operation time periods. Flight operations typically lasted 14 hours per day from 9 a.m. until 11:00 p.m. Sixty noise measurements were taken in eight sleeping locations directly below the flight deck. Berthing areas included in this investigation were located directly below the flight deck and were subject to the noise produced during flight operations and adjacent machinery spaces supporting flight operations. L_{eq} in dBA and noise levels from 16 to 16,000 Hz in dB were measured during flight operations ($L_{eq\,(flt\,ops)}$) and non-flight operations ($L_{eq\,(non-flt\,ops)}$) using 3M™ SoundPro® DL and SE type 1 SLMs with 1/1 octave band analyzers (Quest Technologies, Oconomowoc, WI) set to data log at one-minute intervals. L_{eq} was compared according to sleep area shipboard locations of forward (FWD) $L_{eq\,(FWD)}$, middle (MID) $L_{eq\,(MID)}$, and rear (AFT) $L_{eq\,(AFT)}$. These data were compared to the 70-dBA ACGIH TLV for "effective quiet" areas associated with auditory rest. In addition, these noise measurements were compared to noise levels associated with poor sleep quality and quantity.

The overall mean L_{eq} was 74.6 dBA, $L_{eq\,(flt\,ops)}$ 75.9 dBA, and $L_{eq\,(non-flt\,ops)}$ 69.5 dBA. $L_{eq\,(flt\,ops)}$ in sleeping areas was statistically significant ($p = 0.02$) 6.4 dBA higher than the $L_{eq\,(non-flt\,ops)}$ using a p of 0.05. $L_{eq\,(FWD)}$ was 76.1 dBA, $L_{eq\,(MID)}$ was 75.9 dBA, and $L_{eq\,(AFT)}$ was 60.9 dBA. $L_{eq\,(FWD)}$ and $L_{eq\,(MID)}$ in sleeping areas were statistically significant ($p < 0.01$) 15.2 and 15.0 dBA higher, respectively, than the $L_{eq\,(AFT)}$ noise levels. Mean noise levels at standardized center (1/1) octave bands were highest between 500 and 4,000 Hz ranging from 65.2 to 69.8 dB with SPLs highest at 1,000 Hz. The lowest frequencies (16–63 Hz) corresponded to the lowest overall SPLs ranging from 28.7 to 49.8 dB which suggests high-frequency flight deck noise was the primary noise source compared to low-frequency structure-borne noise. A total of 72% of all area L_{eq} measurements exceeded the 70-dBA ACGIH TLV classified as effective quiet to allow for TTS recovery. When stratifying samples by berthing location, 83% in FWD berthing, 83% in MID berthing, and 0% in AFT berthing exceeded the 70-dBA TLV. Regarding effect on sleep, all mean noise levels exceeded the WHO's

35-dBA threshold of when awakening begins and the 45-dBA threshold where negative effects on sleep begin.

Results suggest that sleeping area location in close proximity to relatively high noise sources and activities occurring on an aircraft carrier (i.e. flight operations) increases noise levels in sleeping areas. In addition, results suggest noise levels in sleeping areas are high enough to evoke negative sleep effects.

11.10 DISCUSSION

Nearly all workers monitored in the previously described investigations exceeded the 80-dBA 24-hour noise limit in populations anticipated to have elevated noise exposures such as flight deck and maintenance personnel and personnel working in professional trades such as administration, medical, and supply (Schaal et al., 2019a, 2019c). However, professional and administrative occupations had noise exposures <85 dBA 8-hour OEL that would trigger placement in an HCP. This information shows that in some environments and among some populations, noise level and exposure duration may hinder recovery from TTSs. Significant differences in 24- and 12-hour on-duty noise exposures between SEGs, despite similar administrative work tasks, suggest primary location of office/work space and proximity to primary noise source may be a better method of constructing SEGs and determining noise exposure in future noise dosimetry measurements than sole reliance on occupational work-tasks accomplished by an SEG. This is important to the concept of TEH because noise exposure occurring outside the workplace, in some cases, may be more important in describing total noise exposure than occupation. Regarding occupations with relatively high occupational noise exposures such as flight deck and aircraft maintenance populations, relatively high non-occupational noise exposures create further challenges with recovering from hearing impairment resulting from occupational exposures. Additionally, the results of the previously described investigations are applicable to a variety of populations working traditional 8-hour work shifts and longer in that the remaining non-occupational 16 hours of a 24-hour day may be filled with a variety of activities. Activities and environments such as concert attendance, personal stereo use, loud restaurant environments, and personal hobbies (i.e. volunteer firefighter, use of weapons at gun ranges, and home wood-working shops, among others) and lead to non-occupational noise exposures in addition to exposures occurring during occupational time periods.

The previously described investigations commonly found noise levels >70 dBA in eating areas, gyms, and social areas (Schaal et al., 2019d). These findings may be applicable to other populations not associated with aircraft carriers because the monitored areas are commonly found in non-occupational environments. Noise levels may be affected by occupancy, area size/design, and individual behavior based on high personnel traffic (i.e. large numbers of personnel gathering and talking after work). Because elevated background noise levels are expected to require a raised voice level to be understood when engaged in conversation, a raised voice is expected to continue to raise overall noise levels.

Additionally, these investigations showed noise levels in sleeping areas were higher than the 45 dBA threshold levels expected to evoke negative effects on sleep (Schaal et al., 2019b). Poor sleep quality and limited sleep duration are associated with sleep disturbance, fragmentation, frequent awakening, difficulty falling asleep, waking too early, alterations in sleep stages, and sleep depth. This is concerning because poor sleep among personnel may lead to fatigue and exacerbate poor decision making resulting in accidents. Personnel that work night shift and sleep during the day may have the greatest risk of sleep disturbance.

11.11 CONCLUSIONS

Personnel assigned to aircraft carriers are typically monitored in a DoD HCP when noise exposures reach 85 dBA or greater as an 8-hour TWA. The 8-hour TWA assumes 16 hours of rest will be available for hearing recovery before the next 8-hour shift begins. An operational aircraft carrier is a unique environment where personnel often work shifts >8 hours. Also, spaces designed for off-duty relaxation may be adjacent to hazardous noise areas, which minimize opportunities for auditory recovery. There are also a limited number of spaces where sailors can spend their off-duty time to provide respite and auditory recovery.

Noise has been a well-studied risk factor for hearing loss; however, only monitoring for noise during 8-hour periods may underestimate and lead to uncharacterized exposures for personnel working extended duration shifts and for personnel that may have elevated noise exposures outside of the workplace. Characterizing 24-hour noise exposures enables occupational and environmental health practitioners to identify segments of time within a 24-hour period that contribute to a worker's risk of incurring noise-induced hearing loss, facilitate hearing loss prevention efforts, as well as employee education, resulting in a more effective HCP.

DISCLAIMER

The views expressed in this chapter are those of the author and do not necessarily reflect the official policy or position of the Department of the Navy, Department of Defense, nor the U.S. Government.

COPYRIGHT STATEMENT

REFERENCES

American Conference of Governmental Industrial Hygienists. (2019). *Threshold Limit Values for Chemical Substances and Physical Agents and Biological Exposure Indices.* Cincinnati, OH: ACGIH, pp. 126.

Babisch, W., Ising, H., Gallacher, J.E., Sweetnam, P.M., and Elwood, P.C. (1999). Traffic noise and cardiovascular risk: the Caerphilly and Speedwell studies, third phase-10-year follow up. *Arch. Environ. Health* 54(3), 210–216.

Banerjee, D., Das, P.P., and Foujdar, A. (2014). Association between road traffic noise and prevalence of coronary heart disease. *Environ. Monit. Assess.* 186(5), 2885–2893.

Basner, M., Babisch, W., Davis, A., Brink, M., Clark, C., Janssen, S., and Stansfeld, S. (2014). Auditory and non-auditory effects of noise on health. *Lancet* 383(9925), 1325–1332.

Berger, E., Royster, L., Royster, J., Driscoll, D., and Layne, M. (2003) *The Noise Manual* (5th Edition). Fairfax, VA: American Industrial Hygiene Association.

Berglund, D., Lindvall, T., and Schwela, D. (1999). *Guidelines for Community Noise*. Geneva: World Health Organization.

Department of Defense. (2019) "DoD Instruction 6055.12 Hearing Conservation Program." Available at https://www.esd.whs.mil/Portals/54/Documents/DD/issuances/dodi/605512p.pdf?ver=2017-10-25-110159-777 (accessed 21 March 2020).

Department of the Navy. (2019). "OPNAVINST 5100.19F: Navy Safety and Occupational Health (SOH) Program Manual for Forces Afloat." Available at https://www.secnav.navy.mil/doni/Directives/05000%20General%20Management%20Security%20and%20Safety%20Services/05-100%20Safety%20and%20Occupational%20Health%20Services/5100.19F.pdf (accessed Aug 11, 2019).

Department of the Navy. (2017). "Report on the Collision between USS Fitzgerald (DDG 62) and Motor Vessel ACX Crystal." Available at https://s3.amazonaws.com/CHINFO/USS+Fitzgerald+and+USS+John+S+McCain+Collision+Reports.pdf (accessed 11 Aug 2019).

Department of Veteran's Affairs. (2019). "Veterans Benefits Administration annual benefits report fiscal year 2018." Available at https://www.benefits.va.gov/REPORTS/abr/docs/2018-compensation.pdf (accessed 11 Aug 2019).

Government Accountability Office. (2018). "GAO-19–225T. Rebuilding Ship, Submarine, and Aviation Readiness Will Require Time and Sustained Management Attention." Available at https://www.gao.gov/products/GAO-19-225T (accessed 11 Aug 2019).

Griefahn, B., Marks, A., and Robens, S. (2006). Noise emitted from road, rail and air traffic and their effects on sleep. *J. Sound Vib.* 295(1–2), 129–140.

Hansell, A.L., Blangiardo, M., Fortunato, L., Floud, S., de Hoogh, K., Fecht, D., … Beevers, S. (2013). Aircraft noise and cardiovascular disease near Heathrow airport in London: small area study. *BMJ* 347, f5432.

Liberman, M.C., and Kujawa, S.G. (2017). Cochlear synaptopathy in acquired sensorineural hearing loss: manifestations and mechanisms. *Hearing Res.* 349, 138–147.

Mills, J.H., Gilbert, R.M., and Adkins, W.Y. (1979). Temporary threshold shifts in humans exposed to octave bands of noise for 16 to 24 hours. *J. Acoust. Soc. Am.* 65(5), 1238–1248.

Picard, M., Girard, S.A., Simard, M., Larocque, R., Leroux, T., and Turcotte, F. (2008). Association of work-related accidents with noise exposure in the workplace and noise-induced hearing loss based on the experience of some 240,000 person-years of observation. *Accident Anal. Prev.* 40(5), 1644–1652.

Schaal, N.C., Lange, K., and Majar, M. (2019b). Noise at sea: characterization of extended shift noise exposures among U.S. Navy aircraft carrier support personnel. *J. Occup. Environ. Hyg.* 16(2), 109–119.

Schaal, N.C., Majar, M., and Hunter, A. (2019d). Sound level measurements in berthing areas of an aircraft carrier. *Ann. Work Exp. Health* 63(8), 918–929.

Schaal, N.C., Salaam, R.A., Stevens, M.E., and Stubner, A.H. (2019a). Living at work: 24-hour noise exposure aboard US navy aircraft carriers. *Ann. Work Exp. Health.* 63(3), 316–327.

Schaal, N.C., Salaam, R.A., Stevens, M.E, and Stubner, A.H. (2019c). Noise characterization of "Effective Quiet" areas on a U.S. navy aircraft carrier. *J. Occup. Environ. Hyg.*
16(5), 329–335.

Tak, S., Davis, R.R., and Calvert, G.M. (2009). Exposure to hazardous workplace noise and
use of hearing protection devices among US workers—NHANES, 1999–2004. *Am. J.
Ind. Med.* 52, 358–71.

World Health Organization. (2009). *Night Noise Guidelines for Europe.* Copenhagen: World
Health Organization Regional Office for Europe. http://www.euro.who.int/__data/
assets/pdf_file/0017/43316/E92845.pdf (accessed 11 Aug 2019).

Yankaskas, K.D. (2013). Prelude: noise-induced tinnitus and hearing loss in the military.
Hearing Res. 295, 3–8.

Yankaskas, K.D., and Shaw, M.F. (1999). Landing on the roof: CVN noise. *Nav. Eng. J.*
111(4), 23–34.

Zaharna, M., and Guilleminault, C. (2010). Sleep, noise and health. *Noise Health* 12(47), 64.

12 Identifying Exposures and Health Outcomes in Former Worker Populations

Jeffrey R. Miller, Ashley Golden,
and Zachariah Hubbell
Oak Ridge Associated Universities

CONTENTS

12.1 INTRODUCTION

The concept of Total Exposure Health (THE) has gained popularity because experts recognize that it binds together multiple disciplines in a common effort to advance disease prevention and human health. Enabling this collaboration is the development of rapid and inexpensive methods for biomonitoring, ubiquitous sensing devices, expansion of electronic health records, and the ability to analyze massive amounts of data. The new frontier in disease prevention is to understand the relationships between lifetime exposure to environmental and workplace agents, individual genetic susceptibility, and the application of precise measures of preventive medicine. This exciting advancement is possible because of recent developments in genomics, toxicology, epidemiology, and exposure science. TEH requires unprecedented collaboration among subject-matter experts in all of these fields. This chapter focuses on the contributions that epidemiologists can make in TEH, primarily through epidemiologic surveillance. It is through surveillance that we obtain a more

DOI: 10.1201/9780429263286-14

complete and accurate understanding of the distribution and determinants of disease and the relationships between exposures and health outcomes.

The universe of exposures to chemical, biological, physical, and radiological agents is referred to as the *exposome*. Rappaport and Smith (2010, 461) defined the exposome as the record of all exposures both internal and external that people receive throughout their lifetime. Understanding the impact of exposures on health outcomes requires knowledge of all exposures from womb to end of life—a daunting assignment. Epidemiologic principles are applied in the study of prenatal and childhood exposures. There are large-scale national programs in the Centers for Disease Control and Prevention (CDC) and the Agency for Toxic Substances and Disease Registry (ATSDR) that are designed to protect communities from harmful health effects related to exposure to natural and man-made hazardous substances. The Childhood Lead Poisoning Prevention Program is administered by the CDC. In addition, the National Institutes of Health (NIH) has programs such as the National Institutes of Environmental Health Sciences Children's Health Exposure Analysis Resource (CHEAR) and Environmental Influences on Child Health Outcomes (ECHO) that examine environmental exposure factors, ranging from air pollution and chemicals in neighborhoods to societal factors such as stress to individual behaviors like sleep and diet.

Understanding occupational exposure during the working years, roughly from ages 18 to 65, is critical to the concept of TEH. Without a quantitative estimate of occupational exposure levels, we would not be able to establish safe exposure limits that drive engineering controls in hazardous workplaces, nor would we be able to establish the relationship between exposure and disease. It is the domain of industrial hygienists to measure occupational exposure and that of occupational physicians and related healthcare providers to establish the presence or absence of disease. Identifying adverse health outcomes, their distribution in the population, and the factors that determine their occurrence requires collaboration between medical providers and epidemiologists. This is the linkage between exposure assessment, disease surveillance, and occupational epidemiology.

When individuals enter the workforce, it is usually the responsibility of the employer to measure and record their exposures. In the United States, regulatory agencies like the U.S. Department of Labor (DOL), Occupational Safety and Health Administration (OSHA) provide oversight and enforcement to help ensure worker protection. Other agencies such as the CDC and National Institute for Occupational Safety and Health (NIOSH) conduct epidemiologic surveillance through programs like the NIOSH Surveillance Program, which aims to improve worker safety and health by identifying and tracking workplace injuries, illnesses, hazards, deaths, and exposures in the United States.

For aging adults, there remains a need to understand exposures that occur after a person retires from the workforce, as well as adverse health outcomes from diseases with long latencies that do not manifest themselves until a person enters retirement. For U.S. military veterans, the U.S. Department of Veterans Affairs (VA) administers the Public Health Surveillance and Research (PHSR) program to provide public health surveillance throughout the VA healthcare system. This is the tool the VA uses to collect data to estimate the health status and behavior of

America's veterans. More often, employers have no organized system for tracking the health status of their retirees. This is one of many issues that surface during one's transition from employed to retired. As Oksanen and Virtanen (2012) noted, health and retirement have a complex relationship. Retirement can occur on time (at official retirement age) or prematurely (*early* retirement from the labor force). Early retirement can take several forms: unemployment, disability, or voluntary early retirement. Evidence points to a range of factors that contribute to retirement decisions. Clarke et al. (2012) found that health status was related to expectations to continue working beyond age 62. Their finding that self-reports of chronic health problems were associated with a lower reported probability of working full time after 62 is in line with evidence showing that poor health is a strong predictor of intent to retire (Harkonmäki et al. 2006).

12.2 BACKGROUND

Epidemiologic surveillance is used to identify changes in the nature or extent of health problems and evaluate the effectiveness of public health interventions. The surveillance process is to collect, manage, analyze, interpret, and report information to prevent and control specific diseases (Rothman et al. 2008, 459). By observing trends in time, place, and persons, changes can be noted or anticipated and appropriate action, including investigation or control measures, can be taken (Porta 2008, 239).

When discussing prevention, it is helpful to distinguish among primary, secondary, and tertiary forms. Primary prevention denotes an action taken to prevent the development of disease in a person who is well and does not (yet) have the disease in question. Secondary prevention involves detecting disease in the early stages and preventing it from getting worse. Tertiary prevention denotes preventing complications in those who have already developed signs and symptoms of illness and have been diagnosed—that is, people who are in the clinical phase of their illness (Gordis 2008, 6–7). The National Supplemental Screening Program (NSSP) is primarily engaged in secondary prevention, though the program occasionally becomes involved in tertiary prevention when its screening results provide information to participants and their primary healthcare providers about the progression of previous diagnoses.

The objectives of epidemiologic surveillance may vary depending on the need. In the case of a newly identified disease or ailment, the objective may be to describe the characteristics and distribution of the disease. An example of this is the surveillance conducted related to the discovery of Popcorn Lung (bronchiolitis obliterans) associated with the exposure of workers in factories manufacturing microwave popcorn to diacetyl (butter flavoring) (Centers for Disease Control and Prevention 2002). The identification of bronchiolitis obliterans as a sentinel health event led to broader studies to further characterize lung disease risk from airborne butter flavoring chemicals. The conclusion of one such study was that microwave popcorn workers at many plants are at risk for flavoring-related lung disease (Kanwal et al. 2006).

Another objective of surveillance may be to provide a bridge to researchers seeking clues to further the investigation of occupational disease. An example of this is the surveillance of chronic beryllium disease (e.g., Eisenbud and Lisson 1983) that contributed to the development of the Beryllium Lymphocyte Proliferation Test (BeLPT) (Kreiss et al. 1989). The BeLPT has proven to be an invaluable tool in the identification of workplace risks in population studies and intervention effectiveness (Kreiss et al. 2007, 261) and has led to the early identification of milder cases of chronic beryllium disease (National Research Council 2008, 11).

At the population level, surveillance may be conducted to provide aggregate data for health program planning as well as to initiate individual preventive or therapeutic action (Rothman et al. 2008, 464). An example of this in an occupational setting is surveillance for the prevalence of chronic diseases like diabetes and obesity within a worker population and using that information to analyze needs for development of the healthcare workforce (Bodenheimer et al. 2009). In their study, Bodenheimer and colleagues (2009) noted that prevention and management of chronic disease are best performed by multidisciplinary teams in primary care and public health. However, the future healthcare workforce is not projected to include an appropriate mix of personnel capable of staffing such teams. To prepare for the growing chronic disease burden, a larger interdisciplinary primary care workforce is needed, and payment for primary care should reward practices that incorporate multidisciplinary teams (Bodenheimer et al. 2009).

Finally, surveillance is a critical tool for evaluating the effectiveness of interventions designed to prevent exposure and thus undesirable health outcomes. As an example, Fahey et al. (1991) measured needle stick injuries and blood exposure among healthcare workers following the establishment of the OSHA Bloodborne Pathogen Standard, which was aimed at controlling the transmission of bloodborne pathogens primarily by means of needle sticks (Occupational Safety and Health Administration, n.d.). These researchers concluded that Universal Precautions training significantly decreased but did not eliminate cutaneous exposures to blood and body substances. The results further suggested that the risk for HIV-1 infection associated with cutaneous exposures is substantially lower than the risk associated with parenteral exposures (Fahey et al. 1991).

The essential elements of an effective epidemiologic surveillance system will be specific to the situation at hand but generally incorporate the following concepts:

- Case definition—A set of criteria (not necessarily diagnostic criteria) that must be fulfilled to identify a person as representing a case of a particular disease. Case definitions can be based on geographic, clinical, laboratory, or combined clinical and laboratory criteria or on a scoring system with points for each criterion that matches the features of the disease (Porta 2008, 32).
- Target population—The collection of individuals, items, measurements, etc., about which inferences are desired. The term is sometimes used to indicate the population or group from which a sample or study population is drawn and sometimes to denote a reference population of interest (Porta 2008, 243).
- Sentinel surveillance—Surveillance based on selected population samples chosen to represent the relevant experience of particular groups. In sentinel surveillance, standard case definitions and protocols must be used to ensure

validity of comparisons across time and sites despite lack of statistically valid sampling (Porta 2008, 228).

- Record linkages—A method for bringing together the information contained in two or more records—e.g., in different sets of medical charts and in vital records such as birth and death certificates—and a procedure to ensure that each individual is identified and counted only once. Record linkages make it possible to relate significant health events that are remote from one another in time and place or to bring together records of different individuals (Porta 2008, 209).

These essential elements are designed into the surveillance system and adjusted as necessary as the system is deployed.

12.3 FOUNDATIONS OF THE U.S. DEPARTMENT OF ENERGY NATIONAL SUPPLEMENTAL SCREENING PROGRAM

One program that demonstrates the ability to track former workers and link occupational exposures to health outcomes is the Department of Energy (DOE) NSSP. The NSSP has provided medical screening examinations for nearly 20,000 former DOE workers since 2005 across the United States and helps them and their healthcare providers identify occupational and non-occupational health conditions that require medical treatment. This program will be used to illustrate how epidemiologists and occupational physicians can collaborate to help fill the data gap associated with health outcomes that occur after a person retires from work.

The NSSP established an integrated approach to health screening and promotion (LaMontagne et al. 2004; National Institute for Occupational Safety and Health 2008; Schill and Chosewood 2013; Sorensen and Barbeau 2004) that is consistent with the CDC/NIOSH Total Worker Health™ initiative (National Institute for Occupational Safety and Health 2018). The DOE Former Worker Program (FWP) was established following issuance by the U.S. Congress of the National Defense Authorization Act, Fiscal Year 1993 (Public Law 102-484), which called for DOE to assist workers in determining whether they have health issues related to their work at a DOE site (102nd U.S. Congress 1993). Medical screening efforts, aimed at identifying latent occupational health conditions, were initiated under the FWP in 1996. In response to a request by DOE in 2004 for applications to create a *nationwide* medical screening program for former DOE workers, the NSSP was established in 2005.

FWP examinations, including those conducted within the NSSP, are provided through cooperative agreements between DOE and university consortia, labor unions, and other organizations and follow the DOE FWP Medical Protocol, which takes into consideration the exposure history of the former worker and their potential exposure toxicity. The NSSP provides exposure-based medical screenings to former DOE workers, facilitated by the use of a web-based relational database management system designed to capture enrollment information, maintain participant correspondence notes, store consent documents and clinical results, securely transfer records, and produce screening result letters. The NSSP collects demographic, occupational exposure, work history, clinical, and health outcome data—over 1,000 data points per initial examination. The NSSP relies on an Integrated Health Model, incorporating a DOE FWP Medical Protocol (Department of Energy 2018) that includes an exposure-based medical examination and rescreening examinations every three years. The NSSP integrated design (Figure 12.1) identifies occupational and non-occupational conditions and extends disease surveillance and health promotion into post-employment.

As a nationwide program, the NSSP accommodates a population with wide geographic dispersal and varying degrees of both the ability and willingness to travel. As such, the program uses a nationwide network of occupational health clinics to allow participants to be screened as near as possible to their residence, regardless of proximity to the site of their former DOE employment site. Through strategic clinic and laboratory partnerships, the NSSP is able to manage health surveillance activities for its more than 20,000 screened participants from a centralized base of operations.

12.4 MEDICAL SCREENING PROGRAM OBJECTIVES

Medical screening programs (such as the NSSP) that seek to adhere to the Total Worker Health™ concept must be designed for the detection of both occupationally and non-occupationally related health conditions (National Institute for Occupational Safety and Health 2018). A context of prior occupational exposures is, of course, essential for identification of occupationally related health conditions. To ensure

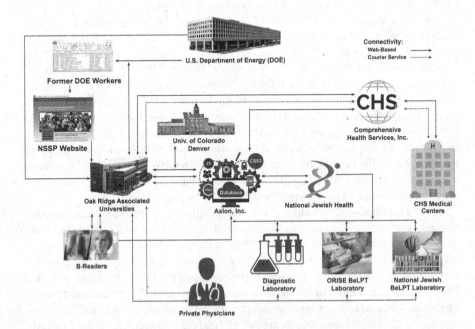

FIGURE 12.1 U.S. Department of Energy National Supplemental Screening Program Conceptual Design.

maximum benefit to participants, medical screening program examination protocols should be regularly evaluated for the practicality and potential utility of adding new medical tests, which can be specifically aimed at assessing either occupational or non-occupational health outcomes.

In early 2017, the NSSP began offering the hemoglobin A1c test to all participants, which provides a three-month average assessment of blood sugar levels and has gained favor among medical professionals as a more accurate indicator of diabetes risk than a simple *snapshot* measure of blood glucose (Nathan et al. 2009). Despite the status of NSSP as a former worker (i.e., occupationally oriented) health surveillance program, the addition of the A1c test to its examination protocol constitutes an intentional effort to bolster the program's non-occupational health screening elements, thereby supporting its goal of promoting Total Worker Health™.

In addition to its primary goal of providing medical screening examinations and their results to DOE former workers, the NSSP also assists participants seeking U.S. Department of Labor Energy Employees Occupational Illness Compensation Program (EEOICP) benefits. The EEOICP program awards compensation and benefits to eligible claimants with illnesses related to hazardous exposures gained during work for federal energy employers—including, but not limited to, DOE (National Institute for Occupational Safety and Health 2000).

Following a set of protocols developed by the NSSP medical team and with adherence to application requirements established by DOL, the NSSP furnishes likely qualified former workers with information about the EEOICP and how to file a claim. Where appropriate, recommendations for contacting the DOL are added to participants' examination result letters. Additionally, NSSP screening results can be and often are used by former workers as support for compensation claims, despite the fact that the NSSP is not affiliated with the DOL or EEOICP and has no role in EEOICP claims evaluations. These efforts, while not directly under the purview of a medical surveillance program, complement the primary objective of the NSSP (and indeed, any health surveillance program) to maximally benefit the wellbeing of its participants.

The DOE FWPs are, by definition, aimed at surveilling participants' health throughout their post-employment years. While a substantial portion of former workers are still in their working years (defined above as roughly ages 18–65), the majority are of retirement age. As such, a priority of the FWPs is the continued monitoring of participants' health throughout post-employment. DOE FWP guidelines allow participants to be screened at three-year intervals, resulting in a large number of former worker participants for whom multiple screening examinations have been performed. Repeated screenings provide valuable context for individualized follow-up recommendations from program medical staff and allow long-term health monitoring of returning participants. The wealth of longitudinal clinical data generated by this approach also affords screening program researchers the opportunity to investigate health outcome trends and quantitatively assess the program's impact on participant health (Hubbell et al., unpublished; Stange et al. 2016). Given adequate resources, current-worker health surveillance programs can achieve similar successes by broadening their scope to follow workers into retirement rather than discontinuation following employee separation.

Since its inception, the NSSP has sought to provide evidence that a nationwide former worker integrated health screening program cannot only reach a large former worker population who may not normally participate in organized health promotion programs but can also provide a basis for improved healthcare and reduced health-care costs. Because the NSSP is available to DOE former workers living anywhere in the United States, common barriers to health surveillance, such as lack of insurance or inability to secure primary care near one's residence, do not impede participants' access. The NSSP does not request information regarding participants' outside health care or health monitoring activities, but it has been observed during enrollments and through other communications that many of its former worker participants are indeed uninsured and do not regularly see a primary care physician, making the NSSP these individuals' only continuing contact with medical professionals.

12.5   NSSP METHODOLOGY

The NSSP approach to former worker medical surveillance is described here as an example of how an integrated screening program contributes to the concept of TEH. The NSSP uses a web-based relational database management system for collection, storage, and transfer of all clinical data—a de facto electronic health record system. The system complies with the Privacy Act of 1974 (Department of Justice 2016), the Health Insurance Portability and Accountability Act (HIPAA) of 1996 (Department of Health and Human Services 1996), and the Federal Information Security Modernization Act (FISMA) of 2014 (Computer Security Resource Center 2014).

The NSSP medical examination protocol begins with the enrollment process, most often completed by telephone, during which information is collected by NSSP staff regarding the enrollee's demographics, work history, and self-reported history of exposures to numerous occupational hazards, including radiation, beryllium, asbestos, silica, diesel exhaust, heavy metals, solvents, miscellaneous chemicals, noise, laser energy, and various respiratory irritants. Due to the self-reported nature of these exposure survey responses, participants' resulting exposure histories can-not be considered to be a complete representation of the occupational hazards they encountered. However, this strategy generally results in an adequate representation of the former workers' exposures.

Each examination is tailored to the individual's medical and occupational exposure history and designed to identify both occupationally and non-occupationally related health conditions. In addition to reported exposure history, medical screening tests offered to enrolled participants take into consideration individuals' former DOE site(s) of employment. Examination components may include a physical examination, an audiogram, vision tests, spirometry, a series of blood and urine tests, a chest X-ray, a BeLPT, and other tests as determined by the exposure-based algorithm and deemed appropriate by program medical staff. As previously discussed, NSSP participants receive their screening examination at a local clinic, rarely traveling more than 50 miles to reach the designated facility—an arrangement made possible by one of the NSSP organizational partners and their nationwide network of clinics.

Every set of medical results undergoes several rounds of quality control checks before the final packet of results and recommendations is sent to the participant. This includes review by two different physicians (not counting the examining clinician), who each review available medical records, exposure histories, and clinical findings to ensure that screening results and recommendations are properly framed within a participant-specific medical context.

Medical screening results and applicable follow-up recommendations are furnished to participants by mail six to eight weeks after the examination. Table 12.1 lists the diagnostic definitions and clinical criteria for occupational and non-occupational conditions. Participants receive a hard copy of the examination results and an accompanying letter summarizing medical findings in *plain language*. While follow-up medical evaluation and treatment are not within the scope of the program, result letters do include brief explanations of the screening findings and recommendations, which may include referral to one of the DOL Resource Centers specializing in EEOICP claims assistance. Result letters also include (when applicable) statements advising participants to seek routine healthcare services (such as immunizations and mammograms), recommending resources to help them quit smoking, and reminding them of their eligibility to be rescreened every three years. The NSSP examination is not intended to be a substitute for private health care, though requests

---

TABLE 12.1

National Supplemental Screening Program Occupational and Non-Occupational Diagnostic Definitions

Occupational	Clinical Criteria
Noise-induced hearing loss, speech frequencies	Audiometry result >25 dB at 500, 1,000, 2,000, 4,000 Hz, worst ear
Asbestosis without pleural disease	Asbestos exposure, B-read: parenchymal abnormalities of shape and location typical for asbestosis (mid and lower lung zone, irregular opacities)
Asbestosis with pleural disease	Asbestos exposure, B-read: parenchymal abnormalities of shape and location typical for asbestosis (mid and lower lung zone, irregular opacities) and pleural abnormalities
Asbestos-related pleural disease	Asbestos exposure, B-read: pleural abnormalities
Lung nodules, nodes, or lesions	B-read: nodules
Pneumoconiosis	B-read: 1/0 or greater, pleural changes
Beryllium sensitization	≥1 abnormal BeLPT
Non-Occupational	**Clinical Criteria**
Above normal body mass index (BMI)	BMI ≥25.0
Hypertension	≥140/90
Fecal occult blood	Positive result
Abnormal thyroid function	TSH <0.40 or >4.50
Elevated hemoglobin A1c	>5.6% (prediabetes), >6.4% (diabetes)

for the secure transfer of NSSP examination results to participants' personal physicians are honored on a regular basis for the purposes of facilitating prompt and relevant medical follow-up. The NSSP examination decision logic and flow chart is illustrated in Figure 12.2.

Occasionally, NSSP medical staff identify abnormal examination results as *urgently abnormal*. These situations typically involve laboratory or chest X-ray findings of a potentially serious and/or time-sensitive nature, of which the participant may be unaware. Participants with urgently abnormal results are contacted immediately by phone by an NSSP medical professional to inform them of the

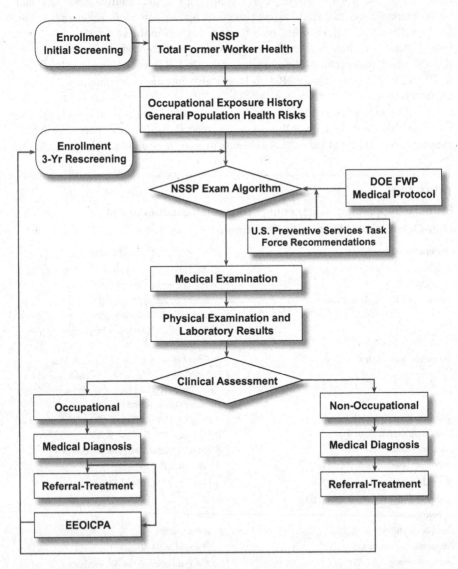

FIGURE 12.2 National Supplemental Screening Program Decision Logic and Flowchart.

finding; a hard copy of the results is also sent by FedEx® to the participant for expedited follow-up with their personal physician. This protocol for urgent results notification allows participants to quickly address potentially significant medical problems without waiting weeks for their complete examination results to be mailed to them.

12.6 SELECTED PROGRAM RESULTS

Between September 1, 2005 and April 30, 2019, 20,632 former DOE workers were enrolled in the NSSP. Of those, females accounted for 5,325 (25.8%) and males 15,307 (74.2%). A total of 18,518 participants completed initial medical screening examinations. Of those, females accounted for 4,668 (25.2%) with an average age of 62 years (range: 22–95 years). Males accounted for 13,850 (74.8%) with an average age of 66 years (range: 21–99 years). Following the initial screening exam, 5,461 participants completed rescreening examinations.

Participants were collectively employed at DOE facilities between the years 1940 and 2019. The duration of DOE employment ranged from less than one year to more than 50 years. The mean duration of employment was 14.0 years, with females working an average of 11.4 years and males working an average of 14.9 years. The median duration of employment was 7.4 years for females and 11.0 years for males.

The geographic distribution of screened NSSP participants is widespread, consisting of people living in every state in the United States. Figure 12.3 shows a map of NSSP initial exam screenings by state of residence. Although the highest concentrations of participants can be found in states containing NSSP *primary* DOE sites (those DOE facilities whose former workers are assigned directly to the NSSP and not to any other FWP), the screening has clearly been utilized by former workers in every corner of the United States over the past 14 years.

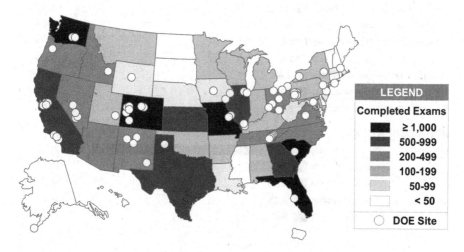

FIGURE 12.3 National Supplemental Screening Program completed initial exams by state of residence.

The most frequently identified occupational condition identified in former workers was noise-induced hearing loss, with more than two-thirds (67.5%) of NSSP participants showing abnormal audiogram results not attributable to natural, age-related hearing loss. The next most common abnormal finding was asbestosis without pleural disease (4.1%). Combined with the findings of asbestosis with pleural disease (1.0%) and asbestos-related pleural disease (1.1%), abnormal asbestos-related lung findings were present in 6.2% of participants. Other abnormal findings included lung nodules, nodes, and lesions (3.4%), pneumoconiosis (3.2%), beryllium sensitization (2.4%), and silicosis (0.2%).

The most common non-occupational finding was elevated body mass index (BMI), with 77.3% of participants considered above normal (BMI of 25.0 or higher) (National Heart, Lung, and Blood Institute n.d.). The second most common non-occupational finding was elevated blood pressure (20.7%), followed by abnormal thyroid function (5.2%), elevated hemoglobin A1c (5.1%), and fecal occult blood (4.7%). Figure 12.4 provides the percentage of participants screened who had abnormal findings for occupational and non-occupational indicators.

A significant proportion of elevated findings for blood pressure (50.3%) and hemoglobin A1c (57.1%) were found in participants who had no prior history of these medical conditions. For these individuals, their NSSP screening results were their first clinical indicator of these medical issues; all individuals were referred to primary care providers for follow-up. Figure 12.5 illustrates the percentage of abnormal findings for these two health outcomes.

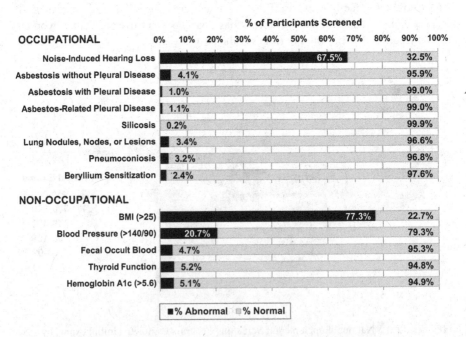

FIGURE 12.4 Occupational and non-occupational conditions identified through screening.

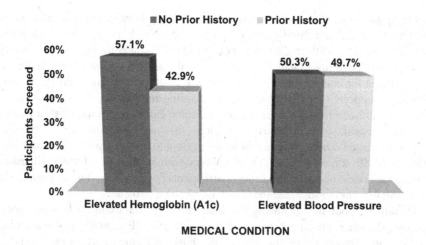

FIGURE 12.5 Medical Conditions with no Prior History Identified by Screening.

12.7 SUMMARY

The NSSP design and methodology overcomes many challenges associated with surveillance of former worker populations, including geographic dispersal of participants, access to clinics, time and budget constraints, health information management, and exposure-medical protocol. These challenges were addressed using a web-enabled, decentralized program model for delivery of occupational and non-occupational screening services to a large population.

Large-scale surveillance for health conditions among former worker populations, as demonstrated by the NSSP, can be a powerful means of secondary and tertiary prevention of occupational and non-occupational disease. Recognition of elevated biomarkers such as hemoglobin A1c informs previously unaware participants of potential health issues and provides them the opportunity to take action to prevent or mitigate disease in the early stages. This is helpful for non-occupational chronic diseases such as diabetes and cardiovascular disease. For occupational diseases, this type of surveillance program identifies cases of long-latency diseases (e.g., asbestosis) that were previously unrecognized. This is important because it helps establish the total burden of occupational disease by filling in gaps related to incidence in retired workers—cases that otherwise might remain undiagnosed and unreported.

The NSSP provides a valuable service to its former worker participants and their families. The Total Worker Health™ model keeps the best interest of the participant at the forefront. Whether abnormal findings are occupational or non-occupational in origin, NSSP healthcare providers seek to inform and educate participants and connect them with the most appropriate resources for their medical situation. The program identifies medical conditions that may have resulted from occupational exposures, positions participants to pursue appropriate medical follow-up, and (where applicable) directs ailing former workers toward potential assistance from the EEOICP (National Institute for Occupational Safety and Health 2000).

Occupational health conditions are commonly seen in participants in all screening phases (initial and three-year follow-up) of the NSSP. Interestingly, combined non-occupational health conditions are observed with greater frequency than strictly occupational conditions, which demonstrates the utility of the NSSP-integrated health model for comprehensive former worker health surveillance and shows how its design supports the TEH objectives of defining the exposome and painting an inclusive picture of health. Cases of diabetes, colon cancer, lung cancer, skin cancer, beryllium sensitization, asbestos-related lung disease, obstructive and restrictive lung disease, and other conditions of various possible origins have been recognized through NSSP screenings in former workers with no history of these illnesses. During the course of operations, many participants have expressed their gratitude to the NSSP for making such health information known to them.

Intuitively, poor health during the later working years can push some workers toward earlier retirement than their healthier peers. Post-employment ongoing medical surveillance programs such as the DOE FWPs are uniquely positioned to investigate such phenomena and potentially develop a more nuanced understanding of the manifestation of interactions between occupational hazards, age- and life-style-related (i.e., non-occupational) ailments, and healthcare intervention. Such insights are well aligned with the goals of TEH. A limitation of the NSSP design is its reliance upon self-reported exposure data, work history information, and medical history. There is no direct linkage to occupational exposures, so these data are subject to recall bias. Thus, there is no record of the frequency, duration, or intensity of exposures. Additionally, there is no substance-specific exposure data that might prove useful in medical evaluation. It also may be unclear as to what new exposures a participant may experience through hobbies or work engagements following separation from the DOE complex. Occasionally, confusion on the part of participants regarding their exact medical diagnoses generates difficulty parsing condition types and linking illnesses to specific exposures. These limitations can be mitigated through the implementation of the concept of TEH.

12.8 ACKNOWLEDGMENTS

The authors greatly appreciate the assistance from Dave Girardi, Eric Adams, and Sherry Atkins in the layout and design of this presentation. The authors would also like to thank the DOE former workers who worked in support of our country and chose to participate in the NSSP. And finally, the NSSP would like to thank the DOE (AU-14) who provided the opportunity to assist in the healthcare management of so many. The NSSP is funded by Cooperative Agreement DE-FC01-05EH04022 between ORAU and the U.S. Department of Energy.

REFERENCES

102nd U.S. Congress. 1993. "National Defense Authorization Act for Fiscal Year 1993, Section 3162, Title 50, Chapter 42, Subchapter VI, Part C 2733. U.S. Senate Bill 3114." Accessed June 4, 2014. https://www.govtrack.us/congress/bills/102/hr5006/text.

Bodenheimer, Thomas, Ellen Chen, and Heather D. Bennett. 2009. "Confronting the Growing Burden of Chronic Disease: Can the U.S. Health Care Workforce Do the Job?" *Health Affairs* 28 (1) (January). doi:10.377/hlthadd.28.1.64.

Centers for Disease Control and Prevention (CDC). 2002. "Fixed Obstructive Lung Disease in Workers at a Microwave Popcorn Factory – Missouri, 2000–2002." *Morb Mortal Wkly Rep* 51 (16): 345–347.

Clarke, Philippa, Victor Marshall, and David Weir. 2012. "Unexpected Retirement from Full Time Work after Age 62: Consequences for Life Satisfaction in Older Americans." *Eur J Ageing* 9 (3): 207–219.

Computer Security Resource Center (CSRC). 2014. "Federal Information Security Modernization Act of 2014 (FISMA) (Public Law 113–283)." Accessed May 30, 2019. https://www.govinfo.gov/content/pkg/PLAW-113publ283/pdf/PLAW-113publ283.pdf.

Department of Energy, Office of Environment, Health, Safety, & Security. 2018. "Former Worker Program Medical Protocol." Accessed May 30, 2019. http://energy.gov/ehss/downloads/former-worker-program-medical-protocol.

Department of Health and Human Services. 1996. "Health Insurance Portability and Accountability Act of 1996." Accessed May 30, 2019. https://aspe.hhs.gov/report/health-insurance-portability-and-accountability-act-1996.

Department of Justice (DOJ), Office of Privacy and Civil Liberties (OPCL). 2016. "The Privacy Act of 1974." Accessed May 31, 2019. http://www.justice.gov/opcl/privacy-act-1974.

Eisenbud, Merril, and Judith Lisson. 1983. "Epidemiological Aspects of Beryllium-Induced Nonmalignant Lung Disease: A 30-Year Update." *J Occ Env Med* 25 (3): 196–202.

Fahey, Barbara J., Deloris E. Koziol, Steven M. Banks, and David K. Henderson. 1991. "Frequency of Nonparenteral Occupational Exposures to Blood and Body Fluids Before and After Universal Precautions Training." *Am J Med* 90 (2): 145–53.

Gordis, Leon. 2008. Epidemiology, 4th Edition. Philadelphia, PA: Saunders, an imprint of Elsevier.

Harkonmäki, Karoliina, Ossi Rahkonen, Pekka Martikainen, Karri Silventoinen, and Eero Lahelma. 2006. "Associations of SF-36 Mental Health Functioning and Work and Family Factors with Intentions to Retire Early Among Employees." *Occup Environ Med* 63: 558–563. doi:10.1136/oem.2005.022293.

Kanwal, Richard, Greg Kullman, Chris Piacitelli, Randy Boylstein, Nancy Sahakian, Stephen Martin, Kathleen Fedan, and Kathleen Kreiss. 2006. "Evaluation of Flavorings-Related Lung Disease Risk at Six Microwave Popcorn Plants." *J Occ Env Med* 48(2):149–157.

Kreiss, Kathleen, Gregory A. Day, and Christine R. Schuler. 2007. "Beryllium: A Modern Industrial Hazard." *Annu Rev Publ Health* 28: 259–277.

Kreiss, Kathleen, Lee S. Newman, Margaret M. Mroz, and Priscilla A. Campbell. 1989. "Screening Blood Test Identifies Subclinical Beryllium Disease." *J Occ Env Med* 31 (7): 603–608.

LaMontagne, Anthony D., Elizabeth Barbeau, Richard A. Youngstrom, Marvin Lewiton, Anne M. Stoddard, Deborah McLellan, L. M. Wallace, and Glorian Sorensen. 2004. "Assessing and Intervening on OSH Programmes: Effectiveness Evaluation of the Wellworks-2 Intervention in 15 Manufacturing Worksites." *Occup Environ Med* 61 (8): 651–660. doi:10.1136/oem.2003.011718.

Nathan, David M., Beverly Balkau, Enzo Bonora, Knut Borch-Johnsen, John B. Buse, Stephen Colagiuri, Mayer B. Davidson, et al. 2009. "International Expert Committee Report on the Role of the A1c Assay in the Diagnosis of Diabetes." *Diabetes Care* 32 (7): 1327–1334. doi:10.2337/dc09–9033.

National Heart, Lung, and Blood Institute. n.d. "Confirming a High Body Mass Index (BMI)." Accessed July 12, 2019. https://www.nhlbi.nih.gov/health-topics/overweight-and-obesity.

National Institute for Occupational Safety and Health (NIOSH). 2000. "Title 42 –The Public Health and Welfare, Chapter 84 – Department of Energy, Subchapter XVI – Energy Employees Occupational Illness Compensation Program, Part A – Establishment of Compensation Program and Compensation Fund." Accessed May 1, 2014. http://www.cdc.gov/niosh/ocas/ocaseeoi.html.

National Institute for Occupational Safety and Health (NIOSH). 2008. "Essential Elements of Effective Workplace Programs and Policies for Improving Worker Health and Wellbeing." Accessed July 15, 2014. https://www.cdc.gov/niosh/TWH/essentials.html.

National Institute for Occupational Safety and Health (NIOSH). 2018. "What is Total Worker Health®?" Accessed May 31, 2019. http://www.cdc.gov/niosh/twh/.

National Research Council (NRC) Committee on Beryllium Alloy Exposures. 2008. *Managing Health Effects of Beryllium Exposure.* Washington, DC: National Academic Press.

Occupational Safety and Health Administration (OSHA). "Code of Federal Regulations, Part 1910: Occupational Safety and Health Standards, Subpart Z: Toxic and Hazardous Substances, Standard Number 1910.1030: Bloodborne Pathogens." Accessed March 28, 2019. https://www.osha.gov/pls/oshaweb/owadisp.show_document?p_id=10051&p_table=STANDARDS.

Oksanen, Tuula and Marianna Virtanen. 2012. "Health and Retirement: A Complex Relationship." *Eur J Ageing* 9 (3): 221–225. doi:10.1007/s10433-012-0243-7.

Porta, Miguel. 2008. A Dictionary of Epidemiology. 5th Edition. Edited for the International Epidemiological Association. Oxford: Oxford University Press.

Rappaport, Stephen M., and Martyn T. Smith. 2010. "Environment and Disease Risks." *Science* 330(6003): 460–461. doi:10.1126/science.1192603.

Rothman, Kenneth J., Sander Greenland, and Timothy L. Lash. 2008. Modern Epidemiology, 3rd Edition. Philadelphia, PA: Lippincott Williams & Wilkins.

Schill, Anita L., and Lewis Casey Chosewood. 2013. "The NIOSH Total Worker Health™ Program: An Overview." *J Occ Env Med* 55 (12S): S8–S11. doi:10.1097/JOM.0000000000000037.

Sorensen, Glorian, and Elizabeth Barbeau. 2004. "Steps to a Healthier U.S. Workforce – Integrating Occupational Health and Safety and Worksite Health Promotion: State of the Science." Presented at the National Institute of Occupational Safety and Health Steps to a Healthier U.S. Workforce symposium, Washington, D.C.

Stange, Bill, John McInerney, Ashley Golden, Wendy Benade, Barbara Neill, Annyce Mayer, Roxana Witter, et al. 2016. "Integrated Approach to Health Screening of Former Department of Energy Workers Detects Both Occupational and Non-Occupational Illness." *Am J Ind Med* 59 (3): 200–211. doi:10/1002/ajim.22554.

13 Personal Environmental Exposure Sensors and the Internet of Things

LeeAnn Racz
US Air Force

CONTENTS

DOI: 10.1201/9780429263286-15

13.1   INTRODUCTION

Full implementation of Total Exposure Health tenets requires extensive data collection of the full spectrum of an individual's exposures. This concept is closely aligned with the exposome, a term coined in 2005 by Wild, which includes all environmental exposures a person experiences from conception throughout his or her entire life. Wild (2012) has divided the exposome into two broad categories: internal and external. The internal exposome includes various processes such as metabolism, circulating hormones, and aging. However, assessing the internal exposome can be problematic as it is difficult to identify the exposure source, account for the route of exposure, and address spatial or temporal variability of exposure (Turner et al. 2017). The external exposome, on the other hand, may be more attainable as we can define and measure exposures prior to the point of entering the body. This chapter focuses on the state of the science in measurements of the external exposome as well as the prospects for incorporating them in the Internet of Things (IoT).

13.2   OVERVIEW OF PERSONAL SENSORS

There is a variety of portable sensors and techniques for assessing personal environmental exposures, especially for air pollution. Whereas concentrations of regulated airborne compounds have conventionally been collected by government agencies using area monitors requiring expensive laboratory analysis, the new paradigm is developing into personal and portable sensors that can be used by communities and individuals. Citizen scientists and those in the "quantified self" movement, a community of people using exposure measurements to understand personal habits and their impact on health, similarly are leveraging advances in exposure sensor technology (Loh et al. 2017). One study successfully employed portable microsensors for land-use regression surfaces for oxides of nitrogen and ozone (Deville Cavellin et al. 2016). Another research group used a drone-based measurement system to assess radiofrequency radiation exposures from cellular telephone base stations. Other personal sensing technology advancements have been applied to noise, temperature, particulates, and organic compounds (Nieuwenhuijsen et al. 2014).

Technology is advancing to a point where use of personal sensors is becoming more practical. In order for personal sensors to be successfully used on a wide scale, they must effectively integrate into one's lifestyle. Loh et al. (2017) defined the following criteria for personal sensor technologies:

1. Unobtrusive to the user (easily worn, carried, or placed).
2. Cost-effective for widespread deployment.
3. Able to collect, store and transmit real-time and high temporal resolution data.
4. Useable by a lay person.
5. Ability to upload data to the internet or download data.
6. Meet quality data constraints such as sensitivity, specificity, and detection limits; low failure rate; precision and accuracy; and stability over time.

Personal sensors are currently not likely to meet reference instrument or "gold standard" criteria. However, they might be able to attain secondary data quality objectives which enable them to collect complementary data (Loh et al. 2017). In this context, it will be important to recognize and account for the uncertainty from widespread use of personal sensors.

13.3 MICRO GAS CHROMATOGRAPHY

One of the most ubiquitous classes of air pollutants, which has a high potential for causing negative health effects, is organic compounds. For decades, one of the practical ways to reliably identify and quantify these compounds is with bench-scale gas chromatography (GC) and a detector. However, since the first successful miniaturization of a GC in 1979 by Terry et al., technology has continued to advance to make micro GC, or µGC, a promising portable sensor.

GC principles are similar in both bench-scale and portable instruments. Both typically pump sample air flow through an injector, a separation column with an oven, and then a detector. In µGC, however, the components are miniaturized to improve portability, decrease power requirements, and increase the efficiency and speed of analysis (Regmi and Agah 2018).

13.3.1 ANALYTE PRECONCENTRATION

For analysis of gases with low concentrations of organic analytes (low parts-per-billion range), conventional methods include using a sorbent tube to collect and preconcentrate the sample. A thermal desorber then desorbs the sample from the sorbent tube before the sample is pumped to the column. Several researchers have made advances in miniaturizing preconcentrator technology, which removes the requirement for the sorbent tube and thermodesorber (Tian et al. 2005, Camara et al. 2011, Akbar et al. 2013, Bourlon et al. 2016). One of the first micro-preconcentrators was a micro hot place coated with a surfactant template sol–gel adsorbent (Manginell et al. 2000). Another approach came from Bourlon et al. (2016) who developed a micro-preconcentrator on a silicon chip measuring 8 mm×21 mm with an inlet and outlet etched only 400 µm deep.

Other advances, referred to as preconcentrator–focuser or preconcentrator–injector, have enabled a preconcentrator to not only concentrate a sample but also narrowly focus the chromatogram using rapid thermal desorption. These devices have also been miniaturized for use in a µGC (Regmi and Agah 2018).

13.3.2 SEPARATION COLUMN

The separation column is arguably the most critical component of a GC system. Bench-scale capillary columns have a circular cross section, whereas µGC columns, or micro-columns, are rectangular. The principles of operation are the same in that both are either coated or packed with materials (stationary phase) that separate analytes from gas mixtures according to their affinity for the materials. However, microcolumns offer several potential advantages. For example, their small size enables high speed and low power to heat the column. They may have a low manufacturing cost as they can be produced in large batches. In addition, their monolithic integration with other components may minimize dead volumes and cold spots (Regmi and Agah 2018).

13.3.2.1 Microcolumn Fabrication

Microelectromechanical systems (MEMS) technology is often used to fabricate microcolumns on silicon wafers. This approach makes channels in the silicon by covering it with a mask (photoresist), transferring the pattern to the mask using photolithography, etching the pattern into the silicon substrate, and hermetically sealing the channels with a glass wafer (Regmi and Agah 2018). Some investigators have also used metal substrates such as nickel (Bhushan et al. 2007a, 2007b, Lewis and Wheeler 2007), steel (Iwaya et al. 2012), and titanium (Raut and Thurbide 2017). For metal substrates, the surfaces have been commonly deactivated by depositing a thin film of silicon. Lewis et al. (2010) successfully fabricated a glass–glass microcolumn using etched glass plates, and some have pursued use of ceramics as a substrate (Darko et al. 2013, Briscoe et al. 2004). Noh et al. (2002) experimented with polymeric materials (parylene) as the microcolumn substrate and found faster heating and cooling rates as well as lower power consumption than silicon-glass columns, but very low experimental plate numbers. In addition to MEMS, laser etching technology (LET) has also become an important fabrication method (Sun et al. 2016).

13.3.2.2 Microcolumn Configuration

Regardless of the substrate used, microcolumn design must consider analysis time, separation efficiency, pressure drop, and sample capacity (Regmi and Agah 2018) just as is done for conventional columns. However, optimization of one parameter may lead to a decrease in performance of another parameter. A longer column will improve chromatogram resolution but will increase the analysis time. Decreasing the width of a column can enhance separation efficiency but will decrease sample capacity. Although use of a bundle of capillaries or a multi-capillary column (MCC) can mitigate sample capacity limitations, they pose a polydispersity effect in which even small changes to the capillary configuration dramatically affects band broadening (Schisla et al. 1993). However, the use of microfabricated pillar-array, or semi-packed, columns may help to overcome the challenges with MCCs (Jespers et al. 2017, Ali et al. 2009).

Although microcolumns may have several advantages, they have their limitations as well. One of these major limitations is the tendency for the stationary phase to accumulate in sharp corners, known as the pooling effect, which leads to band broadening (Wang et al. 2014). Mitigating this effect has been the subject of much research as multiple turns are inevitable when fitting a long separation column (one meter or more) onto a small footprint of just a few square centimeters. For example, Randadia et al. (2009) reduced the pooling effect by rounding the channel walls. The channel configuration is important as well. Of the three common layout patterns (serpentine, circular-spiral, and square-spiral), the serpentine pattern appears to have favorable hydrodynamic flow and more homogeneous stationary-phase coating than the other two and therefore superior separation performance (Radadia et al. 2010). Sun et al. (2012), however, found a spiral pattern had better flow characteristics than the serpentine configuration and therefore better chromatograph resolution.

Several groups have worked toward developing a miniaturized GC×GC, or 2D GC, system. Liu and Phillips (1991) were the first to report success. Whiting et al. (2009) made significant improvements in 2D µGC and were able to separate dimethyl methylphosphonate from three polar interfering compounds in just a few seconds. More recently, Collin et al. (2015) used 2D µGC to separate a mixture of 36 volatile organic compounds in 22 minutes. This approach has continued to evolve into a promising technology.

Correlation chromatography is another technique that has found its way into µGC system research. In correlation chromatography, a pseudorandom sample gas stream is injected into the column, and the chromatogram results from cross-correlation with the output signal (Smit 1970). This approach can significantly improve the signal-to-noise ratio with only moderate increase on the time for analysis (Cheng et al. 2012) and was demonstrated for use in a µGC system by Cesar et al. (2015).

13.3.2.3 Microcolumn Heating

Separation of analytes in an air sample that has been retained onto the stationary phase occurs when differences in temperature drive changes in equilibrium. At low temperatures, molecules weakly retained in the stationary phase pass through the column. More strongly retained compounds require higher temperatures for elution from the column. A temperature profile that changes over time, however, enables separation of the solutes with varying retainability. In bench-scale GCs, the column heating occurs in an oven which demands high power and may have limited temperature gradient rates (Regmi and Agah 2018). These conventional approaches are not suitable for µGC systems.

An alternative resistive heating technology has become widely used in µGC systems (Wang et al. 2012). In some of these approaches, the column material itself is the heating element through which current passes. This requires the column to incorporate conductive metal, such as stainless steel or aluminum, either as the substrate or as a coating material (Staples and Viswanathan 2005, Yost and Hall 1992). Other methods deposit a refractory material or lightly doped semiconductor on the silicon substrate (Regmi and Agah 2018). In each of the successful methods, the heating technique has sufficient thermal time response and reduced power consumption.

13.3.3 DETECTORS

Following separation in the column, a gas comes in contact with a detector for identification and/or quantification. Several detector technologies have been adapted for use in a µGC system. The following is not an exhaustive list but summarizes some of the more common approaches attempted.

13.3.3.1 Thermal Conductivity Detector (TCD)

A TCD detects the thermal conductivity of a compound when compared to a reference cell, such as a carrier gas. TCDs for µGC application have been developed by depositing a thin metal film in microchannels of a silicon substrate (Garg et al. 2015, Dziuban et al. 2004).

13.3.3.2 Surface Acoustic Wave (SAW)

SAW sensors detect changes in the propagation of acoustic waves near the surface of a piezoelectric material. Williams and Pappas (1999) and Frye-Mason et al. (2000) have developed SAW sensors for hand-held GC systems.

13.3.3.3 Photoionization Detector (PID)

PIDs have been a mainstay of GC detectors for many years. A PID uses an ultraviolet lamp to irradiate a gas sample in an ionization chamber. The current generated from the ions is proportionate to the gas concentration. Miniaturization of PIDs has been achieved by reducing the volume of the ionization chamber (Sun et al. 2013, Zhu et al. 2015).

13.3.3.4 Electron Capture Detector (ECD)

ECD has long-been reliable for detection of halogenated, nitroaromatic, organome-tallic, and conjugated compounds (Poole 1982). In this device, beta particles collide with molecules from both the carrier gas, to form a reference current, and the sample gas. After colliding with the beta particles, the sample gas becomes ionized and decreases the current. Klee et al. (1999) have miniaturized an ECD with improved sensitivity and larger dynamic range.

13.3.3.5 Surface Plasmon Resonance Imaging (SPRi)

SPRi detects compounds as the refractive index of a gas changes when passing through a channel. Du et al. (2018) demonstrated good performance of a miniatur-ized SPRi integrated with a microcolumn.

13.3.3.6 Flame Ionization Detector (FID)

FIDs have commonly been used for conventional GCs. A FID uses a hydrogen flame to ionize molecules, which generate a current detected by an electrode. Although there have been attempts to miniaturize FIDs, their need for a large flow of fuel and oxidant have made them less suitable for μGC applications (Zimmermann et al. 2000, Hayward and Thurbide 2008, Lussac et al. 2016).

13.3.3.7 Mass Spectrometry (MS)

MS is a highly sensitive detector that identifies a wide array of organic compounds. Although the bench-scale versions' size, weight, and power requirements have prevented their use outside of laboratory conditions, there has been some effort to produce micro MS detectors. Variants of this technology have included a micro ion-mobility spectrometer (Camara et al. 2011, Luong et al. 2012) and a radiofrequency ion-mobility spectrometer (Eiceman et al. 2001).

13.3.4 PRACTICAL USE OF MICRO GAS CHROMATOGRAPHY

Although there have been impressive advances in technology for μGC systems, there remain challenges to their widespread use in everyday applications. One of the main hindrances to μGC use outside of controlled laboratory conditions is varying climates. Soo et al. (2018) found that with a relative humidity of 75%, a commercially available μGC with a PID had its analytical capability cut by about half for certain compounds when compared to use with a relative humidity of 25%. This performance failed to meet the accuracy criterion by the National Institute for Occupational Safety and Health (NIOSH 2012). These limitations were attributed to humidity interference on the preconcentrator, which was composed of silica gel and absorbs water more readily than most organic compounds (Melcher et al. 1978).

The ideal end state of μGC systems would be their practical use as a wearable device. However, portable systems currently available in the market weigh approximately 13–19 kg or more. Nevertheless, technology continues to advance to possibly make wearable μGC systems a viable option one day. Wang et al. (2016), for example, developed a prototype for a battery-powered μGC system with a preconcentrator–focuser and chemiresistor detector that weighs just 2.1 kg.

13.4 PARTICULATE MATTER MEASUREMENTS

Particulate matter is generated from many different activities, and particulates smaller than 2.5 and 10 μm are well-known for their association with adverse respiratory and cardiovascular health effects. Most portable particulate matter instruments with real-time sensing use an optical method for measurements (Loh et al. 2017). High-end sensors include lasers, and others use a different photodiode to produce light through which particles are counted as they pass.

Currently, available particulate matter sensors are best suited for stationary rather than portable monitoring. Even outdoor applications may be problematic for these instruments where there are higher particulate matter concentrations and relative humidity (Ueberham and Schlink 2018).

13.5 NOISE MEASUREMENTS

Hazardous noise is a direct cause for hearing loss, and it causes other negative health effects such as stress, increased blood pressure, and increased heart rate. For these reasons, in addition to interference with voice communications, it is important to verify noise levels are acceptable.

Noise is one of the most easily measured physical stressors. There are apps, many of which are free, available for smartphones as well as inexpensive devices readily available. However, many of these common measurement tools do not meet standard specifications. For example, most microphones in smartphones are aligned to the human voice (300–400 Hz and 40–60 dB) and may not reliably measure sounds outside those frequencies or sound range (Kardous and Shaw 2014). Furthermore, many apps and devices may not be calibrated, do not provide weighting options (e.g., dBA), or lack the ability to analyze noise frequency. Despite their limitations, they have been useful for citizen scientists and noise mapping projects (Maisonneuve et al. 2009).

13.6 INTERNET OF THINGS

Portability of sensors enables the ability for measurement data to be integrated into internet-linked mobile devices such as smartphones. With such data uploaded to an internet platform, healthcare professionals and researchers may offer possibilities to a world of information at a scale previously unattainable. Not only could physicians monitor environmental triggers for adverse health outcomes such as asthma in individuals, but public health scientists could ascertain trends in environmental exposures, especially if the data is linked to locations with geographic information systems (GIS).

This concept easily aligns with the IoT realm. One definition for IoT is "the networking capability that allows information to be sent to and received from objects and devices using the Internet" (Merriam-Webster 2019). IoT is a global network infrastructure of numerous connected devices that rely on sensory, communication, networking, and information processing technologies (Tan and Wang 2010). Although a foundational technology for IoT is radio-frequency identification (RFID), wireless sensor networks (WSNs) are also key. Barcodes, smartphones, social networks, and cloud computing support IoT as well (Xu et al. 2014).

13.6.1 Data Management

Current environmental exposure measurement systems largely rely on manual processing and analysis of data, which do not leverage real-time data acquisition and communications. One of the main obstacles in making portable environmental exposure sensor data useful is in processing the potentially large data sets and providing salient information in real time (Bae et al. 2013). The volume of data generated from personal sensors could result in intolerant latency, making a significant challenge to deliver important data in a real-time manner (Mukhopadhyay 2015). In order to optimize such a system, the amount of data chosen would need to be robust enough to avoid blind spots, but not so voluminous for practical storage and processing time.

There are established data analysis algorithms that can find patterns, outliers, and classifications. Statistical algorithms, such as Bayesian Item Response Theory and Item Response Theory, can predict the combined effect of spatial-temporal variables on the susceptibility of an individual to a specific health effect (Bae et al. 2013). Bae et al. (2016) also developed a Voroni map method for estimating environmental exposures based on a probabilistic routing aggregation that copes with uncertainty.

13.6.2 Location Tracking

GIS using location tracking such as global positioning system (GPS) technology is a nearly universal feature in smartphones. Linking sensors with these mobile devices would give a valuable dimension to sensor data analysis. Bae et al. (2013) proposed a system in which sensors are interfaced with Android mobile phones, and corresponding GPS data is collected real time, transferred to servers, stored in an extensible markup language (XML) format, and later integrated with other GIS datasets.

13.6.3 SYSTEM ARCHITECTURE

Although an environmental exposure system integrated with mobile internet-enabled devices is not yet a reality, there are certain features the architecture of such a system should include (Bae et al. 2013).

13.6.3.1 Security, Reliability, and Usability

There are potential security concerns for users, especially when exposure data is connected to an individual's personal information. Ethical issues may also be raised when considering that data ownership and protection rules are not clear. If sensor data is collected as part of research, participants must have informed consent and clearly understand the terms of participation and how the data will be used. However, companies that own data can typically deal with data privacy as they wish without consulting users, and data protection laws vary among countries.

13.6.3.2 Extensibility

The IoT universe will continue to grow. An exposome monitoring system will include new algorithms and components that must be accommodated into an existing framework.

13.6.3.3 Performance

In order to be useful, the system must be able to process large data sets and extract meaningful data in a timely fashion. Advances in computing and related disciplines will help usher in this capability.

13.6.3.4 Simplicity and Organization

Ideally, this system will be reasonably simplicity with a high degree of organization. Otherwise, there is a potential for high complexity without a suitable framework. However, simplicity may be elusive given the lack of a widely accepted IoT platform and heterogeneity of its underlying networks (Xu et al. 2014).

13.7 FEASIBLE SYSTEMS FOR TODAY

The possibilities of networked wearable portable sensors connected to GIS data that provide real-time analysis of the external exposome over the internet is a tantalizing prospect. However, work remains to make this scenario a reality. In the meantime, a monitoring system built around a smaller set of portable sensors as well as stationary or publically available sources is a more feasible scenario (Loh et al. 2017). There have also been demonstrated advancements in wearable sensors for single analytes. For example, Li et al. (2019) developed a wearable IoT aldehyde sensor based on an electrochemical fuel cell and integrated with a cloud-based informatics system.

13.8 CONCLUSIONS

Personal sensors for monitoring the external exposome are improving in accessibility, reliability and ease of use, and promise to one day be a practical IoT option.

Coupled with future advances in statistics, data mining techniques, computing power, and careful sharing of data resources while protecting personal data, we may realize a sophisticated and powerful network of environmental exposure sensors.

DISCLAIMER

The views expressed are those of the author and do not necessarily reflect the official policy or position of the Air Force, the Department of Defense, or the U.S. Government.

REFERENCES

Akbar, M.; Wang, D.; Goodman, R.; Hoover, A.; Rice, G.; Heflin, J.R.; Agah, M. (2013) Improved performance of micro-fabricated preconcentrators using silica nanoparticles as a surface template. *J. Chromatog. A*, 1322:1–7.

Ali, S.; Ashraf-Khorassani, M.; Taylor, L.T.; Agah, M. (2009) MEMS-based semi-packed gas chromatography columns. *Sens. Actuators*, 141:309–315.

Bae, W. D.; Alkobaisi, S.; Narayanappa, S.; Liu, C. C. (2013) A real-time health monitoring system for evaluating environmental exposures. *J. Software*, 8(4):791–801.

Bae, W. D.; Alkobaisi, S.; Meyers, W.; Narayanappa, S.; Vojtěchovský, P. (2016) Voroni maps: an approach to individual-based environmental exposure estimation. *The 31st Annual ACM Symposium*, Pisa, Italy, April 2016.

Bhushan, A.; Yemane, D.; Overton, E.B.; Goettert, J.; Murphy, M.C. (2007a) Fabrication and preliminary results for LiGA fabricated nickel micro gas chromatograph columns. *Microelectromech. Syst.* 16(2):383–393.

Bhushan, A.; Yemane, D,; Trudell, D.; Overton, E.B.; Goettert, J. (2007b) Fabrication of micro-gas chromatograph columns for fast chromatography. *Microsys. Technol.* 13:361–368.

Bourlon, B.; Pham Ho, B.-A.; Ricoul, F.; Chappuis, T.; Bellemin Comte, A.; Constantin, O.; Icard, B. (2016) Revisiting gas sampling and analysis with microtechnology: feasibility of low cost handheld gas chromatographs. Conference: IEEE Sensors, 1–3. doi:10.1109/ICSENS.2016.7808672.

Briscoe, C.G.; Yu, H.; Grodzinski, P.; Huang, R.-F.; Burdon, J.W. (2004) *Multilayered Ceramic Micro-gas Chromatograph and Method for Making the Same*. US Patent 6,732,567, 11 May 2004.

Camara, E.H.M.; Breuil, P., Briand, D., de Rooij, N.F.; Pijolat, C. (2011) A micro gas preconcentrator with improved performance for pollution monitoring and explosives detection. *Anal. Chim. Acta*, 688(20):175–182.

Cesar, W.; Flourens, F.; Kaiser, C.; Sutour, C.; Angelescu, Dan E. (2015) Enhanced microgas chromatography using correlation techniques for continuous indoor pollutant detection. *Anal. Chem.*, 87:5620–5625.

Cheng, Y.-K.; Lin, C.-H.; Kuo, S.; Hsiung, S.-Y.; Wang J.-L. (2012) Applications of Hadamard transform-gas chromatography/mass spectrometry for the detection of hexamethyldisiloxane in a wafer cleanroom. *J. Chromatogr. A*, 1220:143–146.

Collin, W.R.; Bondy, A.; Paul, D.; Kurabayshi, K.; Zellers, E.T. (2015) μGC x μGC: comprehensive two-dimensional gas chromatographic separations with microfabricated components. *Anal. Chem.*, 87:1630–1637.

Darko, E.; Thurbide, K.B.; Gerhardt, G.C.; Michienzi, J. (2013) Micro-flame photometric detection in miniature gas chromatography on a titanium tile. *Anal. Chem.*, 85:5376–5381.

Deville Cavellin, L.; Weichenthal, S.; Tack, R; Ragettli, M.S.; Smargiassi, A.; Hatzopoulou, M. (2016) Investigating the use or portable air pollution sensors to capture the spatial variability of traffic-related air pollution. *Environ. Sci. Technol.,* 50(1):313–320.

Du, Z.; Tsow, F.; Wang, D.; Tao, N. (2018) Real-time simultaneous separation and detection of chemicals using integrated microcolumn and surface plasmon resonance imaging micro-GC. *IEEE Sens. J.,* 18(4):1351–1357.

Dziuban, J.; Mroz, J.; Szczygielska, M.; Malachowski, M; Gorecka-Drzazga, A.; Walczak, R., Bula, W.; Zalewski, D.; Lysko, J.; Koxzur, J. (2004) Portable gas chromatograph with integrated components. *J. Sens. Actuators A,* 115:318–330.

Eiceman, G.A., Tadjikov, B., Krylov, E., Nazarov, E., Miller, R.A., Westbrook, J., and Funk, P.A. (2001) Miniature radio-frequency mobility analyzer as a gas chromatographic detector for oxygen-containing volatile organic compounds, pheromones and other insect attractants. *J. Chromatography A,* 917:205–217.

Frye-Mason, G.; Kottenstette, R.; Lewis, P.; Heller, E.; Manginell, R.; Adkins, D.; Dulleck, G.; Martinez, D.; Sasaki, D.; Mowry, C. (2000) Hand-Held Miniature Chemical Analysis System (μChemlab) for Detection of Trace Concentrations of Gas Phase Analytes. In: *Micro Total Analysis Systems,* van den Berg, A., Olthuis, W., Bergveld, P., Eds; Springer, Dordrecht, 229–232.

Garg, A.; Akbar, M.; Vejeranon, E.; Narayanan, S.; Nazhandali, L.; Marr, L.C.; Agah, M. (2015) Zebra GC: A mini gas chromatography system for trace-level determination of hazardous air pollutants. *Sens. Actuators B,* 212:145–154.

Hayward, T.C.; Thurbide, K.B. (2008) Novel on-column and inverted operating modes of a microcounter-current flame ionization detector. *J. Chromatogr. A,* 1200:2–7.

Iwaya, T.; Akao, S.; Sakamoto, T.; Tsuji, T.; Nakaso, N.; Yamanaka, K. (2012) Development of high precision metal micro-electro-mechanical-systems column for portable surface acoustic wave gas chromatograph. *Jpn. J. Appl. Phys.* 51:07GC24.

Jespers, S.; Schlautmann, S.; Gardeniers, H.J.; De Malsche, W.; Lynen, F.; Desmet, G. (2017) Chip-based multicapillary column with maximal interconnectivity to combine maximum efficiency and maximum loadability. *Anal. Chem.,* 89:11605–11613.

Kardous, C.A.; Shaw, P.B. (2014) Evaluation of smartphone sound measurement applications. *J. Acoust. Soc. Am.,* 135:EL186–EL192.

Klee, M.S.; Williams, M.D.; Chang, I.; Murphy, J. (1999) Superior ECD performance through design and application. *J. High Resolut. Chromatogr.,* 22:24–28.

Lewis, A.C.; Hamilton, J.F.; Rhodes, C.N.; Halliday, J.; Bartle, K.D.; Homewood, P.; Grenfell, R.J.; Goody, B.; Harling, A.M.; Brewer, P. (2010) Microfabricated planar glass gas chromatography with photoionization detection. *J. Chromatogr. A,* 1217:768–774.

Lewis, P.R.; Wheeler, D.R. (2007) *Non-Planar Microfabricated Gas Chromatography Colum.* US Patent 7,273,517, 25 September 2007.

Li, B., Dong, Q., Downen, R.S., Tran, N., Jackson, J.H., Pillai, D., Zaghlouol, M., and Li, Z. (2019) A wearable IoT aldehyde sensor for pediatric asthma research and management. *Sens. Actuators B Chem.,* 287: 584–594.

Liu, Z.; Philips, J.B. (1991) Comprehensive two-dimensional gas chromatography using an on-column thermal modular interface. *J. Chromatogr. Sci.,* 29:227–231.

Loh, M.; Sarigiannis, D.; Gotti, A.; Karakitsios, S.; Pronk, A.; Kuijpers, E.; Annesi-Maesano, I.; Baiz, N.; Madureira, J.; Fernandes, E. O.; Jerrett, M.; Cherrie, J. W. (2017) How sensors might help define the external exposome. *Int J. Environ. Res. Public Health,* 14: 434.

Luong, J.; Nazarov, E.; Gras, R.; Shellie, R.A. (2012) Resistively heated temperature programmable silicon micromachined gas chromatography with differential mobility spectrometry. *J. Ion. Mobil. Spectrom.,* 15:179–187.

Lussac, E.; Barattin, R.; Cardinael, P.; Agasse, V. (2016) Review on micro-gas analyzer systems: feasibility, separations and applications. *Crit. Rev. Anal. Chem.,* 46(6):455–468.

Maisonneuve, N.; Stevens, M.; Niessen, M.E.; Stells, L. (2009) NoiseTube: measuring and mapping noise pollution with mobile phones. In *Information Technologies in Environmental Engineering*; Athanasiadis, I.N.; Rissolil, A.E.; Mitkas, P.A.; Gomez, J.M.; Eds.; Springer: Berlin, pp. 215–228.

Manginell, R.P.; Frye-Mason, G.C.; Kottenstette, R.; Lewis, P.R.; Wong, C.C. (2000) *Microfabricated Planar Preconcentrator.* Sandia National Laboratories: Albuquerque, NM.

Melcher, R.G.; Langner, R.L.; Kagel, R.O. (1978) Criteria for the evaluation methods for the collection of organic pollutants in air using solid sorbents. *Am Ind. Hyg. Assoc. J.,* 39(5):349–361.

Merriam-Webster. (2019) https://www.merriam-webster.com/dictionary/Internet%20of%20 Things, accessed 17 May 2019.

Mukhopadhyay, Subhas Chandra. (2015) Wearable sensors for human activity monitoring: a review. *IEEE Sens. J.,* 15(3):1321–1330.

Nieuwenhuijsen, Mark J.; Donaire-Gonzalez, D.; Foraster, M.; Martinez, D.; Cisneros, A. (2014) Using personal sensors to assess the exposome and acute health effects. *Int. J. Environ. Res. Public Health,* 11(8):7805–7819.

National Institute for Occupational Safety and Health. (2012) *NIOSH Technical Report 2012–162: Components for Evaluation of Direct-Reading Monitors for Gases and Vapors,* Cincinnati, OH.

Noh, H.-s.; Hesketh, P.J.; Frye-Mason, G.C. (2002) Parylene gas chromatrographic column for rapid thermal cycling. *J. Microelectromech. Syst.,* 11:718–725.

Poole, C. (1982) The electron-capture detector in capillary column gas chromatography. *J. High Resolut. Chromatogr.,* 5:454–471.

Radadia, A.; Salehi-Khojin, A.; Masel, R.; Shannon, M. (2010) Effect of column geometry on the performance of micro-gas chromatrography columns for chip scale gas analyzers. *Sens. Actuators B,* 150(1):456–464.

Randadia, A.D.; Morgan, R.D.; Masel, R.I.; Shannon, M.A. (2009) Partially buried microcolumns for micro gas analyzers. *Anal. Chem,* 81:3471–3477.

Raut, R.P.; Thurbide, K.B. (2017) Characterization of titanium tiles as novel platforms for micro-flame ionization detection in miniature gas chromatography. *Chromatographia,* 80:805–812.

Regmi, B. P.; Agah, M. (2018) Micro gas chromatography: an overview of critical components and their integration. *Anal. Chem.,* 90:13133–13150.

Schisla, D.; Ding, H.; Carr, P.; Cussler, E. (1993) Polydisperse tube diameters compromise multiple open tubular chromatography. *AIChE J.,* 39:946–953.

Smit, H.C. (1970) Random input and correlation methods to improve the signal-to-noise ratio in chromatographic trace analysis. *Chromatographia,* 3:515–518.

Soo, J.-C.; Lee, E. G.; LeBouf, R. F.; Kashon, M. L., Chisholm, W.; Harper, M. (2018) Evaluation of a portable gas chromatograph with photoionization detector under variations of VOC concentration, temperature, and relative humidity. *J. Occup. Environ. Health,* 15(4): 351–360.

Staples, E.J.; Viswanathan, S. (2005) Ultrahigh-speed chromatography and virtual chemical sensors for detecting explosives and chemical warfare agents. *IEEE Sens. J.,* 5: 622–631.

Sun, J.H.; Cui, D.; Cai, H.Y.; Chen, X.; Zhang, L.L.; Li, H. (2012) Design, modeling, microfabrication and characterization of the micro gas chromatography columns. *Adv. Gas Chromatogr. Prog. Agric. Biomed. Ind. Appl.,* 3:51–66.

Sun, J.H.; Guan, F.; Cui, D.; Chen, X.; Zhang, L.; Chen, J. (2013) An improved photoionization detector with micro gas chromatography column for portable rapid gas chromatography system. *J. Sens. Actuators B,* 188:513–518.

Sun, J.H.; Guan, F.Y.; Zhu, X.F.; Ning, Z.W.; Ma, T.J.; Liu, J.H.; Deng, T. (2016) Micro-fabricated packed gas chromatography column based on laser etching technology. *J. Chromatogr. A.*, 1429:311–316.

Tan, L.; Wang, N. (2010) Future internet: the internet of things. In *Proc. 3rd Int. Conf. Adv. Comput. Theory Eng. (ICACTE)*, Chengdu, China, 20–22 August 2010, pp. V5-376–V5-380.

Terry, S.C.; Jerman, J.H.; Angell, J.B. (1979) A gas chromatographic air analyzer fabricated on a silicon wafer. *IEEE Trans. Electron. Devices*, 26:1880–1886.

Tian, W.-C.; Chan, H.K.L.; Lu, C.-J.; Pang, S.W.; Zellers, E.T. (2005) Multiple-stage microfabricated preconcentrator focuser for micro gas chromatography system. *J. Microelectromech. Syst.*, 14(3):498–507.

Turner, M. C.; Nieuwenhuijsen, M. J.; Anderson, K.; Balshaw, D.; Cui, Y.; Dunton, G.; Hoppin, J. A.; Koutrakis, P.; Jerret, M. (2017) Assessing the exposome with external measures: commentary on the state of the science and research recommendations. *Annu. Rev. Public Health*, 28:215–239.

Ueberham, Maximilian; Schlink, Uwe. (2018) Wearable sensors for multifactorial personal exposure measurements—a ranking study. *Environ. Int.*, 121:130–138.

Wang, A.; Hynynen, S. Hawkins, A.R.; Tolley, S.E.; Tolley, H.D.; Lee M.L. (2014) Axial thermal gradients in microchip gas chromatography *J. Chromatogr.* 1374: 216–223.

Wang, J.; Nuñovero, N.; Lin, Z.; Nidetz, R.; Buggaveeti, S.; Zhan, C.; Kurabayashi, K.; Steinecker, W.H.; Zellers, E.T. (2016) A wearable MEMS gas chromatograph for multi-vapor determinations. *Proc. Eng.*, 168:1398–1401.

Wang, A.; Tolley, H.D.; Lee, M.L. (2012) Gas chromatography using resistive heating technology. *J. Chromatogr. A*, 1261:46–57.

Whiting, J.J.; Fix, C.S.; Anderson, J.M.; Staton, A.W.; Manginell, R.P.; Wheeler, D.R.; Myers, E.B.; Roukes, M.L.; Simonson, R. (2009) In TRANSDUCERS 2009-International Conference on Solid-State Sensors, *Actuators and Microsystems Conference*, IEEE, Denver, CO, 1666–1669.

Wild, C.P. (2005) Complementing the genome with an "exposome": the outstanding challenge of environmental exposure measurement in molecular epidemiology. *Cancer Epidemiol. Biomarkers Prev.*, 14(8):1847–1850.

Wild, C.P. (2012) The exposome: from concept to utility. *Int. J. Epidemiol.*, 41(1):24–32.

Williams, D.; Pappas G. (1999) Rapid identification of nerve agents Sarin (GB) and Soman (GD) with use of a field-portable GC/SAW vapor detector and liquid desorption front-end device. *Field Anal. Chem. Technol.*, 3:45–53.

Xu, L. D.; He, W.; Li, S. (2014) Internet of things in industries: a survey. *IEEE Trans. Ind. Inform.*, 10(4):2233–2243.

Yost, R.A.; Hail, M.E. (1992) Direct Resistive Heating and Temperature Measurement of Metal-clad Capillary Columns in Gas Chromatography and Related Separation Techniques. US Patent 5,114,439, 19 May 1992.

Zhu, H.; Zhou, M.; Lee, J.; Nidetz, R.; Kurabayashi, K.; Fan, X. (2016) Low-power miniaturized helium dielectric barrier discharge photoionization detectors for highly sensitive vapor detection. *Lab Chip*, 15:3021–3029.

Zimmermann, S.; Wischhusen, S.; Mueller, J. (2000) Micro flame ionization detector and micro flame spectrometer. *J. Sens. Actuators B*, 63:159–166.

14 Sensor Platforms and Wireless Networks

Kevin Montgomery
IoT/AI Inc.

CONTENTS

14.1 INTRODUCTION

In order to obtain data from field and industrial locations of interest, one requires some means of acquiring the data and some back-end to store and access the data. This chapter discusses key ideas behind sensor platforms and wireless networks to support Total Exposure Health.

14.1.1 SAMPLING/TRANSMISSION BACKGROUND

Data can be acquired in two different paradigms: logging (with later subsequent download) and transmission (either wired or wireless, perhaps in real time). Objectively, these two paradigms are technologically very similar, and the paradigm selected relates to whether the method of transmission is at the sampling location or at some other (perhaps laboratory) location.

An important concept to note is that there is a difference between the time and frequency that data are sampled (sampling frequency) vs the time which data are transmitted (transmit frequency). For example, a particular sensor could be sampled 100 times per second (100 Hz), but data aggregated in the sensor device would only be transmitted once per hour. Or, in the case of a logging paradigm, data could be sampled over a period of weeks, and the devices manually collected and brought back to a lab for download of data (hence a transmit/download time on the order of weeks). When the sampling time is very close to the transmission time and

DOI: 10.1201/9780429263286-16

individual samples transmitted as acquired, the user terms the data acquisition to be "real time." When the sampling time is similar to the transmission time, the user terms the data acquisition to be "near real time," although this is largely a semantic difference along a spectrum of data acquisition.

It is important to note that the sampling frequency or transmission frequency timing may not be regular. A device could sample a sensor on regular intervals or only upon an external trigger. For example, a light detection sensor could trigger a device to wake up and capture an image. This discussion will term this type of sampling "triggered sampling." Similarly, a device could acquire and store a significant number of samples of data and only transmit them when a condition is met (for example, if those samples indicate an important event such as a threshold exceeded for a particular reading; or, alternatively, a device could transmit only in response to another device requesting its data). This type of sampling will be called "triggered transmission."

Thus, in general, sensors can be sampled on regular intervals (on-schedule sampling), or upon triggering (on-event sampling), or from an external source (on-demand sampling). While a data logging paradigm is important and the predominant method for data acquisition, the rest of this chapter will focus on issues related to data transmission.

14.1.2 Commercial Context

When understanding sensor and data acquisition/transmission technologies, it is also important to understand that they exist within a business or commercial context.

Currently, sensor manufacturers integrate into vertical markets to try to develop solutions to address a particular market need or niche, thus they try to develop a complete solution for the end customer, typically termed "B2C" for Business-to-Customer. This is in contrast to a different business paradigm where the manufacturer develops technologies solely for inclusion into the products created by other companies, termed an "original equipment manufacturer" (OEM) or a Business-to-Business (B2B) paradigm.

Those sensor companies that attempt to develop complete solutions, as stated above, also need to develop a means for data transmission and a back-end to store, process, and derive understanding from that data. Thus, in order to produce solutions, these manufacturers develop their own (typically proprietary, limited) transmission and back-end data storage systems to try to lock in end-users to their business ecosystem. However, sensor manufacturers typically are not experts in data transmission or data storage/databases; they know and are focused on sensors and detection.

Industrial hygiene and other applications, on the other hand, often require the integration of multimodal data from a multitude of sensor modalities. For example, data from noise sensors, air chemistry or particulate sensors, etc., may all be used. If each sensor is developed by a different company that provides a different means of data transmission and back-end, then the end-user is required to cobble together data streams from several proprietary systems and become a systems integrator between incompatible systems. This, in short, is painful, and computer/software system integration is not a typical skillset among the industrial hygiene (IH) end-user community.

Instead, a better idea would be an open, interoperable, common platform across sensor manufacturers so that data integration of other data sources, including personnel exposure monitors, area sensors, even satellite data transmission could be easily integrated. Once this new paradigm for industrial hygiene is chosen using interoperable sensors and open platforms, data fusion across modalities and all sources to obtain a holistic picture of exposure will be possible.

This chapter seeks to present a mental framework for this topic, survey options, and tradeoffs for implementation and provide an insight into the future of complete solutions for IH applications.

14.2 TERMINOLOGY

The following terminology will aid this discussion:

- Detector—samples a single parameter/detects a single agent (e.g., potential hydrogen [pH])
- Sensor—consists of one or more detectors (e.g., multiparameter water anode with pH, oxidation-reduction potential (ORP), and turbidity integrated into one device).
- Sensor platform (aka device)—comprises 0 or more sensors, provides means for data storage, transmission, optional local analytics, etc. (0 sensors = repeater or gateway).
- Station—deployed sensor platform with relevant sensors. Stations can be in fixed locations or mobile vehicle (e.g., unmanned aerial vehicle [UAV], truck) or personal/wearable mounted.
- System—comprises sensors, sensor platforms, along with back-end data storage, analytics, visualization, etc.
- Solution—uses a system to solve a problem, answer a question, distinction=purpose.

14.3 CHALLENGES

A series of challenges exist in the development and deployment of sensor systems, including the following:

- *Size/weight vs transmission power/lifetime*: For wearable/small sensor devices, the devices must be small and lightweight and hence utilize small batteries. This necessarily implies a trade-off of range and/or transmission frequency in order to achieve a sufficient operational duty cycle and battery lifetime. However, these effects can be ameliorated using a hybrid topology network as described below.
- *Competing for location requirements*: Often, the best place to take a reading or sample may not be the best place to mount a device and obtain power, and the best place to mount may not be the best location for transmission.

This can be ameliorated to some small degree: the antenna cables can be placed in an optimal location to radiate and a longer sensor cable can allow the sensor to be placed in the appropriate location so that the sensor device itself may be positioned for the optimal mounting and power location.

- *External dependencies*: Deploying sensor systems with a dependency on external infrastructure (such as cellular or wireless fidelity [Wi-Fi], power, etc.) can all be compromised. Many systems have been deployed which rely on an optimal set of conditions to be met (reliable power, cellular access, etc.), and users have become painfully aware of the fragility of external infrastructure, especially when infrastructures are owned and operated by groups over which the user has little control. Therefore, a redundant, reliable system needs to minimize such dependencies with internal batteries to smooth out and ameliorate unreliable power and wireless transmission systems that employ graceful degradation techniques to maintain and preserve data in the face of communication disruptions.
- *Proprietary vs open*: Many proprietary ecosystems of solutions exist but often are not cost effective nor as innovative. However, open-source systems often prove to be worth their extra cost.

14.4 SENSOR INTERFACES AND PROTOCOLS

Sensors and detectors can be connected to a sensor platform device through many different interface standards (e.g., analog, serial (RS232/485), interface to communicate (I2C), system packet interface (SPI), universal serial bus (USB), ethernet, containing speed/bandwidth, distance, etc.). Options are shown in Table 14.1.

As is evident from the table, each method of interfacing has its own tradeoffs. In general, the thinner the gauge or longer the wire, the harder it is to pass and resolve electronic signals at the other end. A simple voltage will dissipate with distance, so current loop (typically 4–20 mA) analog transmission is used in industrial settings

---

TABLE 14.1

Options for Interface Standards to Connect Sensors/Detectors to Sensor Platform Devices

Interface Type	Bandwidth/Speed	Distance	Circuitry Requirements
Analog (voltage)	Limited by wire	Limited by wire	None
Analog (current loop)	Varies	100 m–1000 m+	Very little
Serial (RS232)	9.6–980 kbps	15 m	Minor
Serial (RS422/485)	Up to 10 Mbps	1200 m	Minor
I2C	100 kbps–3.4 Mbps	1–10 m	Moderate
SPI	1–20 Mbps	3 m (typical)	Moderate
USB (1/1.1/2/3)	1.5/12/480/5000 Mbps	5 m	Greater
Ethernet	10 Mbps–10 Gpbs	100 m	Greater

kbps—Kilobytes per second, Mbps—Megabytes per second, m—Meters.

for longer wire runs. Higher-level protocols and encoding methods present in RS232 (a simple interface of typically two to four wires—send, receive, power, ground) or RS422/485 (similar to RS232 but uses two wires each for send and receive in order to provide for a differential voltage) can extend range significantly. Yet, higher-level protocols and encoding methods as listed in the table can send and receive data even faster, although always with a tradeoff of distance. However, it is important to keep in mind that within the context of sensors, the distances from a hardwired sensor to its platform device is typically very short (on the order of a few meters). More importantly, the interface needed by a particular sensor of interest must be the primary concern when choosing what interface to use.

Beyond the electrical and signaling interfaces described above, a protocol for data acquisition is also layered on top. While the underlying interface may be RS232, a particular serial sensor will perhaps have a command to request its data and a means of encoding that data.

These sensor protocols tend to be very specific and proprietary to individual sensor manufacturers. While there have been many efforts to standardize sensor data transmission protocols, such as Sensor Model Language (SensorML), the vast majority of sensors provide a proprietary interface most appropriate for a target market. In the industrial market, this may be 4–20 milliamperes (mA) current loop as the de facto standard, whereas simple detectors may be analog voltage, and higher-end sensors may provide an ethernet interface with robust signaling protocol (such as Common Chemical, Biological, Radiological Nuclear (CBRN) Sensor Interface (CCSI in the Department of Defense context).

While on the surface this diversity may seem nonsensical, the reason for this lack of sensor interface and communication standardization is not new nor is it arbitrary. Manufacturers desire to provide the simplest and most optimal interface possible to decrease the cost and complexity of a design. Requiring all sensors to provide an ethernet interface would impose an undue cost, complexity, and power burden on a particular sensor and may not be appropriate for all markets and applications.

14.5   SENSOR PLATFORM

A sensor platform (more informally called a sensor device) is designed to acquire time-accurate data from sensors and log or transmit data as required. This section will explore several factors related to the development and deployment of such sensor platforms.

A sensor platform or device may support a multitude of sensors, or it may only allow for one interface. It may have internal sensors such as internal temperature, battery/charging voltages, and other parameters.

One of these internal sensors may provide location information. The Global Positioning System (GPS) is a satellite-based system that has been widely available since the mid-1990s, which uses a constellation of low-earth orbiting (LEO) satellites. The GPS can provide location accuracy to within 4 m horizontally. However, these satellite signals, like any radio frequency (RF) signal, can be reflected and provide inaccurate readings and are subject to spoofing or interference. Additional problems are that GPS signals are usually not available in-buildings or in subterranean environments. Non-GPS localization technologies, such as time difference on arrival (TDOA) and other RF triangulation methods, or inertial "dead reckoning" techniques, have been developed to provide location information in interior, subterranean, or GPS-denied/challenged environments. A robust sensor platform should support a multitude of techniques and provide mitigation against GPS spoofing and denial/challenge environments.

Another important issue in sensor platforms is maintaining accurate time across a multitude of different deployed devices. This is required in order to correlate data samples across several devices. This initially seems like a non-issue, but it is actually quite a bit more complicated. Microprocessor timing is usually derived from an oscillating crystal, and the resonation can be affected by temperature and/or manufacturing differences. In practice, drifts of a few seconds over a few days are possible, leading to increasing imprecision as deployment time continues. In daily use, cell phones and computers sync to a time service (either provided by the cellular carrier, the National Institute of Standards and Technology (NIST), or other authoritative time service) to re-sync their clocks on a daily basis. Similarly, a network of deployed sensors needs to sync timing in order to maintain time accuracy. While the GPS signal can also provide time information, in GPS unavailable/denied/ challenged/spoofed environments, this may not be possible. While many low-cost sensor systems do not address this issue, a reliable sensor platform should provide for an update of valid, authoritative, authenticated/ encrypted time update information on a regular basis to ensure accuracy of the timing of sample acquisition.

Another factor to consider for a sensor platform is power. Options include alternating current (AC) (wall power), direct current (DC) (vehicle or industrial power), internal battery (of some capacity), solar, wind, fuel cell, thermoelectric power generation (TEG), inertial, etc. Typically, sensor devices have a battery in their system to maintain operation even if main power becomes unavailable. A secondary reason for some means of power storage, whether battery or capacitor storage based, is to smooth out fluctuations in power from an unreliable source, or to smooth out power due to uneven load. For example, if a sensor device has a transmitter that pulls quite a bit of current, this power load may be in excess of the capacity of the incoming power.

Battery types are usually separated into two main categories: Primary cells or rechargeable. Primary cells have limited capacity and cannot be recharged. Typical examples include AA, AAA, and 9 volt (9 V) format alkaline batteries, although more specialized primary chemistries exist (including Lithium, Carbon–Zinc, and Zinc–Air). Table 14.2 shows several rechargeable battery options.

When selecting and evaluating battery options for a sensor platform, consideration of the method and capacity of charging, environmental conditions, storage lifetime, cycle life, and other factors are important to ensure a robust system.

Another factor in the development and deployment of sensor devices is the sampling dynamics. A sensor platform should support the regular, timed sampling of a sensor (sample on schedule), but ideally would also provide for collecting a sample when a condition is triggered or met (sampling on event), or when directed to do so from a remote request (sampling on demand). Providing for these sampling dynamics allows a sensor system to support flexible multimodal sampling, so that the output

TABLE 14.2

Rechargeable Battery Options to Support Sensor Technology

Chemistry	Li-Ion/polymer	LiFePO₄	NiCd	NiMH	Sealed Lead Acid (SLA)	Silver oxide
Sizes	18,650 and prismatic sizes	18,650, 26,650, and large prismatic	Widest selection of cylindrical and button sizes	Button and round cells	Large prismatic format	Button cell configurations
Shelf life/self-discharge	≤3% month	≤3% month	20%/month	30%/month	5%/month	Charge retention is over 84% after two years of storage at 70 F (21°C)
Capacity	500 mAh–10,000 mAh	1 Ah to 20 Ah+	11 mAh to 20,000 +mAh	11 mAh to 20,000 +mAh	500 mAh to 100 Ah or more	14 mAh t0 180 mAh
Energy by volume	250 Watt hour/Liter	220 Watt hour/cc	40–60 Watt hour/kg	N/A	30 Watt Hour/kg	60 Wh/lb. (130 Wh/kg)
Energy by weight	120 Watt hour/kg	90+ Watt hour/kg	Watt hour/cubic centimeter	60–80 Watt hour/kg	Watt hour/cubic centimeter	8.2 Wh/cubic inch (500 Wh/l)
Cycle life	500+	2,000–7,000	500–5,000	500	200–500	n/a
Operating temperature range	–20–60°C	–40 to +60°C	–40 to +60°C	–20 to +60°C	–20 to +60°C	–20 to +60°C
Preferred charge method	constant current (CC)/constant voltage (CV)	CC/CV to	Constant current (–D V fast)	DT/dt – peak voltage detect and timer	Constant voltage C/10 to C/4	n/a
Charge temperature	–0 to +45°C	–0 to +45°C	0 to 45°C	0 to 45°C	–20 to 50°C	n/a
Discharge temperature	–20 to 60°C	–20 to 60°C	–20 to 60°C	–20 to 60°C	–20 to 60°C	–20 to +60°C
Charge cutoff voltage	4.2	3.6	Full charge detection by voltage signature	Full charge detection by voltage signature	2.40 Float 2.25	n/a

mAh—milliamp hours.

of one sensor can be used to trigger the sampling of another sensor, perhaps attached to a different type of sensor. An environmental monitoring example of such an application would be a water level sensor being triggered to sample more frequently when a rain gauge sensor detects a rainfall event greater than 1 inch per hour for a flood monitoring application. A personnel exposure monitoring example would be the rapid acquisition of sound level once a threshold value (85 decibels A-weighted [dBA]) is exceeded.

A final factor that should be noted for a sensor platform is its ability to perform analytics "at the edge" (meaning, at the sensor device itself). Many sensors lose sensitivity as time goes on and their reagents are depleted, or as other environmental effects impact the sensitivity or specificity of their acquired data. Providing some amount of processing on the sensor device itself is important in order to provide for sensor drift compensation. Further, analytics on the sensor platform to provide for anomaly detection compared to a background of nominal values is also important for triggering and alerts.

In conclusion, a reliable, robust sensor platform should ideally provide the adequate tradeoffs to support external and internal sensors, location (in GPS and non-GPS environments), time accuracy and drift compensation, appropriate power and energy storage methods, flexible sampling dynamics, and analytics in order to provide reliable and accurate sampling.

14.6   WIRELESS RADIOS, TOPOLOGIES, AND PROTOCOLS

A sensor platform or device as outlined above has the primary function of acquiring data from sensors accurately and in reliable space/time. However, beyond mere logging of data for later collection/download, in situ sensors also often provide a method for wireless transmission of data. This wireless transmission is the topic of this section.

A multitude of Internet of Things (IoT) wireless radio options exists, and others are rapidly being added to the marketplace. Examples are shown in Table 14.3.

Beyond those listed above, other less-deployed options exist, such as Internet Protocol version 6 (IPv6) over Low-Power Wireless Personal Area Networks (6LoWPAN), Thread, HaLow™, narrow band internet of things (NB-IOT), near-field communication (NFC), radio frequency identification (RFID), Ingenu, Weightless, Adaptive Network Topology (ANT), DigiMesh®, MiWi, EnOcean, and Dash. The nuances, details, and tradeoffs of the different wireless radio/protocol options should be the topic of a book by itself, but this discussion will address the tradeoffs below that are most relevant to the IH environment.

It is important to note that the non-cellular radio options tend to operate in the 900 MHz, 2.4 GHz, or 5.8 GHz unlicensed RF bands. Of these, the 2.4 GHz band is unlicensed worldwide (for transmitting powers typically less than 1 w), hence many of the radio options desiring a worldwide usage tend to use this band. However, since many devices may be using this spectrum (from local Wi-Fi at 2.4 GHz to wireless headsets operating at 900 MHz), interference is an increasing issue as radio technologies proliferate. An RF spectrum analyzer can be a handy tool to assess the RF spectrum interference present at a deployment location, and proper RF characterization

TABLE 14.3

Examples of Internet of Things (IoT) Wireless Radio Options

Technology	Frequency (Mega or Giga Herts (MHz, GHz)	Speed (Kilo or Mega Bytes Per Second (Kbps, Mbps))	Range (kilometer (km) or meter (m))	Power	Cost
Cellular (3G/4G-LTE, excluding 5G)	800–900 MHz, 1400–1500 MHz	10–100 Mbps	km+	High	High
802.11 (WiFi)	2.4 GHz/5.8 GHz	1–850 Mbps	km	Medium	Medium
802.15.4 (Zigbee)	2.4 GHz	250 Kbps	100 m	Low	Low
Bluetooth	2.4 GHz	1–3 Mbps	10–100 m	Low	Low
Long Range (LoRa)	<1 GHz	<100 Kbps	2–5 km	Low	Medium
SIGFOX	<1 GHz	<100 Kbps	2–5 km	Low	Medium
Wireless HART	2.4 GHz	250 Kbps	100 m	Medium	Medium
Z-Wave	900 MHz	40 Kbps	30 m	Low	Medium

LTE—Long-Term Evolution, HART—Highway Addressable Remote Transducer Protocol.

and spectrum management is important in the deployment of successful sensor networks. Ideally, radio options should not interfere with other devices, and other devices should guard against similar interference Federal Communications Commission (FCC) Part 15.

Further, deployment of radio options in a metal-rich environment, such as an industrial plant, factory, or distribution warehouse, will create more "multipath interference." This interference occurs when wireless radio signals bounce off a metal surface, reflect, and cancel out the primary wave, resulting in "dead zones" of poor signal-to-noise. Some radio options, such as Long Range (LoRa), that utilize novel encoding methods can be more robust in metal-rich environments and can also provide enhanced immunity from interference.

Another factor to consider in radio options is security. The first aspect is RF detectability (often termed Low Probability of Detection (LPD) or Low Probability of Interference (LPI) that relates to whether the RF signal from a radio can even be detected by a competing system. Beyond LPI/LPD, it is important for a sensor network to provide strong methods for authentication (identifying that a station is valid to be on the network), encryption (to ensure that data cannot be accessed), spoofing detection/prevention (to ensure that an adversary is not impersonating an existing station), and jamming (immunity from interference). Ideally, a sensor system would have low LPI/LPD, strong authentication, encryption (e.g., Advanced Encryption Standard 256 (AES256)), spoofing detection/prevention. Making systems difficult to jam and resistant to interference from other systems is an important part of the overall performance of the sensor system.

For wireless networks, another factor to consider is the wireless topology—in short, how the nodes communicate. A first option is a Star topology where all devices communicate with a single, centralized wireless access point. This is typical of Wi-Fi and other simple wireless technologies. The advantage is that this wireless topology is very easy to configure and implement, but this communication often comes at a cost of range and coverage (since all stations need to communicate directly with the single access point), as well as reliability (the single access point can become a single point of failure). While repeater stations/nodes have been employed to extend coverage, this also tends to increase latency of communication.

A second wireless topology is a mesh or ad-hoc network. In this wireless topology, all stations can communicate directly with others without the need for a centralized node. This topology can be more efficient and more reliable since there is no single point of failure, but simple mesh networks can only communicate with other nodes within range. More sophisticated mesh networks have derived additional techniques to propagate a packet through the mesh to reach nodes beyond direct radio contact. These techniques fall into two main classes: table-driven methods (where all nodes try to determine and maintain routes to all other nodes), and source-initiated methods (where nodes can dynamically broadcast their desire to route to a particular node in order to determine the route on-the-fly as needed). Both methods have their tradeoffs. Table-driven methods do not scale well as all the wireless bandwidths will eventually get taken up just trying to share/maintain routing information. Source-initiated methods have a latency for the first packet as a route is determined and similarly do not scale well or handle dynamically changing topologies well. For these reasons, the most widely used wireless mesh radio networks do not typically scale beyond 100–300 nodes, although compression of data may extend this bandwidth-scalability tradeoff somewhat.

Next-generation hybrid wireless mesh networks attempt to tradeoff the benefits of both methods and provide for improved scalability. These hybrid wireless mesh networks can either be peer-peer (where all nodes are the same but perhaps employ hierarchical or other means of organizing nodes) or multi-tier (where there may be two classes of devices—possibly many lower-cost battery-powered sensor devices transmitting short-range to higher-cost or an AC-powered aggregator sensor device with longer-range radio).

It is important to realize that the wireless networking topology methods could employ static routing (where the connectivity map is fixed and perhaps manually configured) or dynamic routing (where the connectivity map and paths for packets to flow are determined and updated on-the-fly). Clearly, dynamic routing with its self-configuring, self-organizing, and self-healing properties is superior, but topology comes at an increased cost of complexity.

Finally, no matter what method of radio or wireless topology is employed, often one or more stations may provide some means of connectivity to the outside world (typically the Internet). In a Star topology, the wireless access point/router will typically have a method for connecting via wired ethernet and would thus represent a single point of wiring that would be required. However, in other types of networks, one or more of the stations/nodes could provide long-haul connectivity. Options for providing long-haul connectivity are site-specific, meaning that their availability is determined by the location. Options include wired ethernet, Wi-Fi, cellular, satellite (International Mobile Satellite Organization (Inmarsat), Iridium®, Broadband Global Area Network (BGAN), Advanced Research and Global Observation Satellite

(ARGOS), Open System for Communication in Realtime (OSCAR), military (high-frequency satellite communications (HF-SATCOM)), etc. Typically, these uplinks are at a higher cost, so it is more cost effective to have fewer gateway/uplink stations and thus amortize the higher cost across more stations. It is also important to realize that gateway stations depend on external infrastructure such as cellular or satellite, which may become unavailable; so redundancy via multiple gateway nodes and uplink methods may be appropriate to ensure that the ability to store data should an external means of connectivity become unavailable is maintained.

14.7 CONCLUSION

This chapter has explored several factors important to the development and deployment of sensor networks. It has provided an overview of logging vs transmission, commercial factors in sensor systems, terminology, challenges, sensor interfaces and protocols, sensor platform needs and components, wireless mesh networks and topologies, and options for uplink of data. Attention to these important factors will help ensure that the goal of robust and secure sensor networks for acquisition of data is achieved.

ACKNOWLEDGMENTS

The author would like to acknowledge the expert guidance from Dr. Steven Lacey, University of Utah School of Medicine/Chief of the Division of Public Health.

15 Data Integration and Services

Kevin Montgomery
IoT/AI Inc.

CONTENTS

15.1 BACK-END INFRASTRUCTURE/CLOUD SERVICES

In its most basic sense when discussing data integration, data has to flow somewhere. Data acquired from networks of sensors are uplinked through some method to a central system for storage. In modern sensor networks, this system is typically cloud-based where the server infrastructure itself is managed by a service provider. The largest and most advanced provider is Amazon Web Services (AWS), but Microsoft Azure and Google Cloud are other major providers of cloud services. Most of these systems allow for redundancy of servers providing a myriad of services, such as hot backups, automatic restart, and scaling. These providers also offer standardized operating system images and hardware specific to a particular task. For example, AWS provides for a multitude of servers uniquely tuned for Structured Query Language (SQL). These servers are appropriate for structured data that does not change structure such as not only SGL (NoSQL); for unstructured or data that changes structure, such as free text; or ElasticCache®, a high-speed caching/database-like functionality type database. In fact, AWS and others do provide higher-level application programming interfaces (APIs) specific for the storage of sensor data that abstracts and simplifies much of what a user requires. Other open systems such as Collaborate. org provide low-cost or free hosted solutions on top of AWS and other cloud service providers and offer a much more open and less proprietary ecosystem.

While storage of sensor data is important, access to that data is also important. Systems such as those listed above also provide methods for downloading data which has been stored in typical formats, such as spreadsheets (Microsoft Excel) or more generic comma-separated-value (CSV) files. More advanced systems such as "Collaborate" also provide data visualization such as tables, charts, graphs, and

DOI: 10.1201/9780429263286-17

maps, which will be described below; several of the systems also provide open APIs and access for integration of other tools, such as Tableau®, a chart/graph/visualization service.

15.2 DATA INTEGRATION

While data from an individual sensor network may provide insight into one aspect of exposures, the user often needs to integrate data from many other data sources in order to understand the holistic picture. Often this data is from other sensor networks already deployed or may already exist in another area such as a field survey, a report, a personnel database, a satellite or another remote-sensing database. In general, a tremendous amount of data is collected and already available, and most complex exposure and industrial hygiene (IH) problems require the integration of data from multiple sources to obtain true understanding.

Several issues exist in the integration of data from multiple data sources. Temporality of the data (when and how frequently it was collected), spatial accuracy and resolution (over what area is the data valid), confidence (how accurate is the data or individual samples) are only some of many other factors. Overall, the need for maintaining metadata (information about the data and its source, beyond the data itself) is important as well as the need to provide for "drill down" into the data to explore these factors that can impact the use of data from other data sources, especially those over which the user has no control.

Another challenge in data integration is that individual data sources likely provide their data in different formats, units, encodings, or other factors. A non-trivial step in the data integration process is the validation aspect. The user must determine if the data has been converted accurately and if the source of the data is reliable. He also must normalize and re-encode the data into a common format or common units. This step can be difficult and challenging at best due to limited availability and the present digital community's adherence to standard formats and protocols. Moreover, the multimodal aspect of data (sensor data versus human-derived data versus satellite imagery) can produce additional challenges. However, the benefits of data normalization are tremendous because it enables a general framework for future processing, analytics, display, and visualization as outlined in the sections to follow.

Several data integration services or publicly accessible data stores are available. These include AWS Public Data and Google, lesser-known groups like Terbine.io, and non-profit hosted data integration and sharing solutions such as Collaborate.org.

The ultimate goal of this phase is to integrate all relevant data to a problem across multimodal data sources into a common framework and protocol for subsequent processing and visualization.

15.3 ANALYTICS

Once data from relevant data sources are integrated and in a common framework, users often need to derive specific quantitative calculations from the resulting data. Data analytics is the process of transforming data with the goal of deriving higher-level data representing cognitive concepts. Main types include traditional statistical techniques: Artificial Intelligence (AI) and Machine Learning (ML) techniques, and Geospatial Analytics (GA), among others.

Statistical techniques include descriptive statistics, exploratory data analysis (focusing on discovering new features in data), confirmatory data analysis (confirming formerly derived hypotheses), and predictive analytics (focusing on application of statistical models for predicting future states). AI- and ML-based approaches include genetic algorithms, artificial neural networks, and related techniques. GA considers the spatial distribution of data and can include plume modeling, heat maps, and other techniques to interpolate and analyze spatiotemporally derived data. In general, the analytical tools and methods to be used should be derived and driven by the questions to be answered. To learn more on this subject, readers should refer to the extensive literature for data analytics to explore other data decomposition and reduction methods.

In sensor systems, it is also important to note that analytics typically can occur at three different levels: the sensor platform level (sensor drift, anomaly detection), network intelligence (multiple sensor devices working together—baseline background), or central server (multiple integrated data sources). The types of analytics and their output is driven by the data present and available at each of these levels of processing. For example, a sensor drift calculation for an air particulate sensor may occur at the sensor station level while the background air particulate level may occur in a cooperative manner across all stations (network intelligence) in order to derive an anomaly against that background which will be correlated with satellite-based sensor data integrated at the central server.

15.4 VISUALIZATION

While data analytics seeks to derive higher-level values representing cognitive concepts, the goal of visualization is to present the data along with the derived analytics in such a manner as to derive understanding. Note that this process need not be static but is often an interactive exploration of the data and derived analytical values by the user based on the user's intent and the cognitive questions that are sought.

Types of visualization tools include tables, charts, graphs, geospatial (Google Earth, Environmental Systems Research Institute (ESRI®), Arc Graphical Information System (ArcGIS), The National Aeronautics and Space Administration (NASA) WorldWind an open-source virtual globe, etc.), Virtual Reality (VR) or Augmented Reality (AR), among others.

While the goal of visualization is to provide the user with understanding from the data, this presupposes that a single individual is exploring the data, whereas in common practice, a team of individuals is working together to understand and explore the data. Often a Common Operating Picture (COP) paradigm is used where all users can view data and explore in a shared, identical space. While this paradigm has great benefits, it is naïve in its assumption that the platform is static and that all users have the same roles. Instead a Dynamic User-Defined Operating Picture (D-UDOP) is a more advanced concept where interactive exploration of data is possible and presented, perhaps differently to different users, based on their roles and intent at the present time.

15.5 COLLABORATION

The last section focuses on aiding the understanding of data by an individual and ultimately presents the idea that it is even more often the case that groups of people tend to solve more complex problems. Moreover, merely understanding is not enough. Those with valuable insight into a problem wish to disseminate this information, coordinate and take action, form a community of practice, and to affect an impact.

Thus, the final stage of the sensor and data integration pipeline is Collaboration. Collaboration is the means by which impact is made from the decisions derived from the data integrated. While many collaboration tools and platforms are in broad usage, many of these systems are media or modality specific. Examples of collaboration components include videoconferencing (WebEx®, Google Hangouts®, Skype®, Zoom®, Adobe Connect®), file sharing (DropBox®, Box, Gdrive®, OneDrive®, Sharepoint®), chat (Slack®, WhatsApp®, WeChat®, SnapChat®), shared whiteboards (DropBox Paper®), and shared document editing (Google Docs®). As evident from this list, many options exist and are typically "stovepiped" into their respective domains and are not necessarily interoperable. Some larger companies, such as Google, have created ecosystems of toolsets that provide versions of many of the above although the monetization of these platforms has raised privacy concerns and slowed adoption. Collaborate.org is a free, integrated suite of collaboration tools, including data hosting, integration, and visualization, available to the IH which can help the industrial hygiene community integrate the multiple sources of data now so increasingly available.

15.6 CONCLUSION

In the future, industrial hygiene professionals will no longer be data collectors but data scientists, empowered by automated data acquisition from sensor networks and integrating data from multiple sources by data analytics to gain a further understanding of the health needs of each person and using collaboration tools to affect a significant impact on society. This will be the new paradigm of industrial hygiene that will transform and empower the field into the 21st century and beyond.

16 Exposure Health Informatics Ecosystem

Ramkiran Gouripeddi
University of Utah

Philip Lundrigan
Brigham Young University

*Sneha Kasera, Scott Collingwood,
Mollie Cummins, Julio C. Facelli,
and Katherine Sward*
University of Utah

CONTENTS

16.1 DETERMINANTS OF HEALTH

While estimates of the exact contributions vary between studies, at least 50% of a person's health can be attributed to their environment, lifestyle, and behavior (Centers for Disease Control and Prevention 2019, Tarlov 1999, McGinnis, Williams-Russo, and Knickman 2002, Choi and Sonin 2019). A study in England attributed 40% of all disease burden to identifiable risk factors and almost 75% of these to

DOI: 10.1201/9780429263286-18

a combination of individuals' environmental, behavioral, and metabolic profiles (Newton et al. 2015). About one in four deaths worldwide, and a similar proportion of deaths among children under five, are due to modifiable environmental factors (Prüss-Üstün et al. 2016, Landrigan et al. 2018). These 12.6 million deaths are attributed to more than 100 different diseases (World Health Organization 2016a,b).

By itself, air pollution is linked to one in eight deaths globally (World Health Organization 2014, 2017). About two billion children live in areas exceeding the World Health Organization's annual limits for fine particles (United Nations International Children's Emergency Fund 2016). It is noted that 169,250 and 531,000 child deaths are attributable to ambient and household air pollution, respectively (World Health Organization 2017). The global social cost of air pollution is about $3 trillion per year (Erickson and Jennings 2017). Recent studies have provided strong evidence associating air quality with pediatric asthma (Pollock, Shi, and Gimbel 2017). At the same time, there is discussion about our environment being cleaner than ever before and the unprimed nature of our immune systems being responsible for disease manifestation (Richtel 2019). While it is reasonably well understood that continuous exposure to high levels of pollution is unhealthy, much less is known about health effects of low levels, intermittent exposure, and combinations of exposures. Studying the latter requires informatics infrastructures that can aggregate environmental and physiological data from multiple sources at high temporal and spatial resolutions. Research and development of such multi-scale and multi-model informatics infrastructure is just beginning; and in this chapter, we describe the requirement, design, and development activities undertaken to address these issues.

16.2   THE EXPOSOME AND ITS GENERATION

Comprehensive quantification of effects of the modern environment on health requires taking into account data from all contributing environmental exposures and how those exposures relate to health; this is termed the *exposome*, a complementary concept to the genome (Wild 2005, 2012). Measuring the exposome can span a lifetime of exposures starting from conception and includes endogenous processes within the body, biological responses of adaptation to environment, physiological manifestations of these responses, and socio-behavioral factors (Wild 2005, 2012). Generating exposomes at high resolution requires integration of data from wearable and stationary sensors, environmental monitors, personal activities, physiology, medication use and other clinical data, genomic and other biospecimen-derived, person-reported and computational models. Exposomic research is translational in nature, as the exposome includes direct biological pathway alterations, as well as mutagenic and epigenetic mechanisms of environmental influences on the phenome (Miller 2013, Miller and Jones 2014, Lioy and Weisel 2014, NIOSH 2018). The *phenome*, which is an individual's state of well-being and disease, is a result of the interaction between a person's *genome* and their exposome. See Figure 16.1 for a holistic understanding of disease, integration of the exposome, genome, and other factors.

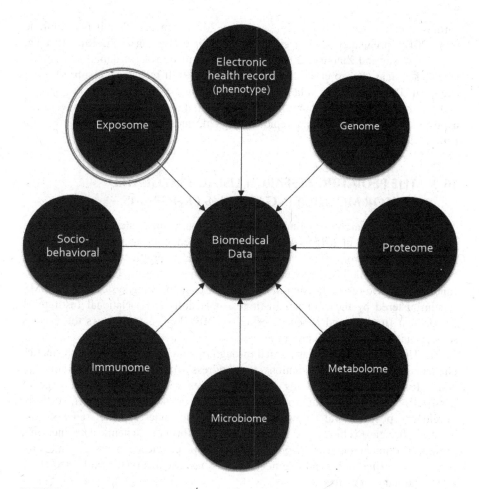

FIGURE 16.1 Holistic understanding of disease requires integration of the exposome with the genome with other biomedical data.

There is a need for understanding an individual's total exposure including simultaneous, cumulative, and latent exposure to multiple environmental species on health (Pollock, Shi, and Gimbel 2017). We refer to any physical (e.g., temperature, humidity), chemical (e.g., particulate matter (PM), ozone), or biological (e.g., pollen, mold) environmental or physiological (e.g., breath rate, forced expiration volume) entity measured by a sensor as a species. Processes to support this aggregation and integration must accommodate variable spatio-temporal resolutions and account for multiple study, experimental and analytical designs. Gaps in measured data may need to be filled with modeled data along with characterization of uncertainties.

The air quality exposome is important to our improved understanding of pediatric asthma and other respiratory conditions (Pollock, Shi, and Gimbel 2017), cardiovascular disease (Lee, Kim, and Lee 2014), cancers (Santibáñez-Andrade et al. 2017), pregnancy (Leiser et al. 2019), suicide (Bakian et al. 2015, Gładka, Rymaszewska, and Zatoński 2018), and its mechanistic role in damage to deoxyribonucleic acid (Bosco et al. 2018, Miri et al. 2019). It includes a combination of chemical (PM, ozone, and volatile organic compounds), biological (pollen, spores) and physical (temperature, humidity) environmental species. Studies involving the exposome can be observational, epidemiological, interventional, or mechanistic in nature (Röhrig et al. 2009).

16.3 THE PEDIATRIC RESEARCH USING INTEGRATED SENSOR MONITORING SYSTEMS PROGRAMS

The Pediatric Research using Integrated Sensor Monitoring Systems (PRISMS) program was launched in 2015 to develop a sensor-based, data-intensive infrastructure for measuring environmental, physiological, and behavioral factors for performing pediatric and adult epidemiological studies (https://www.nibib.nih.gov/research-funding/pediatric-research-using-integrated-sensor-monitoring-systems). PRISMS is administered by the National Institutes of Health (NIH) National Institute of Biomedical Imaging and Bioengineering (NIBIB). Figure 16.2 shows the various projects under the PRISMS program.

The University of Utah was funded through this program to identify informatics challenges and develop solutions to address them (http://prisms.bmi.utah.edu/). Recognizing that solving these challenges will require a wide range of perspectives, the Utah team is a diverse group of faculty, research staff, software developers, post-doctoral fellows, and graduate and undergraduate students from atmospheric science, bioengineering, biomedical informatics, chemical engineering, chemistry, clinical and translational science, computer science, electrical and computer engineering, industrial engineering, nursing, occupational health, pediatrics and pulmonary medicine.

16.4 EXPOSOMIC RESEARCH CHALLENGES AND INFORMATICS SOLUTIONS

Exposomic research requires simultaneous measurement of many types of environmental, physiological, and behavioral factors using sensors. These measurements can be obtained using sensor technologies that are often novel and in various stages of development, evolving to capture measurements of novel species, with improvements in their sensitivity, performance, and validity in measuring different species, in their form factor so that they can be used in personal and mobile settings, and price. In addition, these sensors use diverse device communication protocols and require additional hardware and software modifications for using research studies and for secure data acquisition and transmittal.

Environmental species have spatial and temporal variations and humans are mobile and spend time at home, commuting, at work or school, and in recreation.

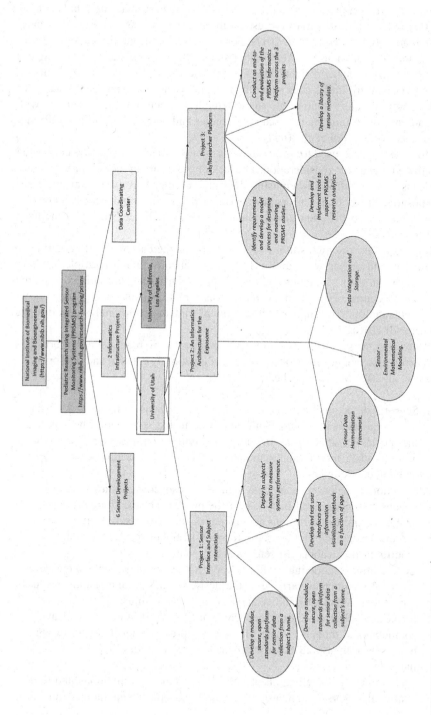

FIGURE 16.2 The PRISMS program and tasks being performed by the University of Utah.

Generation of comprehensive spatio-temporal records of exposures requires collection and integration of data from different types of sensors that might be available at different locations and times corresponding to the locations of the subject under consideration (Gouripeddi et al. 2017). For example, an air quality exposome may require the integration of data from indoor and mobile sensors, stationary regulatory monitors, citizen's networks, and finally supplementation with data from computational models to fill in the gaps when there is an absence of experimental data. All of these would require appropriate spatio-temporal dimensions and resolution with their absence often limiting the quality of studies and potentially leading to erroneous results (Gouripeddi et al. 2017).

Moreover, sensors used for measurements of exposures are not always collocated with the subject under consideration. The lack of proximity of the sensor to the subject leads to uncertainties when using their measurements as exact quantifications of exposures. In addition, sensors have varied capabilities, granularities and resolutions in measuring different environment species, which need to be harmonized prior to analysis.

Total exposure research studies need to be performed across health conditions, age ranges, and sensor types and utilize heterogeneous data at multiple levels of granularities in their semantics and temporalities. Different translational research archetypes require different data, data transformations, data integration workflows, and analytics to support observational and interventional study designs (Gouripeddi 2016).

Addressing these challenges in exposomic research requires an informatics architecture that embeds multiple features that are loosely coupled and interoperable (Sward et al. 2017, Martin Sanchez et al. 2014):

1. Sensor data acquisition: The evolving nature of sensors requires a sensor data acquisition paradigm that is agnostic to the sensor and the type of the species it is measuring. In addition, acquiring these sensor data should accommodate mobile and stationary devices that measure personal and ambient environments.

2. Selection of heterogeneous data sources: Prospective studies require use of sensors that are well-matched for the purposes of the study. Secondary analyses require descriptions about sources and methods including types of sensors used, to support appropriate analysis. In both cases, research teams require metadata about the sensors and the data sources.

3. Computational modeling for filling gaps: It may not be possible to measure every environmental variable at the desired temporal and spatial resolution, either due to availability and/or challenges with use of sensors, cost, privacy, number of sensors needed in large cohort studies, etc. Having computational models to help fill gaps can provide substitutes for or augment sensor-measured environmental factors, activities, and locations of individuals.

4. Uncertainty characterization of data: Understanding limitations and data quality of sensors, their measurements and, similarly, computational models

would enable their proper use within data pipelines, designing appropriate studies, and performing apt analysis. These limitations and uncertainties can be captured and shared as metadata.

5. Generation of a high-resolution spatio-temporal grid of exposures: Exposures are intrinsically tied to location and time. Different sources of exposure data, sensors, and computational model need to be combined to generate a high-resolution grid of personal exposure. These sources could have different granularities and resolution, and their integration would need to support these heterogeneity.

6. Data integration: To support the above requirements, integration of these heterogeneous exposomic data would need to be semantically consistent (Habre et al. 2016) and metadata driven. In addition, the diversity of different objects represented in translational exposomic research require them to be integrated on their spatial and temporal dimensions. Representing data as *events* permits temporal analysis and reasoning around a diverse array of environmental measurements, physiological responses, and conditions. An event-based infrastructure would support multi-scale and multi-omics integration.

7. Presentation and visualization: In order to make meaningful use of the data and processes in exposomic research, there is a need for acceptable and user-friendly interfaces for study participant and investigator interactions. These interfaces will provide feedback, allow participants to be provided instructions for interventions, and a means for participants to input additional requested data. Investigators will be able to manage study processes, assess ongoing data collections, and tailor interventions. There will likely be a need to have these presentation and visualization layer be person-centered and on mobile platforms.

8. Support a diverse set of translational research archetypes: The informatics infrastructure would need to support diverse study types, including observational, epidemiological, interventional, secondary analysis, and mechanistic study. In addition the infrastructure would need to enable reproducibility and transparency of study results with metadata to track data and process provenances.

16.5 EXPOSURE HEALTH INFORMATICS ECOSYSTEM

In order to meet the diverse requirements listed above, we are developing a scalable informatics infrastructure, Exposure Health Informatics Ecosystem (EHIE) (Sward and Facelli 2016, Sward et al. 2017, Gouripeddi et al. 2019b) following an ecosystemic approach. An ecosystem is a collection of loosely coupled software and hardware platforms that co-evolve, interact with one another and with human actors to serve a common business need (i.e., research, in this case), by maintaining symbiotic operational relationships with each other through exchange of data, metadata, knowledge, and process artifacts (Messerschmitt and Szyperski 2003, Jansen, Finkelstein, and Brinkkemper 2009, Lungu 2009, Popp and Meyer 2010,

Jansen, Brinkkemper, and Cusumano 2013, Bala Iyer 2014). Adopting this approach enables researchers to sustain healthy large-scale infrastructures, by having a diversity in tasks performed by different actors within the ecosystem (Manikas and Hansen 2013). In addition, having this diversification in niche components simplifies the management and evolution of the ecosystem as a whole, as each component has its own development cycle managed by a team of experts (Dittrich 2014). Modifications from a specific component can be independently scaled as needed for a particular research use case. Similarly, operational use of the ecosystem paradigm for research studies would have support from several actors with appropriate expertise together providing greater value than on their own (Wnuk et al. 2014).

EHIE is derived from the federally funded National Institutes of Health's (NIH) National Institute of Biomedical Imaging and Bioengineering (NIBIB) Pediatric Research Using Integrated Sensor Monitoring Systems (PRISMS) program (Sward et al. 2016). EHIE addresses the above list of exposomic research challenges by providing informatics solutions at scale, incorporating the latest *Big Data* approaches. The infrastructure is a comprehensive, standards-based, open-source informatics platform that provides semantically consistent, metadata-driven, event-based management of exposomic data. Using an event-driven architecture allows the modeling and storage of all activities related to the study itself and its operations in their primitive form on a timeline as events that can be transformed to higher/analytical models based on use cases. Moreover, its implementation using advanced graph and document store technologies limits semantic dissonance and enables the use of novel Big Data approaches in a natural way. EHIE is aligned with the goals of modern environmental health research supporting meaningful integration of sensor and biomedical data (National Institute of Environmental Health Sciences 2012, Barksdale Boyle et al. 2015, National Institute of Environmental Health Sciences 2018). See Figure 16.3 for an overview of EHIE informatics ecosystem.

Conceptually, all the evolving software and hardware artifacts within EHIE can be grouped into the following components:

1. *Data acquisition pipeline*: Hardware and software tools, wireless networking, and protocols to support easy sensor system deployment and robust sensor data collection.
2. *Participant-facing tools*: Collect and annotate a variety of patient-reported and activity data, as well as inform and provide feedback to study participants on their current clinical and environmental exposure status.
3. *Researcher-facing platforms*: Tools and processes for researchers undertaking exposomic studies for a variety of experimental designs or for clinical care.
4. *Computational modeling platform*: Generate comprehensive spatio-temporal data in the absence of measurements and for recognition of activity signatures from sensor measurements.

Data Acquisition Pipeline

- Hardware and software, wireless networking, and protocols to support easy system deployment for robust sensor data collection in homes, and monitoring of sensor deployments.

Participant Facing Tools

- Annotate participant generated data, display sensor data, and inform participants of their clinical and environmental status.

Researcher Facing Platforms

- Tools and processes for researchers performing exposomic studies of a variety of experimental designs.

Computational Modeling & Uncertainty Characterization

- Generate high resolution spatio-temporal data as well as for recognition of activity signatures from sensor measurements.
- Characterize uncertainties associated with collected or computed data

Central Big Data Integration Platform

- Integrates study-specific, open sensor and computationally modeled data with biomedical information along with characterizing uncertainties associated with these data.

FIGURE 16.3 Exposure Health Informatics Ecosystem (EHIE) and its main components.

5. *Central Big Data federation/integration platform*: Standards-based, open-access infrastructure that integrates measured and computationally modeled data with biomedical information along with characterizing uncertainties associated with using these data.

In the following sections, we describe key features of each of these components.

16.5.1 DATA ACQUISITION PIPELINE

Current *Internet-of-Things (IoT)* solutions are not necessarily designed for health research. Systems are not designed for large study-based deployments wherein the cost and resources required for management of IoT sensors exceeds the cost of the sensors themselves. Research solutions are required to be compliant with pertinent privacy laws applicable at different jurisdictions (e.g., deployment site(s), study site, and/or study sponsor location) for data transmission (Luxton, Kayl, and

Mishkind 2012) and storage. While IoT sensors provide low-cost and smart solutions to measure study participants' environments, they usually use custom software and hardware, require regular maintenance, and have data integrity problems. We, therefore, needed to design an open-source platform that is customizable to different sensors, study designs, and participant requirements. Such a platform would need to have a short deployment time, provide high-quality data, and stream data in real time enabling control loops of feedback and interventions.

In order to meet these needs, we developed a multi-pronged approach for data acquisition. We developed EpiFi (Figure 16.4) (Lundrigan et al. 2018) to overcome these limitations and extend the use of off-the-shelf sensor technologies as IoT solutions for health research. In addition, we developed methods and processes for sensors that can directly transmit data to data acquisition servers, using protocols such as the Message Queuing Telemetry Transport (MQTT) (Hunkeler, Truong, and Stanford-Clark 2008) or HTTP/HTTPS. Our collaborators at Columbia University have adopted AethLabs sensors (www.aethlabs.com) to use these protocols to measure and transmit measurements for PM composition, black carbon, temperature and relative humidity, accelerometry and volatile organic compounds levels (Cox et al. 2019). In order to help investigators choose an appropriate approach, we developed a framework that considers the type of sensors and their transmission, study design, and participant involvement (Tiase et al. 2018). EpiFi provides flexibility in using existing participant home infrastructure and accommodates participant-in-the-loop study designs.

EpiFi brings IoT to health research by providing robustness to consumer applications needed by different study designs. It allows researchers, participants and their families, and clinicians to process data in real time. It simplifies the process of IoT deployment and management in hundreds of participant homes as might be needed in clinical studies. EpiFi consists of a small single-board computer (i.e., Raspberry Pi) gateway and open-source Home Assistant home automation platform (Home Assistant 2019), with custom code to address challenges of using sensors for research data acquisition. It has means to reliably transfer to a remote database using a home WiFi router

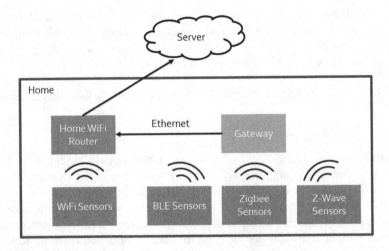

FIGURE 16.4 Overview of EpiFi.

and local storage that can act as a buffer when transmission to the remote database is not available or required. The system architecture of EpiFi is shown in Figure 16.5.

EpiFi (Lundrigan et al. 2018) supports multiple features that make it appropriate for use as an IoT solution in clinical studies:

1. *Device observability*: Allows a remote study manager to know if a WiFi device is functioning or not. It distinguishes between WiFi disruptions and other types of disruptions, so that appropriate troubleshooting can be performed.

2. *Secure WiFi bootstrapping*: Allows secure bootstrapping of WiFi connectivity of multiple devices by making the gateway a temporary access point. By overloading the use of source and destination addresses of an Ethernet frame, the Secure Transfer of Association Protocol (STRAP) (Lundrigan, Kasera, and Patwari 2018) allows a trusted device on the network to send data to unconnected WiFi devices (Figure 16.6). This protocol addresses the challenges of securely connecting new sensors within a home. It protects against eavesdroppers, modified messages, replay attacks, and rogue access point attacks. STRAP also reduces deployment time by needing the entry home WiFi credentials only on EpiFi and eliminating the need of entry by each individual sensor.

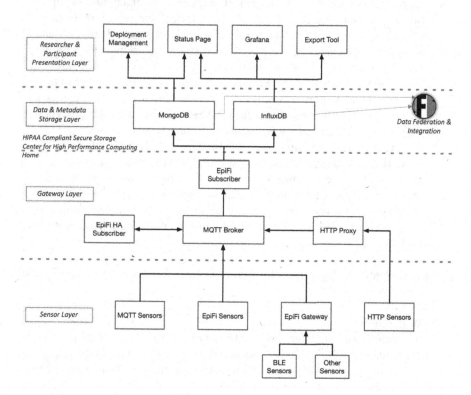

FIGURE 16.5 Architecture of EpiFi.

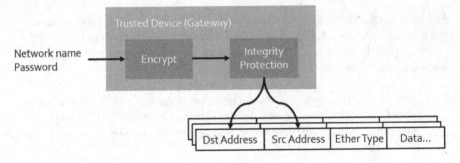

FIGURE 16.6   The Secure Transfer of Association Protocol (STRAP).

3. *Secure sensor reuse*: Tracking of sensors when their location changes and management of backlogged data on sensors. Sensors learn their locations based on network characteristics. A change in network characteristics indicates that the sensor is now in a new location, which then sets off processes to update deployment metadata. Also, each location has a key that is used to encrypt data, which prevents backlogged data from being read by a person at a different location.

4. *Study management tools*: Provides a presentation layer to support a diverse range of tools for study management (Figure 16.5). Integrated bi-directional communications with the gateway device help with remote management and troubleshooting potential sources of signal disruption and apply fixes. We currently use the following study management tools for the PRISMS pilot study (Collingwood et al. 2018, Gouripeddi et al. 2019c):

   a. *Deployment status page*: Provides the status of various deployments.

   b. *Export tool*: Export streaming data in various formats for ad hoc analysis.

   c. *Grafana (2019)*: Streaming data visualization, monitoring, and analytics.

5. *Support of multiple wireless protocols*: Supports among other cellular, Z-Wave (Yassein, Mardini, and Khalil 2016), ZigBee (Farahani 2011), LoRa (Lee and Ke 2018), and HaLow (802.11ah) (Adame et al. 2014).

6. *Data integrity*: Prevents data loss arising due to packet losses, gateway outages, home WiFi router outages, and internet outages by persisting data at every opportunity, deleting persisted data only after acknowledgment of receipt from remote storage, and sending multiple data packets when backlogged.

EpiFi is currently deployed for pilot studies at Utah for facilitating acquisition of data from:

1. WiFi sensors

   a. *Utah Modified Dylos (UMD) (Min et al. 2018, Vercellino et al. 2018, Collingwood et al. 2019)*: PM as PM2.5 (i.e., PM which is 2.5 μm and smaller) and PM10 (i.e., 10 micrometers and smaller), temperature, and humidity.

   b. *AirU (Kelly et al. 2017)*: PM.

2. Bluetooth Low Energy (BLE) sensors
   a. *Wearable air quality sensor from George Washington University (Li et al. 2019)*: Nitrogen dioxide (NO_2), ozone (O_3), ambient temperature, formaldehyde, other aldehydes, and relative humidity.
   b. *Wearable air quality sensor from Arizona State University (Wang and Tao 2017)*: O_3, volatile organic compounds (VOCs), ambient temperature, relative humidity, accelerometry, nitrogen oxides (NOx), formaldehyde (CH_2O), and PM.
   c. *Wearable device from the University of Maryland (Chatterjee et al. 2014, Kukkapalli et al. 2016)*: PM, temperature, transcutaneous partial carbon dioxide (CO_2) pressure, and respiratory rate.

EpiFi has been evaluated in different types of deployment designs, including:

1. *High-resolution air sensing (Min et al. 2018)*: EpiFi acquired data from eight UMDs and AirUs deployed indoors and outdoors, respectively, to create a profile of air quality within a home due to various activities. For example, one of our findings for a home under study showed that, while the furnace fan rapidly improves PM levels in the kitchen, there were short-term increases in PM in other rooms.
2. *Automation of interventions (Min et al. 2018)*: We demonstrated that EpiFi can be integrated into home automated control systems, such as a furnace fan, via an Ecobee thermostat which triggers the furnace fan to switch on when PM levels crossed a present threshold measured by UMDs. This smart control of the furnace fan led to a 70% reduction in power consumption when compared to periodically turning it on.
3. *Requisition of clinical status, feedback, and activity annotation (Collingwood et al. 2018)*: Using EpiFi, we were able to send text notifications to participants when specific thresholds of PM levels were crossed, to acquire participant clinical status, feedback, and log the activities they were performing.
4. *Acquisition heterogeneous sensor data from participant homes*: Including motion sensors, door sensors, tracking smartphones, participant locations, smart light bulbs, WiFi usage, temperature, humidity, energy meters, and any other commercial IoT device to get a sense of participant activities.

Data from EpiFi is stored remotely in a time-series database (Figure 16.5), i.e., InfluxDB (InfluxData 2019). Metadata about the deployments is authored through a graphical user interface into a deployment metadata repository (DMDR) that has been instantiated in a MongoDB database (MongoDB 2019). Together these two stores, along with a set of Software Services (SS), support the presentation layer which provides displays that can be used by participants, researchers, and additional administrative tools. A tracking page was developed to provide the real-time health status of each deployed sensor allowing the administrative team to detect, analyze, and troubleshoot issues in various deployments using established procedures and protocols (Figure 16.7).

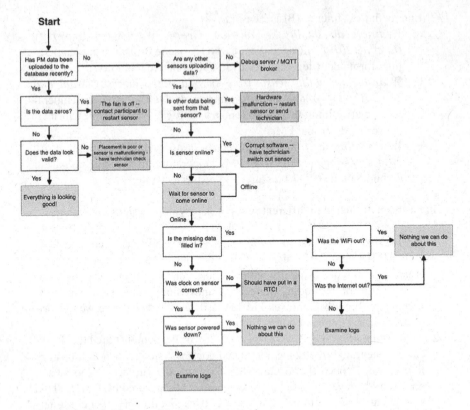

FIGURE 16.7   Example troubleshooting protocol.

In addition to supporting the presentation layer, data and metadata from the time-series database and the DMDR are consumed by the SS of the data federation and integration component for assimilation, generation of exposure records, and study analysis. Software details on EpiFi are available in Lundrigan (2019). We are currently evaluating blockchain approaches for systematically capturing the versioning of sensor deployment metadata as sensors go through life-cycles of deployment and maintenance and to support robust provenance of data arising from these sensors (Sarbhai et al. 2019). Moreover, implementation of blockchain technology will allow us to provide much higher control of data access.

16.5.2   PARTICIPANT-FACING TOOLS

Exposure studies involve multiple stakeholders: participants and their families, clinical coordinators, researchers, sensor developers, and system administrators. In order to meet the needs of all these stakeholders, we utilized user-centered design (UCD) approaches (McMullen et al. 2011) to develop methods for their interactions with EHIE, including data collection, visualization, and analysis. UCD is a multidisciplinary approach rooted in cognitive and behavioral science, based on deep understanding of who will be using the system, their tasks, expectations, and contexts of use. UCD methodologies are congruent with the international standard ISO 9241-210:2010, Ergonomics of Human-System Interaction. In this section, we cover the tools and methods for participant interactions with EHIE.

We use participant-facing tools in exposure health studies to collect participant-reported data prior to the start of a study and during the study phases. We also use these tools to support the collection of data representing participant behavior and environmental sensing, as well as provide feedback and inform participants about interventions for different study designs (Figure 16.8). These interactions could be triggered by environmental and physiological sensor-, clinical-, or participant-reported events.

We developed processes and methods for selection, use, and integration of various types of tools for different study designs. A video titled "Utah PRISMS Informatics Ecosystem" shows these tools in use and can be viewed at https://www.youtube.com/watch?v=FT7Yz5l94fQ. For demonstrative purposes, we used exemplar tools including a generic clinical study tool, a domain-specific exposure health study tool, a visualization tool, and annotation tools:

1. *REDCap (Harris et al. 2009)*: A highly used, open-source study data management tool for designing and administering surveys and data collection. It is a Health Insurance Portability and Accountability Act (HIPAA)–compliant online platform. Participants use REDCap surveys in a PRISMS pilot study for providing their demographics and periodic symptoms. We integrate project-specific data from REDCap using its application programming interface (API).

2. *eAsthmaTracker (eAT) (Nkoy et al. 2012, 2013)*: Integrated asthma patient self-management, education, research and clinician communication platform with alerts developed by the Department of Pediatrics, University of Utah. It collects data on pediatric asthma symptomology through validated instruments to calculate daily and weekly asthma control scores. It also collects participant perceived exposures to asthma triggers (e.g., pollen). In addition, eAT presents participants with air quality indices,

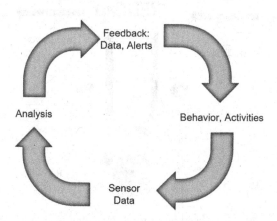

FIGURE 16.8   Uses of participant-facing tools.

pollutant levels from the Environmental Protection Agency (EPA), weather, and pollen counts. We integrate participant symptoms, daily and weekly asthma scores by accessing eAT's MySQL database.

3. *Visualization (Moore et al. 2018)*: We use open-source Grafana software (Grafana 2019) to provide real-time visuals of sensor data to participants in their homes.

4. *Activity annotator (Moore et al. 2018)*: Often, sensor readings require additional information on activities performed by participants or happenings in their environments to provide context to data and its analysis. The activity annotator allows participants to make free-form or prompted annotations, linked to artifacts on the sensor data feed. For example, our participants would note activities such as cooking or cleaning which caused a spike in particulate counts. We examined three approaches to annotation: text messaging, visualization screens (see above), and voice annotations using Google Home. We stored these annotation data into a MongoDB-based annotation document store that then can be consumed for data integration.

5. *Ecological momentary assessments (EMAs) (Shiffman, Stone, and Hufford 2008)*: Obtain participant behaviors and experiences in real time and in their natural environments using short answers to questions. We used EpiFi along with REDCap and Twilio (Twilio 2019) to administer EMAs as text messages that were triggered randomly, periodically at specific dates and times, or by sensor measurement artifacts (e.g., assessments triggered by spikes in sensor readings). See Figure 16.9. Participant responses via text messages were then recorded into REDCap and made available for study data integration, as described above.

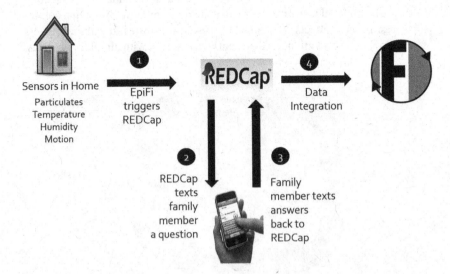

FIGURE 16.9 Ecological momentary assessments administered using text messages and orchestrated by EpiFi, REDCap, and Twilio.

16.5.3 RESEARCHER-FACING TOOLS

Exposure health studies vary widely in design and purpose and, hence, researcher-facing tools must support a wide spectrum of requirements. The studies may range from sensor development projects to highly complex epidemiologic, retrospective observational, or prospective observational designs. Additionally, many of these studies entail real-time interactive data collection (e.g., EMAs) (Gouripeddi et al. 2017, Habre et al. 2016). Both primary and secondary sensor data may be used in studies. The use of primary sensors necessitates collection, storage, and management of real-time data, often with substantial data volume. The sensors may be personal and wearable or stationary, positioned indoors or outdoors, and may measure a wide variety of variables associated with multiple species. If measurements or study interventions must be triggered by sensor values, additional decision support tools are needed to support or automatically initiate the appropriate actions. Secondary sensor data may or may not be pre-processed prior to use, can be high in volume, and details about any pre-processing may be elusive.

The sensor data collected in these studies must often be analyzed jointly with a similarly diverse variety of variables and data types, including patient-reported outcomes, activity annotations, self-reported symptoms, electronic health record data, biospecimen data, computational models, and aggregates of these data types. For this wide variety of data that is used in diverse ways, researchers require support for the collection, monitoring, and integration of data. They also require tools that help them design and monitor studies, with alerting when participants or sensors require attention. In order to achieve the goals of the study, researchers also need additional tools that aid analysis.

Using UCD has allowed us to use some of the same tools used for participants to provide researchers with tools for system interaction. Here, we present examples of researcher-facing tools corresponding to different stages in the life-cycle of an exposomic study:

1. *Study design*: We developed and use process diagram templates (Figure 16.10) for describing study recruitment, sensor deployment, and data integration pipelines that a researcher could design and then can be used by the research administration team to assemble various artifacts.
2. *Sensor selection*: Exposure health studies often use sensors to measure participant environments and physiology. In order to allow researchers to select appropriate sensors, we developed a library that stores detailed descriptions about sensors, which researchers can browse in order to select appropriate sensors for their study needs (Burnett et al. 2018b). The sensor library (Figure 16.11) includes metadata about the owners of the device, methodology used to measure environmental and physiological species, device characteristics (e.g., battery usage), calibration, validation and measurement details, as well as an inventory of number of available devices. We deployed the sensor library using a Neo4j graph database (Neo4j 2019). We are similarly developing a library of computational models.

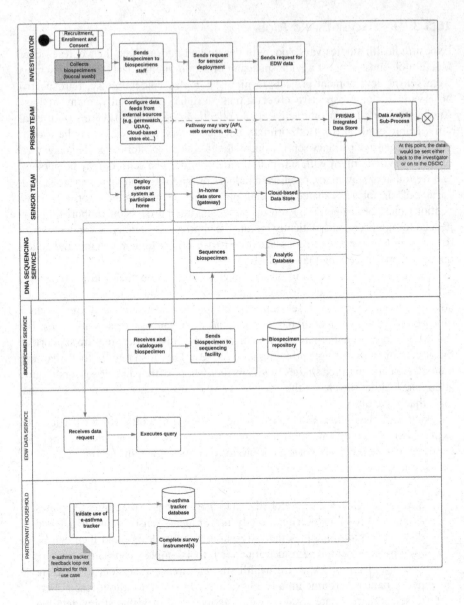

FIGURE 16.10 A high-level process diagram of a pilot study used to evaluate EHIE depicting data streams and their management, including their collection, integration, and final submission.

3. *Data and metadata collection*: At times, the research team itself would need to collect study data, metadata, or other information when performing studies. Using REDCap projects, we can collect:

   a. *Dwelling unit survey (Jacobs et al. 2009)*: Details about home environment including structural characteristics and indoor features such as

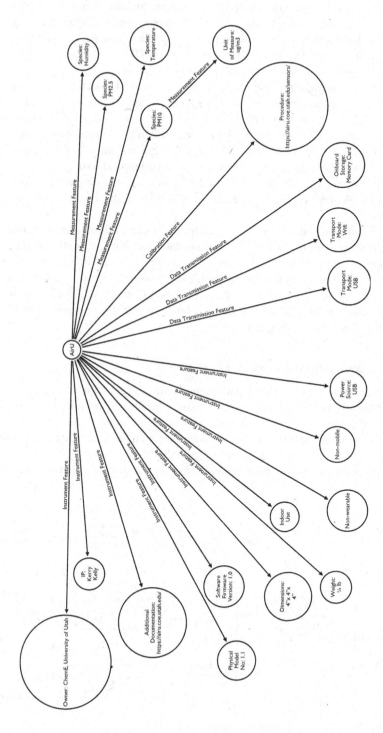

FIGURE 16.11 A section of the metadata about the AirU sensor (Kelly et al. 2017) stored in the sensor library.

carpeting, appliances, heating, ventilation, and air conditions, which can be used for study analysis. Sensor deployment metadata: information about which sensors and where/when they have been deployed is then ingested into the DMDR (i.e., a MongoDB store) (Figure 16.5) for use within the acquisition and integration pipelines.

  b. *Sensor metadata collection (Burnett et al. 2018b)*: Collection of detailed metadata describing sensors (e.g., measurement species, unit of measure, detection limit, sample volume, temperature, humidity) by means of an easy-to-use online tool that can be filled by the sensor owner and then ingested into the Neo4j store of the sensor library. Forms for collecting these metadata are available at http://j.mp/2U3Ixqw.

4. *Study monitoring*: We provide visualizations using the Grafana platform and the deployment status page to get real-time health of each deployed sensor.

5. *Study data analysis*: Various data can be integrated by the central Big Data integration platform. These data are available in different analytical data models or custom formatted databases or as exports. These data can be analyzed by the research team using traditional statistical software (e.g., SAS) or machine learning packages (e.g., R, TensorFlow (Abadi et al. 2016)). They can also be consumed in analytical pipelines as shown in Figure 16.12 or through dashboarding tools.

16.5.4 COMPUTATIONAL MODELING PLATFORM

It is often not possible to measure participant environments with resolution necessary to perform exposure health studies. Also, participants are not always in the proximity of a sensor to measure their environmental exposure. For example, the sparse placement of the EPA air quality monitoring stations in Salt Lake County fails to capture fine-grained variation in air quality due to weather, elevation, and topography. Basic interpolation methods are insufficient for capturing this variation,

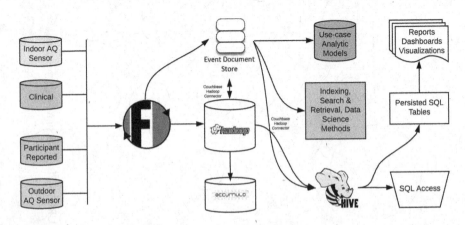

FIGURE 16.12 An example analytic pipeline used in EHIE.

due to geographical and structural irregularities. Increased monitoring (e.g., fine grid or mobile monitoring) is expensive to implement. These limitations can be overcome using computational models to fill gaps in the measured data. In this section, we describe developments within EHIE related to computational modeling:

1. *Activity and location recognition*: While there are multiple models to predict and simulate environmental measurements, a major gap in using these models for exposure health studies is the assignment of either measured or modeled levels of environmental species to participant locations at different times. Human populations are mobile. In addition, situational context of what activities individuals are performing is also important. While it is possible to track locations and activities of participants, there are several major issues, for example, GPS devices do not work reliably in indoor settings, privacy issues complicate activity tracking, and population-scale monitoring is difficult and expensive. To address this, we developed the Spatio-Temporal Human Activity Model (STHAM), which assigns locations and activities to individuals based on their demographic profile. This model can then be integrated with exposure levels to generate comprehensive spatio-temporal records of exposure (Figure 16.13).

STHAM is an agent-based Monte-Carlo model (Sward et al. 2017, Lund, Gouripeddi, and Facelli 2019a,b, Lund et al. 2017). It is semi-empirical and utilizes externally collected datasets: (1) 2010 US Census (US Census

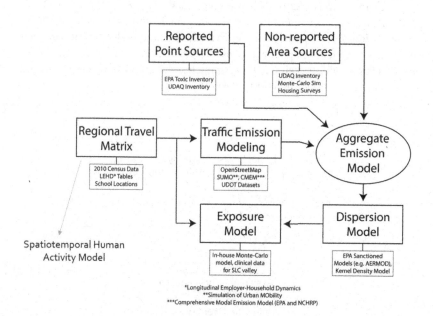

FIGURE 16.13 Overview of the Spatio-Temporal Human Activity Model (STHAM), which integrates simulated activities and locations to develop comprehensive spatio-temporal records of exposures.

Bureau 2010), (2) American Community Survey (US Census Bureau 2017), (3) US Bureau of Labor Statistics American Time Use Survey (ATUS) (U.S. Bureau of Labor Statistics 2017), and (4) Census Bureau Longitudinal Employer-Household Dynamics (LEHD) Origin-Destination Employment Statistics (LODES) (US Census Bureau Center for Economic Studies 2016). Steps taken in building STHAM are summarized in Figure 16.14.

We briefly discuss the use of STHAM for the Salt Lake, Utah, metropolitan area:

a. *Household assignment*: Using data from the census, we assign an age category (0–17, 18–64, 65+ years old) for each household in Salt Lake Valley, based on age of majority of members in that household.

b. *Activity classification*: The ATUS dataset has approximately 10,000 respondents each year and includes their daily activity diaries consisting of about 500 macro activity categories, demographic data, and contextual information for each activity. We performed unsupervised classification using random forests, followed by a dimensionality reduction using t-distributed stochastic neighbor embedding (t-SNE) and, finally, a density-based clustering to result in 90 demographic classes and 40 activity day classes.

c. *Activity sequence construction*: Humans usually follow a schedule, but typically have intra- and inter-person variations. To account for this, we used the activity classes to construct activity windows, probabilistically sorted these windows, and then used a Monte-Carlo based activity generator to construct sequences of activities.

d. *Assessing diurnal patterns*: In the final step, we probabilistically assigned demographic classes to a day type and built activity sequences for each demographic class based on day type. We then assigned these demographic-specific activity sequences at an hourly basis to population distributions at a 500-m grid level.

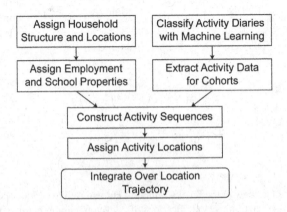

FIGURE 16.14   Schema of steps used in building STHAM.

2. *Indoor activity recognition*: Sensor readings on their own might not always be sufficient to get contexts of triggers leading to changes in environments. We, therefore, have developed methods for participants to annotate sensor data using various approaches as described above. But, often participants are overburdened annotating their activities. In order to automate some of this, we trained machine learning methods with existing annotations and sensor streams to predict activity signatures from the profile of the sensor readings.

3. *Personal exposure modeling (An et al. 2018)*: Estimating exposures at a personal level not only needs to account for the environment, locations, and activities of individuals but also their biological characteristics. We extend our current work from STHAM to such multi-scale models that can then be utilized in research studies.

4. *Modeling metadata of computational models (Lund et al. 2018)*: Many environmental modeling algorithms have been developed by the EPA and other groups (e.g., US Environmental Protection Agency 2016a–c, McMillan et al. 2010, US Environmental Protection Agency 2005, Yanosky et al. 2014). We are also able to accommodate models of different resolutions, such as those available from Mesowest (Horel et al. 2002). All these models have varied capabilities, methods, limitations, deployment needs, inputs and simulated output details. In order to meet the needs of varied exposure health studies, we developed a library of modeling algorithms that can be utilized to generated high spatio-temporal resolution data. This library captures technical details and methodology of each model, their deployment characteristics when used in a particular study, and describes inputs consumed and output generated from these models. Similar to the sensor library, this library of computational models supports selection and use and points to software code that can be executed by workflow engines (Deelman et al. 2015). We implemented the library using a Neo4j graph database platform, along with detailed metadata about each modeling algorithm.

5. *Uncertainty quantification (Gouripeddi et al. 2015, Burnett et al. 2015)*: The computational modeling platform also includes methods to quantify different types of uncertainties that might be present within data or associated with computational models. Uncertainty could be: (1) Inherent: Variations in unknown conditions, (2) Reducible: Associated with the model and input conditions, and (3) Exposure-related: Arising due to differences in person's exposure and true ambient environmental levels (Zeger et al. 2000). For example, STHAM can only provide ranges of activities and expected locations, but not actual behaviors. However, in this example, the model could be validated by proxy, by evaluating simulated traveling numbers against actual measured traffic volumes. Activity or context measurement creates a new and complicated dimension of uncertainty. Multi-agent contributions to activity context also need to be measured or simulated (e.g., two people in the same household contribute to and experience the activity context differently).

16.5.5 CENTRAL BIG DATA INTEGRATION PLATFORM

A key challenge to performing exposomic research is integrating multiple sources of data for generating comprehensive records of exposure. Such an integration of data needs to support the following features (Sward et al. 2017, Gouripeddi et al. 2019a):

1. Generate comprehensive spatio-temporal records of exposures.
2. Semantically consistent metadata-driven integration of heterogeneous data.
3. Maintain spatio-temporal integrity and support reasoning.
4. Associate uncertainties with using data as exact quantifications of exposure.
5. Transform data to support diverse translational research archetypes.

EHIE leverages and extends the OpenFurther (OF) data integration and federation platform (Bradshaw et al. 2009, Livne, Schultz, and Narus 2011, Gouripeddi 2019, Gouripeddi et al. 2012, 2013). Main components of OF include an Ontology/terminology Server (OS); a Metadata Repository (MDR); SS, which can be consumed by various tools; Data Source Adapters (DSA); Administrative and Security Components (ASC); Virtual Identity Resolution on the GO (VIRGO); Quality and Analytics Framework (QAF); a Computational Modeling (CM) and Uncertainty Module; Process-Workflow Module (PWM); a Metadata & Semantics—Discovery and Mapping Service; a Knowledge Repository; and a Federated Query Engine (FQE) that orchestrates queries between the PWM, SS, MDR, OS, DSA, ASC, VIRGO, CM, and QAF. For EHIE, we modified OF with an Event Document Store (EDS) that stores integrated events as events in a Big Data store; and used graphical stores for the MDR. OF supports the selection and integration of heterogeneous data for generating high-resolution spatio-temporal grids of exposures and associates this data with characterized metadata to support their proper utilization. By leveraging characterized metadata and semantic mappings that are stored within a MDR and an OS, respectively, OF provides syntactic and semantic interoperability for dynamically federating data and information. This federation can take place in real time or statically, without requiring data owners to extract and/or transform their data—facilitating integration by retaining data in their native format. Using this approach, OF is able to transform and integrate distributed data across multiple scales, models, and semantics into consumable formats.

In order to meet the above-mentioned requirements for exposomic research, we modified OF as follows:

1. Sensor Common Metadata Specification (SCMS) (Burnett et al. 2017)
   Quantifying exposures and their effects requires integration of multiple sensors that measure the general and personal environments for chemical, physical, and biological species. Even within a given species, there are often differences in their composition profiles based on their source and locations (Yang et al. 2019). Sensors used to measure these species have different instrument characteristics, capabilities, calibrations, and outputs (Williams et al. 2019). Integration of diverse sensor data should be context-aware,

metadata-driven, and semantically consistent. Further, it needs to be sup-plemented with metadata to support appropriate use of data as well as provide a harmonized representation for ease of use in diverse research studies and analytic approaches. In order to support these needs, we developed SCMS by performing a literature review of studies using sensors, reviewing sample data, and iteratively refining it with feedback from sensor experts. SCMS is available at https://github.com/uofu-ccts/prisms-sensor-model for community review and utilization.

The scope of SCMS includes all types of sensors ranging from nanosensors to satellites, measuring physical, chemical, or biological species. These sensors could be personal or mobile, stationary in-home, or ambient monitoring stations. SCMS covers three sensor domains:

- *Instrument*: Physical characteristics of a sensor device.
- *Deployment*: Description of how a sensor device is used in research data collection.
- *Output*: Characteristics of sensor measurements.

The contents of these three domains ensure quality in exposure studies by providing the content and structure for (1) establishing a library of sensors as described in Section 16.5.3, (2) development of a DMDR also described in Section 16.5.1, and (3) the development of data harmonization MDR (described next). Using SCMS, we develop a similar metadata model for interventional devices used in research studies (Morgan, Gouripeddi, and Sward 2019).

2. Metadata management (Gouripeddi et al. 2019b,c, Sward et al. 2017).
   OF's MDR (Bradshaw et al. 2009, Mo et al. 2014) is an Object Modeling Group specification conformant (Object Management Group 2019), FAIR-compliant (Wilkinson et al. 2016), standard-based repository of artifacts and knowledge. It stores metadata artifacts and relationships of data and modular components subscribed by OF. These artifacts include, but are not limited to: (1) logical models, local models, model mappings, (2) administrative information, (3) descriptive information, and (4) translation programs. These are organized as "assets" in a custom-built, highly generic and abstracted entity-relationship model. Assets may have properties and associations to other assets. Stored metadata is shared in various structured and non-proprietary formats using translation programs and made available for consumption by different SS.

   Considering the data and process complexity within exposomic research, we conceptually divided metadata management into three categories:

- *Data metadata*: Metadata that describes data outputs resulting from an observations or measurements. This includes sensor measurements, outputs of computational models, clinical observations, genomic sequence annotations, socio-behavioral data, and participant report data.
- *Process metadata*: Metadata that describes research or data processes within EHIE. This includes sequences of steps followed in different computational models in order to generate outputs, and data

transformation and integration workflows to harmonize source data as events or into analytical models. An example of a research process is sensor deployment.

- *Knowledge resources*: Metadata that describes a source or instrument used to collect, measure, or derive data. This includes sensor devices, electronic medical records, or study-specific data collection instruments.

The SCMS has highly interconnected metadata elements. The labeled property graph provides better support for (1) complex relationships, such as ternary or higher degrees, many-to-many, and self-referencing relationship types, and (2) dynamic schemas (Robinson et al. 2015). Unlike relational stores, graph metadata management does not require deviating from natural relationships representing semantically rich domains in the real world. We, therefore, adopted a graph-based MDR for the instrument and output domains of SCMS which represent data metadata and knowledge resources aspects of metadata categories. Since the deployment domain of the SCMS is fairly simple with one-to-many relationships, we adapted a document store that captures metadata about the deployment processes as described above. We implemented the instrument domain in a Neo4j graph database (Neo4j Graph Platform 2019), which forms the backend store for the sensor library (Burnett et al. 2018a), as described in the participant-facing tools section. OrientDB graph database system (OrientDB 2019) provides better integration with Java classes. We, therefore, used OrientDB for storing data metadata which includes data transformation functions to transform source data into events. Similarly, we have adapted OrientDB for storing data metadata of other data domains such as clinical, biospecimen, socio-behavioral, and participant report which we were originally stored in relational databases. We adapted the MongoDB platform (MongoDB 2019) for the deployment MDR as described in Section 16.5.1.

These new approaches to metadata management limit the introduction of semantic dissonance between conceptual models and their implementation, as it retains complex real-world relationships. Detailed metadata stored in the MDRs provide a spatio-temporal grid of metadata complementing the high-resolution spatio-temporal grid of integrated data, informing end-users of the limitations and uncertainties associated with the data. As a next step, we plan to characterize, develop specifications, consume, and store relevant semantics for the exposome domain (Habre et al. 2016, Mattingly et al. 2016, Burnett et al. 2018a, Kiossoglou et al. 2017, Gouripeddi, Habre, and PRISMS Data Modeling Working 2019, Cummins et al. 2019a, Lopez-Campos et al. 2019) and supplement this metadata work.

3. Event Document Store (EDS)

Exposomic studies require integrity of spatial and temporal dimensions of data in order to ascertain relationships between patient-reported symptoms, physiological measurements, and clinical manifestations, with environmental changes (Gouripeddi et al. 2017). This requirement for generating spatio-temporal records of exposures and the need to provide data in different analytic models and formats led us to transform all data as events occurring in spatio-temporal coordinates. Based on the uncertainty associated with the proximity of data collection to the subject under consideration, and the usage of different data collections in different types of translational research, we classified events into six domains: sensor, clinical, biospecimen-derived, patient-reported, computationally modeled, and aggregates (Figure 16.15) (Gouripeddi et al. 2017). These events are informed by logical models stored in the MDR. Each event is logically a document and we call the aggregation of all these documents an EDS. The EDS is conceptually modeled as events occurring on a timeline and can be implemented in any Big Data store. This primitive storage format allows linkage across different root objects that do not necessarily belong to a person and can be transformed into higher/analytical models based on use cases. Time represented in these events is modeled as (Combi, Keravnou-Papailiou, and Shahar 2010):

- *Unbounded*: Contains upper and/or lower bounds with respect to its order relationship.
- *Dense*: An infinite set of smaller units.
- *Discrete*: Every element has both an immediate successor and an immediate predecessor, if unbounded, and within the bounds, if bounded.
- Instants and intervals (upper and lower time points).
- Finest granularity available with the source.

Similarly, spatial dimensions in these events are continuous and transformable to different reference systems. We stored these events as JavaScript

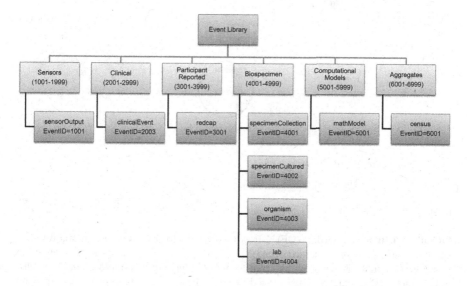

FIGURE 16.15 Conceptual representation of different events implemented with allocated bins of event identifiers.

object notation (JSON) documents in the Couchbase NoSQL platform (Couchbase 2019). The EDS supports (1) natural querying for spatio-temporal reasoning of events and knowledge facts—a critical need for complex and unpredictable diseases in which sequences and locations of events are critical to their understanding and (2) transformation of events into higher/analytical models to support diverse translational research archetypes.

4. Software workflow

OF transforms and stores data from heterogeneous sensors and other health data sources into uniform event-based data structures. In order to facilitate these data transformations, we modified OF to be an event-driven architecture with the following changes (Figure 16.16): First, data services identify user input data criteria for integration. Then, using the contents of the MDR, OF orchestrates querying of data sources which could be web services, database tables and flat files for attributes described in the user's input. OF's SS leverage metadata content in the MDR to inform structural and semantic transformations of selected data to their corresponding events. Using this metadata, OF's services then write events into the EDS. For example, home-based sensor measurements acquired via EpiFi (Lundrigan et al. 2017) are transformed into sensor events and integrated as JSON documents in EDS (Figure 16.15). OF also exposes several services to access and view the documents stored in the EDS.

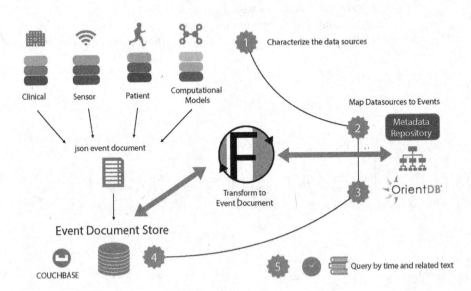

FIGURE 16.16 OpenFurther (OF) software workflow for exposure health studies. Key steps: (1) data sources are characterized, (2) their metadata and mappings to different event types are authored, (3) metadata and transformation functions are stored in an OrientDB-based graph MDR, which is (4) leveraged by OF to generate events stored in a Couchbase event document store, and (5) these events are available for querying by time and other downstream analytic processes.

Data in EDS is stored on a study by study basis. A research study is represented by a study event and consists of one or more integration events that represent periodic data integration runs. We found that the architecture can be scaled for performance. The architectural designs of the infrastructure support a semantically consistent, metadata-driven approach to multi-scale, multi-omics exposomic Big Data integration for diverse translational research ranging from understanding mechanisms of disease to developing preventive and therapeutic interventions. The developed architecture alleviates informatics challenges associated with exposomic data that originate from the characteristics of measurement devices, their deployment, and human behavior.

We index the data using Couchbase's native indexing and with ElasticSearch (Kuc and Rogozinski 2013) to support different spatio-temporal reasoning use cases. In addition, we use a similar metadata-driven approach described above to transform events into higher analytical models depending on the use case, which is then made available via different research-facing tools. We have also submitted the integrated data through data streaming pipelines such as the Kafka (Narkhede, Shapira, and Palino 2017) instance hosted at the PRISMS data coordinating center (Stripelis et al. 2017).

16.6   UTILIZATION OF EXPOSOME IN TRANSLATIONAL STUDIES

We are utilizing EHIE to generate exposomes for two ongoing studies:

1. *PRISMS Pilot (Gouripeddi et al. 2019b,c)*: This study was approved by the University of Utah Institutional Review Board (IRB No._00086107). We adopted an ongoing transient receptor potential pediatric asthma study (Deering-Rice et al. 2015, 2016), where we collected and integrated environmental data with health data for 10 participants residing in Salt Lake, Davis and Utah Counties, Utah, United States, for the period March 1st, 2017 to June 30th, 2018 (study processes depicted in Figure 16.10). A summary of the data used in this study is presented in Table 16.1. We integrated this data into approximately 25 million events for the study period (Figure 16.17). The generated events included participant registration, clinical, survey, sensor output, and sensor deployment events, linked by events representing different integration batches and the study. On evaluation of the quality of the integrated documents, we found the events to be consistent and accurate with the source data. In addition, we were able to perform analysis of these events to ascertain spatio-temporal relationships between various events. We submitted this information to the PRISMS data coordinating center in order to test the PRISMS program concept. Statistical and machine learning analysis results being performed both at the University of Utah and the data coordinating center are pending.

2. *Environmental influences on Child Health Outcomes (ECHO) Study (Collingwood et al. 2018)*: This study was approved by the University of Utah Institutional Review Board (IRB No._00086107). As part of ECHO, we piloted deployment of sensors among urban, rural, frontier, and tribal populations to evaluate the acceptability of low-cost, IoT connected air

TABLE 16.1

Summary of Data Integrated as Events for the Utah PRISMS Pilot Study for the Period from March 1, 2017 to June 30, 2018

Data Stream	Description	Event Count
Participant demographics	Collected using a REDCap questionnaire. Data consumed via the REDCap API (Harris et al. 2009)	10
Participant home assessment	Collected using a REDCap questionnaire. Data consumed via the REDCap API	10
Home sensor deployment	Details about the indoor home sensor deployment. Collected using a REDCap questionnaire. Data consumed via the REDCap API	145
Asthma severity assessment (weekly)	Weekly asthma symptoms and severity scores of participants collected from eAsthmaTracker (eAT) (Nkoy et al. 2012, 2013). Data consumed from MySQL database of eAT	293
Asthma severity assessment (daily)	Daily asthma symptoms and severity scores of participants collected from eAT. Data consumed from MySQL database of eAT	1,160
Particulate matter (PM2.5) for Salt Lake, Davis and Utah Counties, Utah, United States	Environmental Protection Agency's Air Quality Datamart API ("AQS Data Mart I Air Quality System I US EPA" 2019)	73,995
Temperature, humidity for Salt Lake, Davis and Utah Counties, Utah, United States	National Weather Service API (US Department of Commerce 2019)	703,164
Particulate matter (PM2.5) from PurpleAir	Data from Purple Citizen's Network (PurpleAir.Org 2019) aggregated by Mesowest (Horel et al. 2002)	1,738,132
Particulate matter (PM2.5) from Trax light rail in Wasatch front	Mobile Air Quality Assessment from Trax (Mitchell et al. 2015, 2018) aggregated by Mesowest	7,934,529
Indoor particulate matter (PM2.5) measured by Utah Modified Dylos	Data made available through EpiFi (Lundrigan et al. 2017) and consumed from an influx database	14,075,201
Total		**24,526,639**

quality measurement devices varied populations. With good results in our pilot testing, we deployed multiple sensors in homes of participants recruited via a geographic random sampling protocol whereby the primary inclusion criteria was a women of childbearing age residing in the home. To date, we have deployed multiple sensors in 28 homes of participants and collected in excess of 50,000,00 sensor readings measuring PM2.5 using AirU devices (Kelly et al. 2017) through EHIE over a 1-year period.

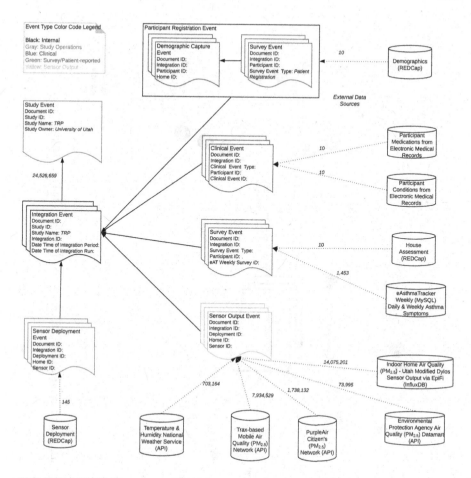

FIGURE 16.17 Different types of events generated by integrating sensor and clinical datasets in the Utah PRISMS pilot study. Data from ten participants for the period March 1st 2017 to June 30th, 2018 and residing in Salt Lake, Davis and Utah Counties, Utah, United States, were integrated resulting in a total of 24,526,659 events. Source data consisting of participant registrant data (bottom right to left) including participant demographics and criteria of their eligibility to the study, clinical data, home assessment surveys, asthma symptoms, indoor and outdoor air quality sensor readings, weather and detailed sensor deployment data. These events are linked via integrated events and study events. Counts of events integrated from each source are indicated on top of arrows connecting them to their corresponding event types.

Ongoing investigations relative to these environmental sensors include in-home air quality variation, relationship between indoor/outdoor & housing characteristics, individual sensor measurement variation (drift), and home-based air quality influences on urinary markers of inflammation. Future work will expand the deployment to more than 200 AirU sensors and in 60 additional homes. In addition, the measurement capability of the AirU's

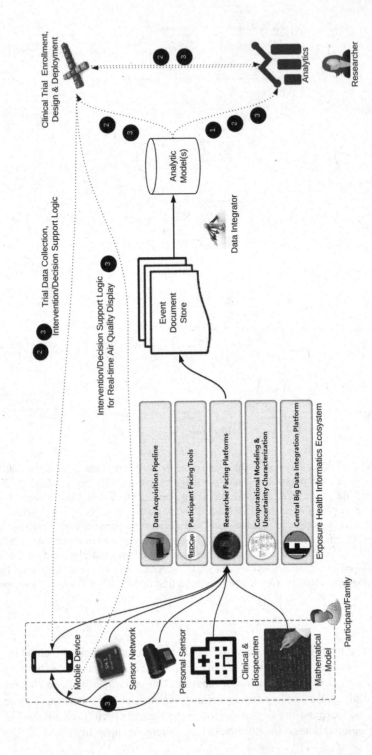

FIGURE 16.18 Diverse translational exposomic research use cases supported by EHIE leveraging IoT Devices and Big Data methods.

will be enhanced by embedding ozone and volatile organic compound (VOC) sensors into the unit, using EHIE for management of deployment processes, and integration of data arising from over 250 sensors.

Our initial results from these pilots show that it is feasible to use informatics ecosystems like EHIE to perform sensor-based longitudinal cohort studies (Collingwood et al. 2018, Gouripeddi et al. 2018, Sward 2019, Cummins et al. 2019b). While different sensors capture data at different time resolutions and have varying spatial distributions, it is possible to generate spatio-temporal grids of exposures and relate to symptoms and clinical observations. Most participants were supportive of using their personal WiFi for sensor data transmission, but there is a need for flexible data transmission and storage methods to account for limitations in home networks. Preliminary statistical analysis of the data using mixed modeling approaches shows that particular matter (PM) levels were generally lower indoors compared to outdoors ($p < 0.001$). Indoor PM counts were not related to asthma control test (ACT) scores and rescue medication usage ($p > 0.05$). Outdoor PM2.5 was related to worsened ACT scores and increases in asthma treatment ($p < 0.001$), but outdoor PM10 counts were not related ($p = 0.52$).

16.7 DISCUSSION AND CONCLUSION

In this chapter, we discussed challenges and data needs for performing total exposure health research (Sward et al. 2017). These include (1) acquisition of sensor data, (2) selection of heterogeneous data sources, (3) filling gaps in measurements using computational modeling, (4) characterization of uncertainties associated with data, (5) generation of high-resolution spatio-temporal grids of exposures, (6) integration of data, (7) presentation and visualization of data, and (8) support for diverse set of translational research archetypes. In order to address these needs, we developed a loosely coupled, scalable informatics infrastructure called EHIE that consists of (1) data acquisition pipeline, (2) participant-facing tools, (3) researcher-facing platforms, (4) a computational modeling platform, and (5) a central Big Data federation/integration platform. For each of the above components, we provide an introduction and discuss their subcomponent architecture. The ECHO and PRISMS pilot are examples of demonstrative studies utilizing EHIE to generate exposomes for research.

EHIE is a generalizable, multi-scale, and multi-omics platform providing robust pipelines for reproducible exposomic research that uses real-time, low-cost sensors to provide spatio-temporal records of environmental exposures. Using this component-based ecosystem, we are able to support the deployment and performance of sensor-based studies, and the integration, processing, visualization, and secure transmission of study data for most research designs. EHIE provides an effective, flexible, and open access approach to collecting, managing, and analyzing high-resolution data from sensors. Because the infrastructure is based on logical data models for clinically relevant exposomes (environmental exposures such as air quality, which have health impacts), the infrastructure is flexible and adaptable to many translational research scenarios (Figure 16.18). The infrastructure also provides mechanisms for integrating exposure profiles (exposomes) with clinical, self-reported, behavioral, and other research data. In addition, EHIE supports supplementation of direct measurements with computationally-modeled data for exposures, activities and locations that can then easily be assimilated into comprehensive spatio-temporal records.

We have formalized the development and sustenance of this ecosystem and our team of collaborators as a Center of Excellence for Exposure Health Informatics (CEEHI) (http://ceehi.ccts.utah.edu/). CEEHI serves as a collaborative for continuing investigations and development of state-of-the-art informatics methods for exposomics. It is a go-to center for researchers interested in conducting sensor-based, mobile, and virtual studies that include measurements of the environment, physiology, and behavior of participants by providing expertise, guidance, infrastructure, and other resources to the total exposure health research community.

CEEHI provides a key infrastructure that accommodates diverse types of future studies, including general and personal environmental exposure monitoring, activities, and physiological responses to the environment. From an infrastructure perspective, CEEHI seeks to evaluate the ecosystemic health (Jansen 2014) of EHIE. We will then advance it as an ultra-large-scale infrastructure with integrated sensor health monitoring systems and with added abilities to perform studies using mobile sensors during real-life activity and location trajectories of participants (Bill Pollak 2006, Friedman et al. 2014). We will advance the use of novel sensors (Wang and Tao 2017, Li et al. 2019, Mirowsky et al. 2013), sensing paradigms (Schivo et al. 2013, McCartney et al. 2017, Hichwa and Davis 2018), and sensor networks and architectures (Kasera 2019). We will improve upon the science of using appropriate resolutions of data for different use cases by testing different data resolutions as available from the measured and modeled data available in networks such as Mesowest (Horel et al. 2002). We will add robust support for management of research processes and data for activities related to the study and its operations.

On a health research front, CEEHI is working with multiple researchers at the University of Utah and elsewhere to perform studies that seek to understand mechanistic, health outcomes, interventional aspects of exposure, and diverse disease conditions. Our current pediatric collaborators are interested in pediatric asthma and children with complex medical conditions in improving care, better self-tracking with environmental changes (Nkoy et al. 2012, 2013) and pharmacogenomics in relation to the environment (Deering-Rice et al. 2015, 2016). The Utah Children's Project, part of the ECHO Consortium (Stanford and Collingwood 2017), is continuing a longitudinal cohort study of children starting from pre-conception with plans to follow them through 20 years of age while measuring a broad array of environmental exposures. These include examining effects of diverse exposures (chronic and intermittent) on health and human development; investigating basic mechanisms and gene-environment interactions of developmental disorders and environmental factors (both risk and protective) that influence health and developmental processes; indoor and outdoor air sampling; home evaluations; questionnaires; and a diverse array of biomarkers including microbiome, serum antibodies, and others. In addition, components of the data acquisition platform are being used to investigate exposures in occupational environments (industry and military organizations), as well as environmental exposures of underserved populations (frontier and rural families). Other total exposure health conditions being studied include adult pulmonary disease (Pirozzi et al. 2015, 2017), sleep apnea (Sundar, Daly, and Willis 2013, Zanobetti et al. 2010, Weinreich et al. 2015, Billings et al. 2019), chronic kidney disease (Bowe et al. 2018, Kaskel et al. 2014), diabetes and metabolic disorders (Riches et al. 2019), aging and neurological conditions. In addition, at a mechanistic level, we are planning studies that look at the interaction of the microbiome with the exposome in asthma (Gouripeddi 2019a), and the role of PM chemical constituents in pulmonary health (Kitt et al. 2019). We are working on quantifying the digital exposome (Lopez-Campos, Merolli, and Martin-Sanchez 2017) and relating it with effects on health. Lastly, we are expanding the integration and real-time assimilation capabilities of the platform to obtain objective measures of autonomic nervous system physiology to detect real-time status of different conditions, such as impaired awareness of hypoglycemia (Groat et al. 2019, Mehta et al. 2019) and neuropathic pain (Singleton et al. 2008, 2014), and use them to develop interventions for managing these conditions.

ACKNOWLEDGMENTS

This research is supported by the Utah PRISMS Informatics Center (NIH/NIBIB U54EB021973), the Utah Center for Clinical and Translational Science (NCATS UL1TR001067), and the Utah ECHO Program (NIH UG3OD023249). Content is the sole responsibility of authors and does not necessarily represent official views of the NIH. Computational resources were provided by the Utah Center for High Performance Computing, which has been partially funded by the NIH Shared Instrumentation Grant 1S10OD021644-01A1. The authors acknowledge the contributions of all the team members affiliated with the Utah PRISMS Informatics Center grant, collaborators from the NIH PRISMS program, and the Program for Air Quality, Health, and Society, University of Utah.

REFERENCES

Abadi, Martin, Paul Barham, Jianmin Chen, Zhifeng Chen, Andy Davis, Jeffrey Dean, Matthieu Devin, et al. 2016. "TensorFlow: A system for large-scale machine learning." In *12th {USENIX} Symposium on Operating Systems Design and Implementation ({OSDI} 16)*, 265–283, Savannah, GA. https://www.usenix.org/conference/osdi16/technical-sessions/presentation/abadi.

Adame, Toni, Albert Bel, Boris Bellalta, Jaume Barcelo, and Miquel Oliver. 2014. "IEEE 802.11AH: The WiFi approach for M2M communications." *IEEE Wireless Communications* 21 (6): 144–152. doi:10.1109/MWC.2014.7000982.

An, Soyoung, Albert Lund, Nicole Burnett, Le-Thuy Tran, Peter Mo, Randy Madsen, Katherine Sward, R.K. Gouripeddi, and Julio Facelli. 2018. "Utah PRISMS ecosystem: An infrastructure for personal exposomic research." In *Ygnite* 2018, Washington, DC. http://yg.ksea.org/faq.html.

"AQS Data Mart I Air Quality System I US EPA." 2019. https://aqs.epa.gov/aqsweb/documents/data_mart_welcome.html.

Bakian, Amanda V., Rebekah S. Huber, Hilary Coon, Douglas Gray, Phillip Wilson, William M. McMahon, and Perry F. Renshaw. 2015. "Acute Air Pollution Exposure and Risk of Suicide Completion." *American Journal of Epidemiology* 181 (5): 295–303. doi:10.1093/aje/kwu341.

Iyer, Bala. 2014. "Understanding Software Ecosystems." Business, April 4. https://www. slideshare.net/balaiyer/software-ecosystem-visualization-methodology.

Boyle, Barksdale, Elizabeth, Nicole C. Deziel, Bonny L. Specker, Scott Collingwood, Clifford P. Weisel, David J. Wright, and Michael Dellarco. 2015. "Feasibility and informative value of environmental sample collection in the National Children's Vanguard Study." *Environmental Research* 140 (July): 345–353. doi:10.1016/j.envres.2015.04.006.

Billings, Martha E., Diane Gold, Adam Szpiro, Carrie P. Aaron, Neal Jorgensen, Amanda Gassett, Peter J. Leary, Joel D. Kaufman, and Susan R. Redline. 2019. "The association of ambient air pollution with sleep apnea: The multi-ethnic study of atherosclerosis." *Annals of the American Thoracic Society* 16 (3): 363–370. doi:10.1513/AnnalsATS.201804-248OC.

Bosco, Liana, Tiziana Notari, Giovanni Ruvolo, Maria C. Roccheri, Chiara Martino, Rosanna Chiappetta, Domenico Carone, et al. 2018. "Sperm DNA fragmentation: An early and reliable marker of air pollution." *Environmental Toxicology and Pharmacology* 58 (March): 243–249. doi:10.1016/j.etap.2018.02.001.

Bowe, Benjamin, Yan Xie, Tingting Li, Yan Yan, Hong Xian, and Ziyad Al-Aly. 2018. "Particulate matter air pollution and the risk of incident CKD and progression to ESRD." *Journal of the American Society of Nephrology* 29 (1): 218–230. doi:10.1681/ASN.2017030253.

Bradshaw, Richard L., Susan Matney, Oren E. Livne, Bruce E. Bray, Joyce A. Mitchell, and Scott P. Narus. 2009. "Architecture of a federated query engine for heterogeneous resources." *AMIA Annual Symposium Proceedings* 2009: 70–74.

Burnett, Nicole, Ram Gouripeddi, Mollie Cummins, Julio Facelli, and Katherine Sward. 2018a. "Towards a molecular basis of exposomic research." In *AMIA 2018 Informatics Summit*, San Francisco, CA. https://knowledge.amia.org/amia-66728-tbi2018-1.4078408/t004-1.4078844.

Burnett, Nicole, Ram Gouripeddi, Naresh Sundar Rajan, Randy Madsen, Peter Mo, and Julio C. Facelli. 2015. "A framework for validating modeled air quality data for use in biomedical research." http://www.airquality.utah.edu/files/2015/01/Burnette_Poster.pdf.

Burnett, Nicole, Ram Gouripeddi, Jingran Wen, Peter Mo, Randy Madsen, Ryan Butcher, Katherine Sward, and Julio C. Facelli. 2017. "Harmonization of sensor metadata and measurements to support exposomic research." In *2016 International Society of Exposure Science*, Research Triangle Park, NC. http://www.intlexposurescience.org/ISES2017.

Burnett, Nicole, Ramkiran Gouripeddi, Julio Facelli, Peter Mo, Randy Madsen, Ryan Butcher, and Katherine Sward. 2018b. "Development of sensor metadata library for exposomic studies." *ISEE Conference Abstracts* 2018 (1). https://ehp.niehs.nih.gov/doi/10.1289/isesisee.2018.P01.0320.

Centers for Disease Control and Prevention. 2019. "Frequently Asked Questions | Social Determinants of Health | NCHHSTP | CDC." https://www.cdc.gov/nchhstp/socialdeterminants/faq.html.

Chatterjee, Madhubanti, Xudong Ge, Yordan Kostov, Leah Tolosa, and Govind Rao. 2014. "A novel approach toward noninvasive monitoring of transcutaneous CO_2." *Medical Engineering and Physics* 36 (1): 136–139. doi:10.1016/j.medengphy.2013.07.001.

Choi, Edwin, and Juhan Sonin. 2019. "Determinants of Health Visualized." https://www.goinvo.com/vision/determinants-of-health/.

Collingwood, Scott, Ramkiran Gouripeddi, Bob Wong, and Katherine Sward. 2018. "Environmental influences on health outcomes-integrating real-time exposure measures from homes into longitudinal cohort studies: Lessons from the field." *ISEE Conference Abstracts* 2018 (1). https://ehp.niehs.nih.gov/doi/10.1289/isesisee.2018.P02.0860.

Collingwood, Scott, Jesse Zmoos, Leon Pahler, Bob Wong, Darrah Sleeth, and Rodney Handy. 2019. "Investigating measurement variation of modified low-cost particle sensors." *Journal of Aerosol Science* 135 (September): 21–32. doi:10.1016/j. jaerosci.2019.04.017.

Combi, Carlo, Elpida Keravnou-Papailiou, and Yuval Shahar. 2010. *Temporal Information Systems in Medicine*, 1st edition. New York: Springer.

Couchbase. 2019. https://www.couchbase.com/.

Cox, Jennie, Seung-Hyun Cho, Patrick Ryan, Kelechi Isiugo, James Ross, Steven Chillrud, Zheng Zhu, Roman Jandarov, Sergey A. Grinshpun, and Tiina Reponen. 2019. "Combining sensor-based measurement and modeling of PM2.5 and black carbon in assessing exposure to indoor aerosols." *Aerosol Science and Technology*: 1–13. doi:10. 1080/02786826.2019.1608353.

Cummins, Mollie, Ramkiran Gouripeddi, Flory Nkoy, Julio Facelli, and Katherine Sward. 2019a. "Utah PRISMS Center: Sensor-based, data intensive science." In *Council for the Advancement of Nursing Science 2019 Advanced Methods Conference: The Expanding Science of Sensor Technology in Research*, Washington, DC. https://www.nursing-science.org/events/2019advancedmethods.

Cummins, Mollie, Rima Habre, Ramkiran Gouripeddi, Flory Nkoy, Julio Facelli, and Katherine Sward. 2019b. "Compatibility of sensor study data elements with ECHO." In *Council for the Advancement of Nursing Science 2019 Advanced Methods Conference: The Expanding Science of Sensor Technology in Research*, Washington, DC. https:// www.nursingscience.org/events/2019advancedmethods.

Deelman, Ewa, Karan Vahi, Gideon Juve, Mats Rynge, Scott Callaghan, Philip J. Maechling, Rajiv Mayani, et al. 2015. "Pegasus, a workflow management system for science automation." *Future Generation Computer Systems* 46 (May): 17–35. doi:10.1016/j. future.2014.10.008.

Deering-Rice, Cassandra E., Darien Shapiro, Erin G. Romero, Chris Stockmann, Tatjana S. Bevans, Quang M. Phan, Bryan L. Stone, et al. 2015. "Activation of transient receptor potential Ankyrin-1 by insoluble particulate material and association with asthma." *American Journal of Respiratory Cell and Molecular Biology* 53 (6): 893–901. doi:10.1165/rcmb.2015-0086OC.

Deering-Rice, Cassandra E., Chris Stockmann, Erin G. Romero, Zhenyu Lu, Darien Shapiro, Bryan L. Stone, Bernhard Fassl, et al. 2016. "Characterization of Transient Receptor Potential Vanilloid-1 (TRPV1) Variant Activation by Coal Fly Ash Particles and Associations with Altered Transient Receptor Potential Ankyrin-1 (TRPA1) Expression and Asthma." *Journal of Biological Chemistry* 291 (48): 24866–24879. doi:10.1074/jbc. M116.746156.

Dittrich, Yvonne. 2014. "Software engineering beyond the project: Sustaining software ecosystems." *Information and Software Technology, Special Issue on Software Ecosystems* 56 (11): 1436–1456. doi:10.1016/j.infsof.2014.02.012.

Erickson, Larry E., and Merrisa Jennings. 2017. "Energy, transportation, air quality, climate change, health nexus: Sustainable energy is good for our health." *AIMS Public Health* 4 (1): 47–61. doi:10.3934/publichealth.2017.1.47.

Farahani, Shahin. 2011. *ZigBee Wireless Networks and Transceivers*. Oxford: Newnes.

Friedman, Charles, Joshua Rubin, Jeffrey Brown, Melinda Buntin, Milton Corn, Lynn Etheredge, Carl Gunter, et al. 2014. "Toward a science of learning systems: A research agenda for the high-functioning learning health system." *Journal of the American Medical Informatics Association*. doi:10.1136/amiajnl-2014-002977.

Gładka, Anna, Joanna Rymaszewska, and Tomasz Zatoński. 2018. "Impact of air pollution on depression and suicide." *International Journal of Occupational Medicine and Environmental Health* 31 (6): 711–721. doi:10.13075/ijomeh.1896.01277.

Gouripeddi, Ramkiran. 2016. "An informatics architecture for an exposome." In *American Medical Informatics Association Spring 2016*. https://www.amia.org/jointsummits2016/implementation-informatics-track-sessions.

Gouripeddi, Ramkiran. 2019. OpenFurther, http://Openfurther.Org/ and Utah Center for Clinical and Translational Science, http://openfurther.org/.

Gouripeddi, Ramkiran, Nicole Burnett, Mollie Cummins, Julio Facelli, and Katherine Sward. 2017. "A conceptual representation of exposome in translational research." In *AMIA 2017 Annual Symposium*, Washington, DC. https://amia2017.zerista.com/speaker/print?order=company&speaker_page=16.

Gouripeddi, Ramkiran, Nicole Burnett, and Julio Facelli. 2015. "Data, modeling, uncertainty and integration: The informatics of an air quality exposome." In *2015 International Society of Exposure Science Annual Meeting*, Henderson, NV. http://www.ises2015.org/Images/ISES-progam-DRAFT1.pdf.

Gouripeddi, Ramkiran, Scott C. Collingwood, Bob Wong, Mollie Cummins, Julio Facelli, and Katherine Sward. 2018. "The Utah PRISMS informatics ecosystem: An infrastructure for generating and utilizing exposomes for translational research." In *Total Exposure Health Conference 2018*, Bethesda, MD. http://www.cvent.com/events/total-exposure-health-2018/event-summary-f5ae5c586a414ceb84a7fb594789dd7b.aspx?lang=en.

Gouripeddi, Ramkiran, Rima Habre, and PRISMS Data Modeling Working Group. 2019. "Developing a specification for representing exposure health semantics." In *The International Societies of Exposure Science (ISES) and Indoor Air Quality and Climate (ISIAQ) 2019 Conference*, Kaunas, Lithuania.

Gouripeddi, Ramkiran, Andrew Miller, Karen Eilbeck, Katherine Sward, and Julio C. Facelli. 2019a. "Systematically integrating microbiomes and exposomes for translational research." *Journal of Clinical and Translational Science* 3 (s1): 29–30. doi:10.1017/cts.2019.71.

Gouripeddi, Ramkiran, N Dustin Schultz, Richard L. Bradshaw, Peter Mo, Randy Madsen, Phillip B. Warner, Bernard A. LaSalle, and Julio C Facelli. 2013. "FURTHeR: An infrastructure for clinical, translational and comparative effectiveness research." In *American Medical Informatics Association* 2013 *Annual Symposium*, Washington, DC. http://knowledge.amia.org/amia-55142-a2013e-1.580047/t-10-1.581994/f-010-1.581995/a-184-1.582011/ap-247-1.582014.

Gouripeddi, Ramkiran, Le-Thuy Tran, Albert Lund, Randy Madsen, Julio Facelli, and Sward Katherine. 2019b. "The Utah PRISMS informatics ecosystem: An infrastructure for generating and utilizing exposomes for translational research." In *AMIA 2019 Informatics Summit*, San Francisco, CA. https://informaticssummit2019.zerista.com/event/member/543073, Presentation: https://uofu.box.com/s/t7ehydznuwx5muka6ctof1dcu7aecfcv.

Gouripeddi, Ramkiran, Le-Thuy Tran, Randy Madsen, Tanvi Gangadhar, Peter Mo, Nicole Burnett, Ryan Butcher, Katherine Sward, and Julio Facelli. 2019c. "An architecture for metadata-driven integration of heterogeneous sensor and health data for translational exposomic research." In *2019 IEEE EMBS International Conference on Biomedical and Health Informatics (BHI) (IEEE BHI 2019)*, Chicago, IL.

Gouripeddi, Ramkiran, Phillip B. Warner, Peter Mo, James E. Levin, Rajendu Srivastava, Samir S. Shah, David de Regt, Eric Kirkendall, Jonathan Bickel, and E. Kent Korgenski. 2012. "Federating clinical data from six pediatric hospitals: Process and initial results for microbiology from the PHIS+ consortium." In *AMIA Annual Symposium Proceedings*, 281. http://www.ncbi.nlm.nih.gov/pmc/articles/PMC3540481/.

Grafana - The Open Platform for Analytics and Monitoring. 2019. https://grafana.com/.

Groat, Danielle, Ram Gouripeddi, Yu Keui Lin, and Julio C. Facelli. 2019. "Measuring the autonomic nervous system for translational research: Identification of non-invasive methods." *Journal of Clinical and Translational Science* 3 (s1): 28–28. doi:10.1017/cts.2019.68.

Habre, Rima, Jose-Luis Ambite, Alex Bui, Mollie Cummins, Michael Dellarco, Sandrah Eckel, Ramkiran Gouripeddi, and Katherine Sward. 2016. "Pediatric Research Using Integrated Sensor Monitoring Systems, Data Modeling Working Group." In *26th Annual International Society of Exposure Science (ISES) Meeting*, Utrecht, The Netherlands. https://www.intlexposurescience.org/Public/Annual_Meeting/ Past_Meetings/26th_Annual_Meeting/Public/Annual_Meeting/PastMeetings/2016_ Meeting.aspx?hkey=9ae9d30a-6e0b-4177-98d5-95e58a1f64fb.

Harris, Paul A., Robert Taylor, Robert Thielke, Jonathon Payne, Nathaniel Gonzalez, and Jose G. Conde. 2009. "Research Electronic Data Capture (REDCap): A metadata-driven methodology and workflow process for providing translational research informatics support." *Journal of Biomedical Informatics* 42 (2): 377–381. doi:10.1016/j.jbi.2008.08.010.

Hichwa, Paul, and Cristina E Davis. 2018. "Modern application potential of miniature chemical sensors." In Kevin Yallup and Laura Basiricò (Eds.), *Sensors for Diagnostics and Monitoring*, 295–314. Boca Raton, FL: CRC Press.

Home Assistant. 2019. https://www.home-assistant.io/.

Horel, J., M. Splitt, L. Dunn, J. Pechmann, B. White, C. Ciliberti, S. Lazarus, J. Slemmer, D. Zaff, and J. Burks. 2002. "Mesowest: Cooperative mesonets in the Western United States." *Bulletin of the American Meteorological Society* 83 (2): 211–226. doi:10.1175/1520-0477(2002)083<0211:MCMITW>2.3.CO;2.

Hunkeler, U., H. L. Truong, and A. Stanford-Clark. 2008. "MQTT-S: A publish/subscribe protocol for wireless sensor networks." In *2008 3rd International Conference on Communication Systems Software and Middleware and Workshops (COMSWARE'08)*, 791–798. doi:10.1109/COMSWA.2008.4554519.

InfluxData (InfluxDB) | Time Series Database Monitoring & Analytics. 2019. https://www. influxdata.com/.

Jacobs, David E., Jonathan Wilson, Sherry L. Dixon, Janet Smith, and Anne Evens. 2009. "The Relationship of housing and population health: A 30-year retrospective analysis." *Environmental Health Perspectives* 117 (4): 597–604. doi:10.1289/ehp.0800086.

Jansen, Slinger. 2014. "Measuring the health of open source software ecosystems: Beyond the scope of project health." *Information and Software Technology, Special Issue on Software Ecosystems*, 56 (11): 1508–1519. doi:10.1016/j.infsof.2014.04.006.

Jansen, Slinger, Sjaak Brinkkemper, and Michael A. Cusumano. 2013. *Software Ecosystems: Analyzing and Managing Business Networks in the Software Industry*. Cheltenham, UK and Northampton, MA: Edward Elgar Publisher.

Jansen, Slinger, Anthony Finkelstein, and Sjaak Brinkkemper. 2009. "A sense of community: A research agenda for software ecosystems." In *2009 31st International Conference on Software Engineering: Companion Volume*, 187–190, Vancouver, BC, Canada: IEEE. doi:10.1109/ICSE-COMPANION.2009.5070978.

Kasera, Sneha Kumar. 2019. "Powder: Platform for open wireless data-driven experimental research." https://powderwireless.net/.

Kaskel, Frederick, Daniel Batlle, Srinivasan Beddhu, John Daugirdas, Harold Feldman, Maria Ferris, Lawrence Fine, et al. 2014. "Improving CKD therapies and care: A national dialogue." *Clinical Journal of the American Society of Nephrology* 9 (4): 815–817. doi:10.2215/CJN.12631213.

Kelly, K.E., J. Whitaker, A. Petty, C. Widmer, A. Dybwad, D. Sleeth, R. Martin, and A. Butterfield. 2017. "Ambient and laboratory evaluation of a low-cost particulate matter sensor." *Environmental Pollution* 221 (February): 491–500. doi:10.1016/j. envpol.2016.12.039.

Kiossoglou, Phillip, Ann Borda, Kathleen Gray, Ferdinando Martin-Sanchez, Karin Verspoor, and Guillermo H. Lopez Campos. 2017. "How well do existing ontologies represent exposome literature?" In *AMIA 2017 Informatics Summit*, San Francisco, CA. https://knowledge.amia.org/amia-64484-tbi2017-1.3520073/t004-1.3520463.

Kitt, Jay, Randall Martin, Krishna Sundar, Cheryl Pirozzi, Ramkiran Gouripeddi, Joel Harris, and Facelli Julio. 2019. "Informatics and chemistry: Examining the impact of particulate matter chemical composition on pulmonary disease outcomes." In *The Air We Breathe: A Multidisciplinary Perspective on Air Quality*, Salt Lake City, UT.

Kuc, Rafal, and Marek Rogozinski. 2013. *Elasticsearch Server*. Birmingham: Packt Publishing Ltd.

Kukkapalli, R., N. Banerjee, R. Robucci, and Y. Kostov. 2016. "Micro-radar wearable respiration monitor." In *2016 IEEE Sensors*, 1–3. doi:10.1109/ICSENS.2016.7808741.

Landrigan, Philip J., Richard Fuller, Nereus J. R. Acosta, Olusoji Adeyi, Robert Arnold, Niladri (Nil) Basu, Abdoulaye Bibi Baldé, et al. 2018. "The Lancet Commission on pollution and health." *The Lancet* 391 (10119): 462–512. doi:10.1016/S0140-6736(17)32345-0.

Lee, Byeong-Jae, Bumseok Kim, and Kyuhong Lee. 2014. "Air pollution exposure and cardiovascular disease." *Toxicological Research* 30 (2): 71–75. doi:10.5487/TR.2014.30.2.071.

Lee, H., and K. Ke. 2018. "Monitoring of large-area IoT sensors using a LoRa wireless mesh network system: Design and evaluation." *IEEE Transactions on Instrumentation and Measurement* 67 (9): 2177–2187. doi:10.1109/TIM.2018.2814082.

Leiser, Claire L., Heidi A. Hanson, Kara Sawyer, Jacob Steenblik, Ragheed Al-Dulaimi, Troy Madsen, Karen Gibbins, et al. 2019. "Acute effects of air pollutants on spontaneous pregnancy loss: A case-crossover study." *Fertility and Sterility* 111 (2): 341–347. doi:10.1016/j.fertnstert.2018.10.028.

Li, Baichen, Quan Dong, R. Scott Downen, Nam Tran, J. Hunter Jackson, Dinesh Pillai, Mona Zaghloul, and Zhenyu Li. 2019. "A wearable IoT aldehyde sensor for pediatric asthma research and management." *Sensors and Actuators B: Chemical* 287: 584–594.

Lioy, Paul, and Clifford Weisel. 2014. *Exposure Science: Basic Principles and Applications*, 1st edition. Amsterdam and Boston, MA: Academic Press.

Livne, Oren E., N. Dustin Schultz, and Scott P. Narus. 2011. "Federated querying architecture with clinical & translational health IT application." *Journal of Medical Systems* 35 (5): 1211–1224. doi:10.1007/s10916-011-9720-3.

Lopez-Campos, Guillermo, Christopher Hawthorn, Philip Kiossoglou, Ramkiran Gouripeddi, Ann Borda, Kathleen Gray, Fernando Martin-Sanchez, and Karin Verspoor. 2019. "Characterising the scope of exposome research: A generalisable approach." In *2019 Exposome Symposium*, Brescia, Italy.

Lopez-Campos, G., M. Merolli, and F. Martin-Sanchez. 2017. "Biomedical informatics and the digital component of the exposome." *Studies in Health Technology and Informatics* 245: 496–500.

Lund, Albert, Nicole Burnett, Ram Gouripeddi, and Julio Facelli. 2017. "An agent-based model for estimating human activity patterns on the wasatch front." In *Air Quality: Science for Solutions*, Salt Lake City, UT. http://harbor.weber.edu/Airqualityscience/abstracts/default.html.

Lund, Albert, Ram Gouripeddi, Nicole Burnett, Le-Thuy Tran, Peter Mo, Randy Madsen, Mollie Cummins, Katherine Sward, and Julio Facelli. 2018. "Enabling reproducible computational modeling: The Utah PRISMS Ecosystem." In *Conference: Building Research Integrity Through Reproducibility*, Salt Lake City, UT. campusguides.lib.utah.edu/UtahRR18/abstracts.

Lund, Albert M., Ramkiran Gouripeddi, and Julio C. Facelli. 2019a. "Generation and classification of activity sequences for spatiotemporal modeling of human populations." ArXiv:1911.05476 [Cs], November. http://arxiv.org/abs/1911.05476.

Lund, Albert, Ramkiran Gouripeddi, and Julio C. Facelli. 2019b. "STHAM: An agent based model for simulating human exposure across high resolution spatiotemporal domains." *Journal of Exposure Science and Environmental Epidemiology*, In press. doi.org/10.1038/s41370-020-0216-4.

Lundrigan, Philip. 2019. VDL-PRISM. https://github.com/VDL-PRISM.

Lundrigan, Philip, Sneha Kumar Kasera, and Neal Patwari. 2018. "STRAP: Secure TRansfer of Association Protocol." In *2018 27th International Conference on Computer Communication and Networks (ICCCN)*, 1–9. doi:10.1109/ICCCN.2018.8487333.

Lundrigan, Philip, Kyeong Min, Neal Patwari, Sneha Kasera, Kerry Kelly, Jimmy Moore, Miriah Meyer, et al. 2017. "EpiFi: An In-Home Sensor Network Architecture for Epidemiological Studies." *ArXiv:1709.02233 [Cs]*, September. http://arxiv.org/abs/1709.02233.

Lundrigan, Philip, Kyeong T. Min, Neal Patwari, Sneha Kumar Kasera, Kerry Kelly, Jimmy Moore, Miriah Meyer, et al. 2018. "EpiFi: An in-Home IoT Architecture for Epidemiological Deployments." In *2018 IEEE 43rd Conference on Local Computer Networks Workshops (LCN Workshops)*, 30–37. doi:10.1109/LCNW.2018.8628482.

Lungu, Mircea. 2009. "Reverse Engineering Software Ecosystems," September, 208.

Luxton, David D., Robert A. Kayl, and Matthew C. Mishkind. 2012. "MHealth data security: The need for HIPAA-compliant standardization." *Telemedicine and E-Health* 18 (4): 284–288. doi:10.1089/tmj.2011.0180.

Manikas, Konstantinos, and Klaus Marius Hansen. 2013. "Software ecosystems: A systematic literature review." *Journal of Systems and Software* 86 (5): 1294–1306. doi:10.1016/j.jss.2012.12.026.

Martin-Sanchez, Fernando, Kathleen Gray, Riccardo Bellazzi, and Guillermo Lopez-Campos. 2014. "Exposome informatics: Considerations for the design of future bio-medical research information systems." *Journal of the American Medical Informatics Association* 21 (3): 386–390. doi:10.1136/amiajnl-2013-001772.

Mattingly, Carolyn J., Rebecca Boyles, Cindy P. Lawler, Astrid C. Haugen, Allen Dearry, and Melissa Haendel. 2016. "Laying a Community-Based Foundation for Data-Driven Semantic Standards in Environmental Health Sciences." *Environmental Health Perspectives* 124 (8). doi:10.1289/ehp.1510438.

McCartney, Mitchell M., Yuriy Zrodnikov, Alexander G. Fung, Michael K. LeVasseur, Josephine M. Pedersen, Konstantin O. Zamuruyev, Alexander A. Aksenov, Nicholas J. Kenyon, and Cristina E. Davis. 2017. "An easy to manufacture micro gas preconcentrator for chemical sensing applications." *ACS Sensors* 2 (8): 1167–1174. doi:10.1021/acssensors.7b00289.

McGinnis, J. Michael, Pamela Williams-Russo, and James R. Knickman. 2002. "The case for more active policy attention to health promotion." *Health Affairs (Project Hope)* 21 (2): 78–93. doi:10.1377/hlthaff.21.2.78.

McMillan, Nancy J., David M. Holland, Michele Morara, and Jingyu Feng. 2010. "Combining numerical model output and particulate data using Bayesian space–time modeling." *Environmetrics* 21 (1): 48–65. doi:10.1002/env.984.

McMullen, C. K., J. S. Ash, D. F. Sittig, A. Bunce, K. Guappone, R. Dykstra, J. Carpenter, J. Richardson, and A. Wright. 2011. "Rapid assessment of clinical information systems in the healthcare setting: An efficient method for time-pressed evaluation." *Methods of Information in Medicine* 50 (4): 299–307. doi:10.3414/ME10-01-0042.

Mehta, Maitrey, Danielle Groat, Yu Kuei Lin, Ramkiran Gouripeddi, and Julio Facelli. 2019. "Classifying impaired awareness of hypoglycemia with convolutional neural networks." In *2019 IEEE EMBS International Conference on Biomedical & Health Informatics (BHI) (IEEE BHI 2019)*, Chicago, IL.

Messerschmitt, David G., and Clemens Szyperski. 2003. *Software Ecosystem: Understanding an Indispensable Technology and Industry*. Cambridge, MA: The MIT Press.

Miller, Gary W. 2013. *The Exposome: A Primer*, 1st edition. Amsterdam and Boston, MA: Academic Press.

Miller, Gary W., and Dean P. Jones. 2014. "The nature of nurture: Refining the definition of the exposome." *Toxicological Sciences* 137 (1): 1–2. doi:10.1093/toxsci/kft251.

Min, Kyeong T., Philip Lundrigan, Katherine Sward, Scott C. Collingwood, and Neal Patwari. 2018. "Smart home air filtering system: A randomized controlled trial for performance evaluation." *Smart Health*. doi:10.1016/j.smhl.2018.07.009.

Miri, Mohammad, Milad Nazarzadeh, Ahmad Alahabadi, Mohammad Hassan Ehrampoush, Abolfazl Rad, Mohammad Hassan Lotfi, Mohammad Hassan Sheikhha, Mohammad Javad Zare Sakhvidi, Tim S. Nawrot, and Payam Dadvand. 2019. "Air pollution and telomere length in adults: A systematic review and meta-analysis of observational studies." *Environmental Pollution (Barking, Essex: 1987)* 244 (January): 636–647. doi:10.1016/j.envpol.2018.09.130.

Mirowsky, Jaime, Christina Hickey, Lori Horton, Martin Blaustein, Karen Galdanes, Richard E. Peltier, Steven Chillrud, et al. 2013. "The effect of particle size, location and season on the toxicity of urban and rural particulate matter." *Inhalation Toxicology* 25 (13): 747–757. doi:10.3109/08958378.2013.846443.

Mitchell, L., E. Crosman, B. Fasoli, L. Leclair-Marzolf, A. Jacques, J. Horel, J. C. Lin, D. R. Bowling, and J. R. Ehleringer. 2015. "Spatiotemporal patterns of urban trace gases and pollutants observed with a light rail vehicle platform in Salt Lake City, UT." *AGU Fall Meeting Abstracts* 23 (December): A23P-06.

Mitchell, Logan E., Erik T. Crosman, Alexander A. Jacques, Benjamin Fasoli, Luke Leclair-Marzolf, John Horel, David R. Bowling, James R. Ehleringer, and John C. Lin. 2018. "Monitoring of greenhouse gases and pollutants across an urban area using a light-rail public transit platform." *Atmospheric Environment* 187 (August): 9–23. doi:10.1016/j. atmosenv.2018.05.044.

Mo, Peter, N. Dustin Schultz, Richard L. Bradshaw, Ryan Butcher, R. Gouripeddi, Phillip B. Warner, Randy Madsen, Bernard A. LaSalle, and Julio C. Facelli. 2014. "Real-time federated data translations using metadata-driven XQuery." In *AMIA 2014 Summit on Clinical Research Informatics*, San Francisco, CA. http://knowledge.amia. org/amia-56636-cri2014-1.977698/t-004-1.978136/a-089-1.978209/a-089-1.978210/ ap-085-1.978211.

MongoDB | The Most Popular Database for Modern Apps. 2019. https://www.mongodb.com/ index.

Moore, Jimmy, Pascal Goffin, Miriah Meyer, Philip Lundrigan, Neal Patwari, Katherine Sward, and Jason Wiese. 2018. "Managing in-home environments through sensing, annotating, and visualizing air quality data." *Proceedings of the ACM on Interactive, Mobile, Wearable and Ubiquitous Technologies* 2 (3): 28. doi:10.1145/3264938.

Morgan, Taylor, Ramkiran Gouripeddi, and Katherine Sward. 2019. "Characterizing metadata of e-devices for interventional translational research." In *AMIA 2019 Informatics Summit*, San Francisco, CA. https://www.amia.org/summit2019.

Narkhede, Neha, Gwen Shapira, and Todd Palino. 2017. *Kafka: The Definitive Guide: Real-Time Data and Stream Processing at Scale*, 1st edition. Sebastopol, CA: O'Reilly Media.

National Institute of Environmental Health Sciences (NIEHS). 2012. "National Institute of Environmental Health Sciences Strategic Plan 2012–2017." https://www.niehs.nih.gov/ about/strategicplan/strategicplan2012/index.cfm.

National Institute of Environmental Health Sciences (NIEHS). 2018. "National Institute of Environmental Health Sciences Strategic Plan 2018–2023: Advancing Environmental Health Sciences, Improving Health." https://www.niehs.nih.gov/about/strategicplan/ index.cfm.

National Institute for Occupational Safety and Health (NIOSH). 2018. CDC - Exposome and Exposomics - NIOSH Workplace Safety and Health Topic. https://www.cdc.gov/niosh/ topics/exposome/default.html.

Neo4j Graph Platform – The Leader in Graph Databases. 2019. https://neo4j.com/.

Newton, John N., Adam D. M. Briggs, Christopher J. L. Murray, Daniel Dicker, Kyle J. Foreman, Haidong Wang, Mohsen Naghavi, et al. 2015. "Changes in health in England, with analysis by English regions and areas of deprivation, 1990–2013: a systematic analysis for the Global Burden of Disease Study 2013." *Lancet (London, England)* 386 (10010): 2257–2274. doi:10.1016/S0140-6736(15)00195-6.

Nkoy, Flory L., Bryan L. Stone, Bernhard A. Fassl, Karmella Koopmeiners, Sarah Halbern, Eun H. Kim, Justin Poll, Joseph W. Hales, Dillon Lee, and Christopher G. Maloney. 2012. "Development of a novel tool for engaging children and parents in asthma self-management." *AMIA Annual Symposium Proceedings* 2012 (November): 663–672.

Nkoy, Flory L., Bryan L. Stone, Bernhard A. Fassl, Derek A. Uchida, Karmella Koopmeiners, Sarah Halbern, Eun H. Kim, et al. 2013. "Longitudinal validation of a tool for asthma self-monitoring." *Pediatrics* 132 (6): e1554–e1561. doi:10.1542/peds.2013–1389.

Object Management Group (OMG). 2019. https://www.service-architecture.com/articles/web-services/object_management_group_omg.html.

OrientDB - Distributed Multi-Model and Graph Database. 2019. http://orientdb.com/orientdb/.

Pirozzi, Cheryl S., Barbara E. Jones, James A. VanDerslice, Yue Zhang, Robert Paine, and Nathan C. Dean. 2017. "Short-term air pollution and incident pneumonia. A case–crossover study." *Annals of the American Thoracic Society* 15 (4): 449–459. doi:10.1513/AnnalsATS.201706-495OC.

Pirozzi, Cheryl, Anne Sturrock, Hsin-Yi Weng, Tom Greene, Mary Beth Scholand, Richard Kanner, and Robert Paine Iii. 2015. "Effect of naturally occurring ozone air pollution episodes on pulmonary oxidative stress and inflammation." *International Journal of Environmental Research and Public Health* 12 (5): 5061–5075. doi:10.3390/ijerph120505061.

Pollak, Bill, ed. 2006. *Ultra-Large-Scale Systems the Software Challenge of the Future.* Pittsburgh, PA: Software Engineering Institute Carnegie Mellon.

Pollock, Jenna, Lu Shi, and Ronald W. Gimbel. 2017. "Outdoor environment and pediatric asthma: An update on the evidence from North America." *Canadian Respiratory Journal* 2017: 8921917. doi:10.1155/2017/8921917.

Popp, Karl, and Ralf Meyer. 2010. *Profit from Software Ecosystems.* Norderstedt: Books on Demand.

Prüss-Üstün, Annette, J. Wolf, C. Corvalán, Robert Bos, and M. Neira. 2016. *Preventing Disease through Healthy Environments: A Global Assessment of the Burden of Disease from Environmental Risks*, 2nd edition. Geneva, Switzerland: World Health Organization.

PurpleAir.Org. 2019. http://www.purpleair.org/.

Riches, Naomi, Ramkiran Gouripeddi, Kevin Perry, and Rod Handy. 2019. "Informatics methods for characterizing multi-pollutant air quality exposure on health." In *The Air we Breathe: A Multidisciplinary Perspective on Air Quality*, Salt Lake City, UT.

Richtel, Matt. 2019. *An Elegant Defense: The Extraordinary New Science of the Immune System: A Tale in Four Lives*, Larger Print edition. New York: HarperLuxe.

Robinson, Ian, Jim Webber, and Emil Eifrem. 2015. *Graph Databases: New Opportunities for Connected Data*, 2nd edition. Beijing: O'Reilly Media.

Röhrig, Bernd, Jean-Baptist du Prel, Daniel Wachtlin, and Maria Blettner. 2009. "Types of study in medical research." *Deutsches Arzteblatt International* 106 (15): 262–268. doi:10.3238/arztebl.2009.0262.

Santibáñez-Andrade, Miguel, Ericka Marel Quezada-Maldonado, Álvaro Osornio-Vargas, Yesennia Sánchez-Pérez, and Claudia M. García-Cuellar. 2017. "Air pollution and genomic instability: The role of particulate matter in lung carcinogenesis." *Environmental Pollution* 229 (October): 412–422. doi:10.1016/j.envpol.2017.06.019.

Sarbhai, Aarushi, Ramkiran Gouripeddi, Philip Lundrigan, Pavithra Chidambaram, Aakansha Saha, Julio C. Facelli, Katherine Sward, and Sneha Kumar Kasera. 2019. "Managing sensor metadata in exposomic studies using blockchain." In *The Air We Breathe: A Multidisciplinary Perspective on Air Quality*, Salt Lake City, UT.

Schivo, Michael, Felicia Seichter, Alexander A. Aksenov, Alberto Pasamontes, Daniel J. Peirano, Boris Mizaikoff, Nicholas J. Kenyon, and Cristina E. Davis. 2013. "A mobile instrumentation platform to distinguish airway disorders." *Journal of Breath Research* 7 (1): 017113. doi:10.1088/1752-7155/7/1/017113.

Shiffman, Saul, Arthur A. Stone, and Michael R. Hufford. 2008. "Ecological momentary assessment." *Annual Review of Clinical Psychology* 4 (1): 1–32. doi:10.1146/annurev.clinpsy.3.022806.091415.

Singleton, John Robinson, Billie Bixby, James W. Russell, Eva L. Feldman, Amanda Peltier, Jonathan Goldstein, James Howard, and A. Gordon Smith. 2008. "The Utah early neuropathy scale: A sensitive clinical scale for early sensory predominant neuropathy." *Journal of the Peripheral Nervous System* 13 (3): 218–227. doi:10.1111/j.1529-8027.2008.00180.x.

Singleton, John R., Robin L. Marcus, Justin E. Jackson, Margaret K. Lessard, Timothy E. Graham, and Albert G. Smith. 2014. "Exercise increases cutaneous nerve density in diabetic patients without neuropathy." *Annals of Clinical and Translational Neurology* 1 (10): 844–849. doi:10.1002/acn3.125.

Stanford, Joseph, and Scott Collingwood. 2017. "Utah's Children's Project." https://healthcare.utah.edu/.

Stripelis, D., J. L. Ambite, Y. Chiang, S. P. Eckel, and R. Habre. 2017. "A scalable data integration and analysis architecture for sensor data of pediatric asthma." In *2017 IEEE 33rd International Conference on Data Engineering (ICDE)*, 1407–1408. doi:10.1109/ICDE.2017.198.

Sundar, Krishna M., Sarah E. Daly, and Alika M. Willis. 2013. "A longitudinal study of CPAP therapy for patients with chronic cough and obstructive sleep apnoea." *Cough* 9 (1): 19. doi:10.1186/1745-9974-9-19.

Sward, Katherine. 2019. "Making the connection: Integrated sensor systems research." In *52nd Annual Communicating Nursing Research Conference*, San Diego, CA. https://www.winursing.org/2019-researchconference/.

Sward, Katherine, Alex Bui, Jose-Luis Ambite, Michael Dellarco, Julio Facelli, and Frank D. Gilliland. 2016. "Pediatric Research Using Integrated Sensor Monitoring Systems (PRISMS): Applying sensor technology and informatics to better understand asthma." In *2016 American Medical Informatics Association Annual Symposium*, Chicago, IL. https://www.amia.org/amia2016.

Sward, Katherine, and Julio Facelli. 2016. "Pediatric Research Using Integrated Sensor Monitoring Systems (PRISMS): Utah Informatics Center Federated Integration Architecture." In *2016 International Society of Exposure Science Annual Meeting*, Utrecht, The Netherlands. https://ises2016.org/.

Sward, Katherine, Neal Patwari, Ramkiran Gouripeddi, and Julio Facelli. 2017. "An infrastructure for generating exposomes: Initial lessons from the Utah PRISMS platform." In *2017 International Society of Exposure Science Annual Meeting*, Research Triangle Park, NC. https://intlexposurescience.org/ISES2017/default.aspx.

Tarlov, A. R. 1999. "Public policy frameworks for improving population health." *Annals of the New York Academy of Sciences* 896: 281–293.

Tiase, Victoria, Ram Gouripeddi, Nicole Burnett, Ryan Butcher, Peter Mo, Mollie Cummins, and Katherine Sward. 2018. "Advancing study metadata models to support an exposomic informatics infrastructure." In *2018 ISES Annual Meeting, Ottawa*, Canada. http://www.eiseverywhere.com/ehome/294696/638649/?&t=8c531cecd4bb0a5efc6a0045f5bec0c3.

Twilio: Communication APIs for SMS, Voice, Video and Authentication. 2019. Accessed June 1. https://www.twilio.com.

United Nations International Children's Emergency Fund. 2016. "Clear the Air for Children." https://www.unicef.org/publications/index_92957.html.

US Bureau of Labor Statistics. 2017. *American Time Use Survey*. https://www.bls.gov/tus/.

US Census Bureau. 2010. *Decennial Census by Decades*. https://www.census.gov/programs-surveys/decennial-census/decade.html.

US Census Bureau. 2017. *American Community Survey (ACS)*. https://www.census.gov/programs-surveys/acs.

US Census Bureau Center for Economic Studies. 2016. US Census Bureau Center for Economic Studies Publications and Reports Page. https://lehd.ces.census.gov/data/.

US Department of Commerce, NOAA. 2019. *National Weather Service*. http://www.weather.gov/.

US Environmental Protection Agency. 2005. "Revision to the guideline on air quality models: Adoption of a Preferred general purpose (flat and complex terrain) dispersion model and other revisions." Federal Register. https://www.federalregister.gov/documents/2005/11/09/05-21627/revision-to-the-guideline-on-air-quality-models-adoption-of-a-preferred-general-purpose-flat-and.

US Environmental Protection Agency. 2016a. "Model Clearinghouse Information Storage and Retrieval System I Support Center for Regulatory Atmospheric Modeling I Technology Transfer Network I US EPA." https://cfpub.epa.gov/oarweb/MCHISRS/.

US Environmental Protection Agency. 2016b. "Air Quality Data for the CDC National EPHT Network I Human Exposure and Atmospheric Sciences I US EPA." https://archive.epa.gov/heasd/archive-heasd/web/html/cdc.html.

US Environmental Protection Agency. 2016c. "Support Center for Regulatory Atmospheric Modeling (SCRAM)." *Data and Tools*. https://www.epa.gov/scram.

Vercellino, Robert J., Darrah K. Sleeth, Rodney G. Handy, Kyeong T. Min, and Scott C. Collingwood. 2018. "Laboratory evaluation of a low-cost, real-time, aerosol multi-sensor." *Journal of Occupational and Environmental Hygiene* 15 (7): 559–567. doi:10.1080/15459624.2018.1468565.

Wang, Di, and Nongjian Tao. 2017. A New Take on Asthma Sensors Offers Breath of Fresh Air: The State Press. https://www.statepress.com/article/2017/04/spscience-prisms-air-quality-watch.

Weinreich, Gerhard, Thomas E. Wessendorf, Noreen Pundt, Gudrun Weinmayr, Frauke Hennig, Susanne Moebus, Stefan Möhlenkamp, et al. 2015. "Association of short-term ozone and temperature with sleep disordered breathing." *The European Respiratory Journal* 46 (5): 1361–1369. doi:10.1183/13993003.02255-2014.

Wild, Christopher Paul. 2005. "Complementing the genome with an 'exposome': The outstanding challenge of environmental exposure measurement in molecular epidemiology." *Cancer Epidemiology and Prevention Biomarkers* 14 (8): 1847–1850. doi:10.1158/1055-9965.EPI-05-0456.

Wild, Christopher Paul. 2012. "The exposome: From concept to utility." *International Journal of Epidemiology* 41 (1): 24–32. doi:10.1093/ije/dyr236.

Wilkinson, Mark D., Michel Dumontier, IJsbrand Jan Aalbersberg, Gabrielle Appleton, Myles Axton, Arie Baak, Niklas Blomberg, et al. 2016. "The FAIR guiding principles for scientific data management and stewardship." *Scientific Data* 3 (March): 160018. doi:10.1038/sdata.2016.18.

Williams, R., R. Duvall, V. Kilaru, G. Hagler, L. Hassinger, K. Benedict, J. Rice, et al. 2019. "Deliberating performance targets workshop: Potential paths for emerging PM2.5 and O_3 air sensor progress." *Atmospheric Environment* X 2 (April): 100031. doi:10.1016/j.aeaoa.2019.100031.

Wnuk, Krzysztof, Per Runeson, Matilda Lantz, and Oskar Weijden. 2014. "Bridges and barriers to hardware-dependent software ecosystem participation: A case study." *Information and Software Technology, Special issue on Software Ecosystems*, 56 (11): 1493–1507. doi:10.1016/j.infsof.2014.05.015.

World Health Organization. 2014. "WHO | 7 Million Premature Deaths Annually Linked to Air Pollution." https://www.who.int/mediacentre/news/releases/2014/air-pollution/en/.

World Health Organization. 2016a. "WHO | By Category | Deaths Attributable to the Environment: Data by Country." http://apps.who.int/gho/data/node.main.162.

World Health Organization. 2016b. "An Estimated 12.6 Million Deaths Each Year Are Attributable to Unhealthy Environments." https://www.who.int/news-room/detail/15-03-2016-an-estimated-12-6-million-deaths-each-year-are-attributable-to-unhealthy-environments.

World Health Organization. 2017. WHO | Inheriting a Sustainable World: Atlas on Children's Health and the Environment. http://www.who.int/ceh/publications/inheriting-a-sustainable-world/en/.

Yang, Yang, Zengliang Ruan, Xiaojie Wang, Yin Yang, Tonya G. Mason, Hualiang Lin, and Linwei Tian. 2019. "Short-term and long-term exposures to fine particulate matter constituents and health: A systematic review and meta-analysis." *Environmental Pollution* 247 (April): 874–882. doi:10.1016/j.envpol.2018.12.060.

Yanosky, Jeff D., Christopher J. Paciorek, Francine Laden, Jaime E. Hart, Robin C. Puett, Duanping Liao, and Helen H. Suh. 2014. "Spatio-temporal modeling of particulate air pollution in the conterminous United States using geographic and meteorological predictors." *Environmental Health* 13 (1): 63. doi:10.1186/1476-069X-13-63.

Yassein, M. B., W. Mardini, and A. Khalil. 2016. "Smart homes automation using Z-wave protocol." In *2016 International Conference on Engineering MIS (ICEMIS)*, 1–6. doi:10.1109/ICEMIS.2016.7745306.

Zanobetti, Antonella, Susan Redline, Joel Schwartz, Dennis Rosen, Sanjay Patel, George T. O'Connor, Michael Lebowitz, Brent A. Coull, and Diane R. Gold. 2010. "Associations of PM10 with sleep and sleep-disordered breathing in adults from seven U.S. Urban Areas." *American Journal of Respiratory and Critical Care Medicine* 182 (6): 819–825. doi:10.1164/rccm.200912-1797OC.

Zeger, S. L., D. Thomas, F. Dominici, J. M. Samet, J. Schwartz, D. Dockery, and A. Cohen. 2000. "Exposure measurement error in time-series studies of air pollution: Concepts and consequences." *Environmental Health Perspectives* 108 (5): 419–426. doi:10.1289/ehp.00108419.

Section III

Bioethics

17 Bioethics and Precision Medicine
Focus on Information Technology

Kenneth W. Goodman
University of Miami

CONTENTS

17.1 INTRODUCTION

The thrusts of science regularly confound the parries of ethics and public policy. From organ transplantation and genetic testing to end-of-life care and, now, *precision medicine*, the history of medical technology is often the history of tools whose use predates guidance for their appropriate uses and users. Precision medicine poses several interesting and important challenges for ethics, in part because it embodies or relies on a suite of once disparate technologies: genetics/genomics, cellular and immunotherapies and health information technology, or biomedical informatics. Precision medicine would be neither possible, nor *precise*, in the absence of tools to manage large amounts of health data and information. There are many sources of such data and information, but precision medicine begins with the electronic health record (EHR).

Though the use of computers to collect, store, analyze and share health information is not new and, indeed, is well established, the EHR systems available continue to challenge, if not vex, clinicians. Getting the ethics of precision medicine right will require that we get the ethics of EHRs right. In doing so, we will reaffirm the links between and among quality, standards and ethics.

DOI: 10.1201/9780429263286-20

17.2   FROM PAPYRUS TO SILICON: PRECISION MEDICINE AND THE HISTORY OF THE MEDICAL RECORD

The world's oldest existing medical texts are believed to be a Sumerian clay tablet in Philadelphia and an Egyptian papyrus in London. The latter, on women's health, is hybridized: hints of information about cases, recipes for pain management, improbable concoctions for contraception, and so on. It was not until the 5th century BCE when cases, apparently preserved by students, made their way into the Hippocratic corpus and made clear that, if nothing else, patients' stories could be instructive (Goodman 2016).

The 17th-century physician, Thomas Sydenham, known as the "English Hippocrates," synthesized cases into disease profiles—arguably, an important initial recognition of precision in medical documentation. A century later, the Board of Governors of the Society of the New York Hospital approved the first hospital rules under which the apothecary prepared and delivered a monthly report of the "Names and Diseases of the Persons, received, deceased or discharged in the same, with the date of each event, and the Place from whence the Patients last came." This is an early, if not the first, appreciation of the potential utility of metadata in medical documentation.

René Laennec, whose 19th-century discovery of the (more-or-less) modern stethoscope, is credited—or blamed—for shifting the focus of the case history from reports of patients' observations to those of physicians. Compare this change to current acknowledgment of the utility and importance of patient-reported outcomes in clinical research.

Perhaps the greatest foreshadowing of contemporary emphases on the careful collection and analysis of data and information occurs in the work of Pierre-Charles-Alexandre Louis, whose analysis of bloodletting cases led to the "numerical method" and, indeed, the demise of bloodletting: His scrutiny of outcomes demonstrated that it simply did not work. Subsequently, in the 19th and 20th centuries, cases from medical records achieved a key role in medical education, such that in 1910, Massachusetts General Hospital began weekly conferences to review cases and analyze "clinical logic" of patient management. In 1915, the hospital began publishing the cases and analyses, which became a regular feature of the *Boston Medical and Surgical Journal* (renamed in 1928 as *The New England Journal of Medicine*) (Reiser 1991).

The past century has seen information from individual cases used for education and, more importantly, information aggregated and distilled from many cases for research. The growth of patient-reported outcomes, pragmatic clinical trials and analyses of data and information in EHRs have, in some respects, changed, if not transformed, the way we try to increase biomedical knowledge.

Moreover, in the case of precision medicine, the role of concatenated information and data about individuals and their genomes will be of at least as much use as the result of traditional randomized, blinded trials. This reliance on data and information comes at a price: risks are now shaped by inapt, biased or faulty programs and algorithms; by poorly designed, "buggy" and incomplete databases and by a failure to identify and maintain standards in the use of decision support systems. After several millennia, the medical record is more important than ever.

17.3 ETHICAL ISSUES

Though precision medicine raises many interesting and challenging issues in genetics and genomics, emphasis here is focused on information technology issues. Much of what follows will apply to *bioinformatics* or the use of computers and related tools for the storage and analysis of genetic and genomic data and information. Ethical issues raised by information technology are too often neglected in precision medicine and, therefore, are the focus of this chapter.

17.3.1 CLINICAL DECISION SUPPORT

Clinical decision support (CDS) systems and tools help clinicians in many ways:

- *Reminders and alerts*: From simple memory aids ("Did you check the creatinine?") to notices that something might be a miss (a sound or alarm if blood pressure or pulse changes significantly) to queries about intent ("Did you mean to prescribe that dose?"), these tools prevent mistakes, educate and, if poorly designed or implemented, are sources of vexing distraction.
- *Diagnostic support*: A CDS system can generate and rank a list of differential diagnoses, recommend tests to narrow the list, suggest associated therapies, etc. Computers can provide a wide range of decision aids and guidance for clinicians.
- *Prognostic scoring*: Predicting the course of a malady, or a malady given various treatments, could be useful to help decide whether an intervention is worthwhile, identify a more appropriate treatment and, generally, improve the consent process.

Construed broadly, decision support is essential for successful precision medicine. Traditional medical tradecraft, celebrating the judgments of individual humans, is increasingly inadequate in an environment shaped by vast amounts of data and the probabilistic inferences drawn from large datasets. In many respects, medicine has always required nuanced judgments under uncertainty. We cannot yet say how long it will take before the digital engines of precision medicine are strong or clever enough to reduce that uncertainty.

What is clear is that automated decision support will play an increasing role. Advances in genomics and human genetics have enabled a more detailed understanding of the impact of genetics in a disease and its treatment. In addition to a patient's clinical signs and symptoms, physicians can now, or in near future, consider genetic data for their diagnosis and treatment decisions. This new information source, based on genome and gene expression analysis, makes clinical decision processes even more complex. Beyond that, behavioral and environmental aspects should also be considered in order to realize personalized medicine. Given these additional information sources, the need for support in decision-making is increasing (Denecke and Spreckelsen 2013, Castaneda et al. 2015).

Perhaps the greatest ethical challenges for the use of decision support are framed by the following questions: What is an appropriate use and who is an appropriate user (Miller et al. 1985, Goodman 2016)? It is important to acknowledge what has come to be known as the "Standard View," which refers to the use of intelligent machines by clinicians, namely, that a computer, however smart, is no substitute for a human (Miller 1990). There are several reasons for this, including that the practice of medicine and nursing are not, and have never been, exclusively about mere calculations. Rather, these professions require nuanced communication, empathy and understanding of social and economic context. No artificial intelligence or machine learning system can do any of that, yet.

Stated differently, a decision support system is a tool not unlike others in the clinician's armamentarium. It still requires a human to practice effective medicine and nursing. It is implied that, at a minimum, there be a human, perhaps an expert, between the machine and the patient. Such a "learned intermediary" helps ensure (albeit, not guarantee) that what happens to any patient is overseen or governed by what we know so far to be the most competent to practice medicine or nursing—a human.

Should patients use CDS tools? This question has, in many respects, become moot given the ubiquity of online CDS apps and gadgets. From cancer nomograms to prognostic scoring systems, patients already have access to CDS programs. More and more, patients are using these CDS programs to compare against their doctors' and nurses' analyses. This trend will likely persist as precision medicine nomograms continue to evolve (Kattan et al. 2016).

What seems necessary for both clinicians and patients is the development and elucidation of ethical standards and education for their appropriate use. This might include the following:

- Know your software and its limitations.
- Take special and additional precautions' when a decision support machine produces counterintuitive or surprising guidance.
- In general, do not be beguiled by a machine's processing speed or capacity.

Health information technology continues to introduce tools whose availability suggests an obligation to develop, adapt and use them more widely. Further, what is needed now is to apply CDS insights from clinical practice to precision medicine. To do this, an approach called "Progressive Caution" might be followed—it is the idea that "Medical informatics is, happily, here to stay, but users and society have extensive responsibilities to ensure that we use our tools appropriately. This might cause us to move more deliberately or slowly than some would like" (Goodman 1998). Moreover, with a focus on bioinformatics,

> It might be that the tools and uses of computational biology will eventually offer ethical challenges—and opportunities—as important, interesting and compelling as any technology in the history of the health sciences. Significantly, this underscores the importance of arguments to the effect that attention to ethics must accompany attention to science. Victories of health science research and development will be undermined by any failures to address corresponding ethical challenges. We must strive to identify, analyze and resolve or mitigate important ethical issues.

(Goodman and Miller Forthcoming)

This also makes clear that the proper contribution of ethics in assessing the role of CDS in precision medicine is not adversarial or negative. Rather, it embodies the idea that the correct position is not to say "no," but, rather, "here's how."

17.3.2 SOFTWARE ENGINEERING

It is now common to worry that artificial intelligence algorithms are or might be biased. Bias in software is as much an empirical confounder as other forms of bias in science. To the extent that such bias is racial, ethnic or sexual, it is especially troublesome as decisions about health and public policy are at stake.

Consequently, the first order of ethical business is to ensure that datasets used to train or tune algorithms are scrutinized for bias and other confounders. It is worth mentioning that all forms of bias based on flawed or narrow sampling will reduce the accuracy and effectiveness of the software used to support clinical decisions. Additional challenges arise when empirical data are flawed, dirty or even absent. What statisticians call "missingness" is too often overlooked as an ethical challenge.

Both basic statistical and machine learning algorithms raise issues linking standards or best practices to safety and error reduction. Four such issues merit consideration (Goodman 2016):

1. *Proper annotation*: Computer programmers customarily document or annotate their code. These comments make explicit what was changed and why. One might note why something was not changed or was changed trivially.
2. *Reporting of provenance*: It can be essential to high-quality software writing. Code is often reused, adapted and shared. Making explicit its origins and sources helps subsequent programmers and those who are trying to debug or improve software. Depending on the source, there might be intellectual property or copyright issues to address.
3. *Fitness for use* is a kind of promise or attestation that the program applied to a purpose is suitable and will work as intended. Code written to support precision medicine in oncology might not work in cardiology, even with changes in the lexicon or ontology.

Last, *version control*—familiar to anyone who has discovered that more than one member of a team has been working on the same document at the same time—is important in software engineering ethics as a strategy to prevent divergent or incompatible versions of a program (perhaps with the same annotation) to be used.

It has been suggested that attention to these and perhaps other standards might be useful in addressing the problem of reproducibility (Breining 2017). This suggestion is, at least, a hypothesis to be tested. Moreover, and to the extent that laboratory scientists and clinicians create or customize software for precision medicine, such standards might be useful for error reduction. Still in its youth, precision medicine's evolution will help guide us in efforts to adopt existing standards and best practices, or to develop and test new ones as needed.

17.3.3 Big Data, Machine Learning and Learning Healthcare Systems

The idea of a learning healthcare system is inspired in part by the recognition that healthcare institutions and systems generate vast amounts of data which, traditionally, are either lost or, if retained, are in EHRs not designed or intended for subsequent analysis. Given that every clinical and hospital encounter generates data, and that at least some of it is valuable, then such health systems can improve care if they do a better job of collecting data in formats that lend themselves to knowledge generation—which in turn is used to improve patient care (Budrionis and Bellika 2016, Guise et al. 2018). Precision medicine constitutes an excellent use-case for learning healthcare systems.

Indeed, precision medicine is not possible without the apt collection and storage and robust and accurate analysis of a great deal of data. (It also makes clear that Big Data is often constituted by many collections of small data.)

The ability to gather and analyze more data to improve patient care entails both that we ought to try to do so and that we carefully scrutinize that effort. Whereas ethics is too often seen or thought to be about hindering, slowing or impeding biomedical progress, this is an example of how such scrutiny serves the mission: Not "stop," but "here's how." It is among the better consequences of adopting the principle of Progressive Caution.

Ethical issues raised by the collection, storage and use of Big Data in Learning Healthcare Systems are still being identified. In addition to designating the proper role of decision support systems and the need for ethically optimized software, meeting challenges of privacy and general governance is an increasingly urgent task.

Often ranked first among ethical challenges in the domain of health information technology, privacy and confidentiality are too frequently wheeled out as obstacles or, worse, showstoppers: There is just too much personal data, the tools of informed consent are meek safeguards and patients are presumed to have little interest in advancing the goals of biomedical research. Some of these concerns are well motivated, but some are either mistaken or overstated.

There is good reason to believe that ordinary citizens actually both want to and believe they have an obligation to contribute to the health systems they rely on (Marquard and Brennan 2009, Meslin and Goodman 2010). Though no one would seriously dispute the need for robust privacy-protection laws, everyone who works in a hospital has seen those laws invoked hyperbolically, unnecessarily and even inaccurately. An ancient challenge—how to make it easy for clinicians and others who need patient information to access it, while simultaneously making it difficult or impossible for those with no credible purpose to do so—has never before been more salient.

Successful precision medicine in a Learning Healthcare System might as plausibly consider the concepts of tacit or latent consent (Goodman 2016), disclose that information will be studied and, crucially, institute better security and data protection protocols and policies. Rarely has a competent and successful public health system, for instance, sought consent for information analysis from all the citizens in its jurisdiction, and countless lives have been saved and bettered as a result.

To be sure, this requires the trust of those one seeks to protect. Trust is earned and sustained in many ways, and a health department is likely to enjoy more trust than a for-profit health system in which proprietary interests might guide personalized medicine and other research-intensive pursuits. Some of this variability is dependent on jurisdiction: countries (1) with well-functioning health systems, (2) which do not penalize people for getting sick and (3) do not permit financial ruination caused by healthcare costs are more likely to succeed than others.

There is, in any case, a greater need to protect health information from evil doers, profiteers and extortionists than there is from legitimate researchers trying to improve the health of populations.

In addition to smart and nimble privacy laws, we should require structures to oversee all other aspects of information technology deployed in patient care and research. From development and use of artificial intelligence and machine learning tools to the management of uncertainty and probabilistic data in patient care, there will be an increased need to ensure that efforts to improve and expand precision medicine enjoy the confidence and trust of those being treated.

It has been suggested that clinical software applications might plausibly be overseen by "autonomous software oversight committees, in a manner partially analogous to the institutional review boards that are federally mandated to oversee protection of human subjects in biomedical research" (Miller and Gardner 1997a,b). Such governance, envisioned nearly a quarter-century ago for clinical software systems, could be developed to guide the more highly advanced digital information tools used in precision medicine.

Whatever steps are taken will lead and need to address several major challenges faced by contemporary healthcare systems. These include the problem of interoperability of computer systems, including EHRs; the hybridized nature of those systems, which are mostly developed by for-profit vendors largely unregulated by the government; and the fact that most clinicians learn to use information technology tools in an ad hoc and unstructured way.

There might even be a role for institutional ethics committees. These committees, whose existence and role in hospitals and nursing homes is entailed by Joint Commission accreditation standards, deal mostly with disagreements in the context of end-of-life care, but they could find a role in contributing to better software hygiene and use. That would require additional education, but there is a growing body of work in, and opportunities for, curriculum development at the intersection of ethics and health information technology.

17.4 CONCLUSION

From organ transplantation and genetics to end-of-life care and assisted reproduction, the role of applied ethics in the education and daily life of clinicians and students has been well established. That role has been expanded to the world of precision medicine (Fiore and Goodman 2016), including its use of powerful information technologies. A robust ethics presence can contribute the following:

- Identification and balancing of conflicting rights, and of rights and duties
- Identification and justification of duties
- Consultation regarding measured and proportionate governance tools.

Applied ethics provides support for patients, clinicians and institutional leaders in managing challenges raised by new technologies; it is a crucial resource for policy makers. Both precision medicine and health information technology are rich sources of ethical issues and challenges. If we are to make the most of these technologies, and to use them appropriately, there is an unparalleled opportunity—indeed, obligation—to make plain the ethically optimized standards needed for EHRs, decision support systems and the computer code that undergirds them.

REFERENCES

Breining, G. 2017. Addressing the research replication crisis. *AAMC News*, December 12, https://news.aamc.org/medical-education/article/academic-medicine-research-replication-crisis/.

Budrionis, A., and J. G. Bellika. 2016. The learning healthcare system: Where are we now? A systematic review. *Journal of Biomedical Informatics* 64:87–92.

Castaneda, C., K. Nalley, C. Mannion, P. Bhattacharyya, P. Blake, A. Pecora, A. Goy, and K. S. Suh. 2015. Clinical decision support systems for improving diagnostic accuracy and achieving precision medicine. *Journal of Clinical Bioinformatics* 5:4.

Denecke, K., and C. Spreckelsen. 2013. Personalized medicine and the need for decision support systems. *Studies in Health Technology and Informatics* 186:41–45.

Fiore, R. N., and K. W. Goodman. 2016. Precision medicine ethics: Selected issues and developments in next-generation sequencing, clinical oncology, and ethics. *Current Opinions in Oncology* 28:83–87.

Goodman, K. W. 1998. Outcomes, futility, and health policy research. In *Ethics, Computing, and Medicine: Informatics and the Transformation of Health Care*, ed. K. W. Goodman, 116–138. Cambridge: Cambridge University Press.

Goodman, K. W. 2016. *Ethics, Medicine and Information Technology: Intelligent Machines and the Transformation of Health Care*. Cambridge: Cambridge University Press.

Goodman, K. W., and R. A. Miller. Forthcoming. Ethics in biomedical and health informatics: Users, standards, and outcomes. In *Biomedical Informatics: Computer Applications in Health Care and Biomedicine*, eds. E. H. Shortliffe, and J. Cimino, Fifth Edition. New York and London.

Guise, J. M., L. A. Savitz, and C. P. Friedman. 2018. Mind the gap: Putting evidence into practice in the era of learning health systems. *Journal of General Internal Medicine* 33:2237–2239.

Kattan, M. W., K. R. Hess, M. B. Amin, Y. Lu, K. G. M. Moons, J. E. Gershenwald, P. A. Gimotty, J. H. Guinney, S. Halabi, A. J. Lazar, A. L. Mahar, T. Patel, D. J. Sargent, M. R. Weiser, and C. Compton. 2016. American Joint Committee on Cancer acceptance criteria for inclusion of risk models for individualized prognosis in the practice of precision medicine. *CA: A Cancer Journal for Clinicians* 66:370–374.

Marquard, J. L., and P. F. Brennan. 2009. Crying wolf: Consumers may be more willing to share medication information than policymakers think. *Journal of Health Information Management* 23:26–32.

Meslin, E. M., and K. W. Goodman. 2010. Bank on it: An ethics and policy agenda for biobanks and electronic health records. *Center for American Progress, Science Progress*, February 25, 2010, http://scienceprogress.org/2010/02/bank-on-it/#_edn25.

Miller, R. A. 1990. Why the standard view is standard: People, not machines, understand patients' problems. *The Journal of Medicine and Philosophy* 15:581–591.

Miller, R. A., and R. M. Gardner. 1997a. Summary recommendations for the responsible monitoring and regulation of clinical software systems. *Annals of Internal Medicine* 127:842–845.

Miller, R. A., and R. M. Gardner. 1997b. Recommendations for responsible monitoring and regulation of clinical software systems. *Journal of the American Medical Informatics Association: JAMIA* 4:442–457.

Miller, R. A., K. F. Schaffner, and A. Meisel. 1985. Ethical and legal issues related to the use of computer programs in clinical medicine. *Annals of Internal Medicine* 102:529–536.

Reiser, S. J. 1991. The clinical record in medicine. Part 1: Learning from cases. *Annals of Internal Medicine* 114:902–907.

18 Unresolved Ethical Questions Raised by Genomic Sequencing Research

Benjamin E. Berkman[1]
National Human Genome Research Institute,
National Institutes of Health

CONTENTS

18.1 INTRODUCTION

Over the past decade, new genomic sequencing technology has emerged that would have been unimaginable to previous researchers (Mardis 2011). Previously, creating the genetic sequence was the "bottleneck"; the first genome, sequenced by the Human Genome Project, took billions of dollars over decades of work (Collins et al. 2003). Since that historic achievement, massively parallel platforms have emerged, translating to an exponential improvement in the speed and efficiency of our sequencing capacity. Now, an individual's entire genome can be mapped in a matter of days, for around $1,000 (Wetterstrand 2019, Collins and Hamburg 2013, Feero et al. 2010). The promise of personalized medicine has long felt like a distant goal, but our emerging ability to generate massive amounts of sequence data has emerged as a powerful tool to help move us more quickly toward that goal (Teer and Mullikin 2010). Further, sequencing has also begun to play an increasingly important role

---

[1] The opinions expressed herein are the author's own and do not reflect the policies and positions of the National Institutes of Health, the U.S. Public Health Service, or the U.S. Department of Health and Human Services. This research was supported by the Intramural Research Program of the National Human Genome Research Institute, National Institutes of Health.

DOI: 10.1201/9780429263286-21

in clinical care (Collins 1999, Manolio et al. 2013, Taber et al. 2014, Green and Guyer 2011).

New technologies often raise new questions and it is not surprising that the emergence of genomic sequencing as a powerful research and clinical tool has raised a series of fascinating, if not contentious, ethical problems. The greatest questions have swirled around the problem of incidental findings, which research ethicists and genomic researchers have argued about for the past decade (Jackson et al. 2012, President's Commission for the Study of Bioethical Issues 2013). Traditionally, doctors and researchers have only ordered the targeted test(s) required to answer their clinical or scientific questions (Kohane et al. 2006). Producing massive amounts of genomic data can help answer scientific questions, but it can also incidentally reveal clinically relevant information. An *incidental finding* is often defined as a piece of medical information "concerning an individual research participant that has potential health or reproductive importance and is discovered in the course of conducting research, but is beyond the aims of the study" (Wolf et al. 2013). As sequencing technology becomes increasingly ubiquitous, the routine availability of data on functional variants in virtually all protein-coding genes raises complicated questions about the management of incidental findings—including a determination of how, to whom, and under what circumstances to return results. Questions about the disclosure of results become more complicated as the number of potential results generated increases, which is precisely what is happening as whole exome and genome sequencing (WES/WGS) technologies continue to supplant targeted genetic research techniques.

These questions are particularly important because WGS challenges some of the core assumptions that have long been made about the ethics of returning results to participants (Tabor et al. 2011, McGuire et al. 2008). First, there has long been an assumption that genetic research will not produce clinically relevant information. This was true when researchers were utilizing methodologies that only interrogated targeted genetic regions because it was extremely unlikely that these small slices of the genome would contain clinically significant information beyond that which the researchers were actively seeking. WGS, however, explodes this assumption. If there is access to a patient's entire genome, one could theoretically learn a large number of important medical facts about the individual; every person's genome has flaws if you look hard enough. As a result, it is no longer appropriate to assume that genetic research projects will not produce incidental findings. The data are there, but the question is what obligations researchers have toward those data.

There has long been a second, related assumption that researchers do not have an obligation to act as clinicians and actively look for incidental findings. This might have been true when it was very difficult to search through genetic data for clinically relevant findings or when there weren't many findings to search for, but recent advances have called that into question. Researchers are constantly discovering new relationships between genotypes and phenotypes; our understanding of the relationship between genetic variants and diseases is increasing exponentially. Furthermore, this expanding body of knowledge is increasingly easy to interrogate, as analytic tools become increasingly sophisticated and powerful. As we get closer to a world where looking for incidental findings only requires pushing an extra button, it becomes more difficult to embrace a "don't ask, don't tell" approach (Tabor et al. 2011).

This chapter will explore this vigorous debate, with the goal of identifying the extant ethical issues that remain unresolved. How can one define the contours of the obligation to return information to patients and research participants whose genomes are being sequenced? Given that researchers and clinicians have different obligations to participants and patients, to what extent should researchers devote time and resources toward the return of clinical information unrelated to their scientific aims (Jarvik et al. 2014)? Is there a duty to actively interrogate sequencing data to look for incidental findings as the difficulty of doing so decreases (Gliwa and Berkman 2013)? Does an obligation to disclose clinically relevant information extend to relatives of participants or patients, particularly after the death of the proband (Chan et al. 2012)? Is there any risk of liability for failing to disclose clinically relevant incidental findings (Pike et al. 2014)?

This chapter describes the terminological distinction that the President's Commission for the Study of Bioethical Issues drew between *incidental* and *secondary findings*. The term *incidental findings* has somewhat dominated the bioethics discussion and represents a broader category of findings that could be uncovered by a research or clinical test but is unrelated to the purpose of that test. Some incidental findings can be anticipated ("Practitioner aims to discover A, but learns B, a result known to be associated with the test or procedure at the time it takes place") or unanticipated ("Practitioner aims to discover A, but learns C, a result not known to be associated with the test or procedure at the time it takes place"). In contrast, *secondary findings* represent the narrow category of unrelated findings that are actively sought ("Practitioner aims to discover A, and also actively seeks D per expert recommendation"). Both terms are important to understand and, therefore, appear throughout this chapter.

18.2 AN EMERGING OBLIGATION TO RETURN SECONDARY FINDINGS

The field of genomic medicine is rapidly evolving. New associations between genotypes and phenotypes are uncovered each week and the understanding of how genetics influences human disease continues to increase. But, one of the side effects of a rapidly evolving area of science is that the standard of care is extremely difficult to define. Specifically, even after a decade of debate about the ethics of incidental and secondary findings, it remains unclear whether there is an obligation to return genetic results.

One major effort to define the standard of care was undertaken by the American College of Medical Genetics and Genomics. In their controversial position statement ("ACMG Recommendations for Reporting of Incidental Findings in Clinical Exome and Genome Sequencing"), they sought to begin a conversation about how to define the standard for addressing the anticipatable array of findings that were going to result from the increasingly prominent role that genomic sequencing was playing in clinical care (Green et al. 2013). They suggested that whenever a clinically indicated test is undertaken, the lab should actively interrogate the resulting genomic data to look for a defined list of variants. They defined this list narrowly, only including "unequivocally pathogenic mutations in genes where pathogenic variants lead to disease with very high probability and where evidence strongly supports the benefits of early intervention" such that the information "would likely have medical benefit for the patients and families of patients undergoing clinical sequencing" (Green et al. 2013). In arguing for this standard of care, they appealed to the notion of *opportunist screening* and to the idea that there is a fiduciary duty to look for this high-value genetic information, at least in the clinical sequencing context. While these recommendations were not universally accepted, it was largely because of concerns about the related proposal to not ask patients whether they wanted these findings—a topic that will be explored in the right-not-to-know section below.

These guidelines, along with other commentaries and policy initiatives, indicate movement toward a standard of care where there is an obligation to look for and return secondary findings in clinical care. But since most genomic sequencing is still being done in the research setting, more work is needed to explore the obligations to research participants. Along with the publication of the ACMG recommendations, there is perhaps an obligation to actively look for secondary findings in a research context. This argument builds on the ancillary care debate as part of research ethics. *Ancillary care* is the idea that clinical researchers, particularly in low-resource settings, will sometimes be presented with subjects who have acute medical needs unrelated to the research aims or methods. For example, researchers conducting parasite (e.g., hookworm) research in a tropical area where malaria is endemic will predictably have subjects who present with the infectious disease. The ethical question is whether researchers have an obligation to provide ancillary care to these subjects. Commentators have argued that ancillary care should be provided in cases where (1) there is an opportunity to provide a large benefit to the individual; (2) providing the care would not unduly burden the research enterprise; and (3) the researchers are in a unique position to help.

As recent as 2013, there seemed to be no obligation to look for secondary findings as it was still burdensome for researchers to actively interrogate genomic data and because there was only limited benefit due to our limited understanding of genetic influence on disease. Since then, it could be argued that there is a duty to look for secondary findings when the three criteria outlined above are met and this seems to be happening more and more. There now are curated lists of high-value variants and analytic tools have advanced to the point that actively searching is not burdensome. Yet, our medical system has not fully integrated genomics into clinical practice, so researchers remain in a unique position to provide potentially life-saving information.

Evidence suggests an emerging notion that it is standard of care to look for and return some results to patients and research participants (Ormond et al. 2019). This is further supported by empirical data. A survey of institutional review board (IRB) members and staff found that 78% of respondents believed that there was always or sometimes an obligation to return genetic incidental findings discovered in the course of research (Gliwa et al. 2016). Respondents generally did not endorse the idea that researchers' additional time and effort, or lack of resources, were valid reasons for diminishing a putative obligation, further supporting my argument that the burden on researcher counter-argument is becoming harder to assert.

But contours of that obligation remain unclear, in large part because the justification for the obligation cannot be agreed upon. The bioethics literature is full of asserted theories about why there might be an obligation to return incidental or secondary genetic research findings. Proposed justifications have included beneficence, autonomy of participants, the right-to-know information about oneself, a duty to warn, professional responsibility, reciprocity, maintaining trust in the research enterprise, maintaining an institution's reputation, and fear of legal liability. In our survey of IRBs, the respondents did not clearly endorse a single justification for returning results, suggesting that conceptual confusion remains. The three justifications with the strongest support were duty to warn (84%), autonomy (80%) and beneficence (79%). Other reasons also gained majority support but at significantly lower levels.

The lack of clear consensus is important because these principles conflict in the breadth of their implied obligation. For example, relying on the duty to warn would only require disclosing findings that would potentially provide significant health benefit. In contrast, beneficence would imply disclosing all potentially useful findings, without appeal to any minimum significance threshold. Autonomy would suggest offering to return whichever findings participants decided were important given their circumstances. Given the confusion about why it is important to return incidental or secondary findings, it should not be surprising that there is trouble defining the contours of the obligation.

Arguably, it has been difficult to come to consensus about the shape of a return of results obligation because of terminological confusion in the literature (Eckstein et al. 2014). When commentators discuss researchers' obligation to return genetic findings, they often appeal to terms like actionability, clinical relevance/utility/significance, clinical validity, and analytic validity. By using these concepts, the hope is to delineate the threshold above which findings need to be disclosed. While intuitively appealing, the problem with this approach is that there is significant variability in the way that these concepts are used by bioethics scholars. What seems at first glance to represent a convergence of thinking is actually contributing to confusion in the field.

For example, *actionability* is often used to suggest that researchers only have an obligation to return findings when they can lead to some sort of intervention. Unfortunately, commentators often use this term without being clear about the kind(s) of actions that should count. In a narrow sense, *actionability* could be limited only to clinically indicated medical or preventative interventions (e.g., enhanced cancer screening) that could mitigate the course of a disease. However, in a broader sense, actionability could include a broader set of medical-adjacent decisions (e.g., reproductive planning). And at the highest level of generality, actionability could include any life-planning decision that might be influenced by knowledge of future disease risk (e.g., early spending of retirement funds). Without further specification, *actionability* could include any of these meanings, and the literature's confusion is, at least in part, due to our inability to come to a shared understanding of commonly used terms.

Given the conceptual and definitional confusion inherent to the return of results debate, perhaps it should not be surprising that after more than a decade of debate, we still do not have a clear standard of care. There is an emerging notion that the standard of care is to look for and return secondary findings, but it remains difficult to say that this is the clear consensus position.

18.3   RETURNING RESULTS IN DIFFERENT KINDS OF STUDIES

Even if there is an obligation to return findings, should it apply universally to all research projects? In other words, how much does the research context matter? Some commentators have argued that return of results obligations will be a function of the characteristics of the research study and research subject population (Beskow and Burke 2010). Relevant characteristics might include (1) the nature of the study (e.g., clinical, basic science); (2) whether the study has resources to return results; (3) investigator expertise (e.g., medical geneticist, physician, non-clinician); (4) specific aims of the study and methods employed; and (5) feasibility of recontact. Relevant characteristics of the study population could include (1) whether the subjects have alternative access to the information; (2) vulnerability of the subjects; (3) depth and nature of the relationship; and (4) whether the finding is actionable for that person or group. Depending on how one weighs these various considerations in a particular context can help to determine whether it is more or less appropriate to return results in a given research context (Darnell et al. 2016).

One of the most difficult emerging questions has to do with whether or not to return findings in low-resources settings (Sullivan and Berkman 2018). This issue is becoming increasingly pressing as investigators are rapidly expanding genomic research into transnational settings. Until recently, genetic research has been limited primarily to US and European settings. Similarly, the incidental findings debate has primarily focused on research conducted in high-income countries. But this kind of research raises the "actionability problem" inherent to research conducted in low-resource settings. The actionability problem refers to the idea that actionability can vary across populations, particularly in low-resource settings where there is minimal access to standard medical care. For example, in some countries, there are extremely limited numbers of mammography machines and treatment for breast cancer is not available. In those settings, finding out one's BRCA (i.e., BReast CAncer gene) status is arguably not clinically useful since there are no available screening or treatment options.

The ethical question is whether this reality should alter the way we think about when and why incidental findings should be offered to research participants. On the one hand, diverting research resources toward the return of incidental or secondary findings is generally predicated on the assumption that the results have clear medical value. Without that obvious value, perhaps returning results is not justified. On the other hand, justice requires that we treat similarly situated populations the same. Is it fair to deprive already vulnerable people potentially important medical information because they do not have access to medical services?

It can be argued that while genetic research in low-resource settings is valuable and necessary, there is a tension between the reduced benefit of returning incidental findings in low-resource settings and not wanting to perpetuate inequality in access to healthcare. An expanded concept of the duty to rescue represents an obligation to return incidental findings and its conditions and creates a framework that can help researchers and ethicists decide when it is obligatory to return medically actionable incidental findings. Specifically, there is an obligation to provide ancillary care when (1) a person is in a life or health-threatening situation, (2) the proposed action is necessary to prevent or mitigate that threat, (3) the action will likely succeed in preventing or mitigating the threat, and (4) the benefit to the threatened person greatly outweighs the burden on the rescuer. It is argued that some commentators have been too quick to discount the possibility of benefit or overstate the potential for harm from disclosure of genetic findings in low-resource settings. Using this framework, it is concluded that while it remains possible that the risk/benefit calculus is different in such settings, there are good reasons to justify disclosure in many cases.

18.4   RECONSENT AND RESEARCH WITH STORED SAMPLES

There is a growing problem in the research world, related to the increasing tendency for researchers to store samples indefinitely (i.e., "the freezer problem"). When researchers want to use new technologies and methodologies to conduct research on these samples, when is it necessary to obtain specific consent for research approaches that were not anticipated in an original consent form? Take the following case:

> A research study on genetic causes of asthma that incorporated targeted genetic tests was initiated several years ago. In the original consent, participants allowed "genetic analysis" of their samples, but next-generation sequencing (NGS) was not explicitly mentioned as it was not an option at the time. Now that NGS is less expensive, researchers would like to use it as part of their study to increase their chances of discovering genes related to asthma. Is it necessary to obtain new consent from the subjects who donated these samples before sequencing them? If the investigators make a good faith effort to recontact a participant, but fail to locate him/her, can their specimen still be sequenced?

On the one hand, there are ethically relevant characteristics of genomic sequencing that differentiate it from older targeted genetic testing. The scope of clinically relevant (and potentially sensitive) information that can be generated by sequencing might make some people feel differently about participating in that kind of research activity, such that new consent might be required. On the other hand, often these consent forms contained broad language (e.g., "genetic tests") that can be interpreted to perhaps include sequencing. Additionally, given that samples might have been stored in a freezer for years, or even decades, the difficulty of requiring new consent might practically preclude using these samples.

When researchers made an explicit promise to only use samples in a particular way, it can be argued that they are bound by that promise. But the above considerations can prove difficult to balance in cases where consent language is vague. At the very least, it seems prudent for researchers to be required to articulate a compelling scientific reason for sequencing legacy samples when there has not been explicit consent. They should also be able to explain why these samples are of particular value, such that they could not be easily replaced by newer samples.

But assuming that researchers can make these arguments, one can argue for the ethical appropriateness of sequencing older samples. This view is based on an emerging sense that genetic exceptionalism is unwarranted, and that the oft-cited worries about the dangers associated with genetic testing have yet to be borne out. It has been argued elsewhere that the advent of genomic sequencing technology necessitates a fundamental reassessment of how risks and benefits associated with genetic information are being characterized and understood (Prince and Berkman 2018). Until now, conceptions of risks and benefits have been generally static, arising out of the early ethical, legal, and social implications (ELSI) studies conducted in the context of targeted genetics. But the increasing availability of genetic information is changing views about risks and benefits. As genomics proliferates, it is becoming clear that there is very little robust empirical evidence of psychosocial harms, necessitating a rethinking of long-held assumptions about the ethics of genomic research. Perhaps people should not be overly concerned with sequencing legacy samples that were collected with ambiguous consent language.

18.5 THE RIGHT-NOT-TO-KNOW GENETIC INFORMATION ABOUT ONESELF

The influential ACMG recommendations (discussed above) controversially argued against soliciting patient preferences about receiving (or not receiving) incidental findings. They did not think that it was appropriate to give patients a choice not to learn about clinically important and actionable findings, advancing the claim that clinicians have a fiduciary duty to warn patients about high-risk variants where an intervention is available (Green et al. 2013).

The recommendation against soliciting patient preferences for not knowing genetic information ignited an extended (and often quite spirited) debate within the research ethics community about the right-not-to-know ("RNTK") genetic information about oneself. A relatively small set of commentators tried to defend the call for mandatory disclosure of high-value incidental findings (Berkman and Hull 2014, McGuire et al. 2013). The overwhelming majority view, however, was extremely critical of the recommendation, holding that patients have a strong, autonomy-based RNTK, and that any abrogation of that right was inappropriate (Burke et al. 2013, Wolf et al. 2013). As one paper put it, the ACMG statement was "an instance of paternalistic overreach" that should be "widely rejected as inconsistent with the ethical and legal duties of clinicians" (Trinidad et al. 2015). Even more interesting was the fact that these pro-RNTK views were often couched in relatively absolute terms. These pro-RNTK commentators were not blind to the fact that strongly preferencing the RNTK meant that some patients might not receive information that could save their lives.

Though the backlash to the ACMG argument was fierce, it can be argued that the debate has not yet been resolved. Here, the widely accepted view that an individual has a strong RNTK genetic information about him or herself is challenged. Challenging the majority view that the RNTK is sacrosanct, this chapter pushes back against that vigorously held (although not always rigorously defended) position, in defense of the idea that we should abandon the notion of a strong RNTK. The view here is that we should have a default policy of returning high-value genetic information without asking about a preference not to know.

Several points are made to support this alternative view (Berkman 2017). First, the idea often presented by pro-RNTK advocates that a strong autonomy-based RNTK has a long history of support is dismissed. Upon examining the RNTK philosophical literature, it becomes apparent that the concept is on much more analytically shaky ground than many contemporary commentators acknowledge. The RNTK genetic information is a relatively new idea, first appearing in the literature in the 1970s and 1980s, but not gaining much traction until the 1990s (Laurie 1999, 2000, Takala 1999). A substantial body of work developed in the subsequent decade, concurrent with the gradual incorporation of genetic testing into clinical medicine. While there appears to be significant recent support for the RNTK, a robust examination of the concept reveals a much more controverted and nuanced history.

Interestingly, there does not seem to be overwhelming support in the foundational RNTK literature for a strong, autonomy-based RNTK. There are a few scholars who support such a view, but the weight of the literature is squarely against a strong concept of the RNTK. Many scholars argued for a much narrower concept of the RNTK, suggesting a much more limited version that only applies in certain contexts and that can be overridden by factors like strong medical benefits associated with the information. Another block of scholars advocated against the notion of an RNTK altogether. This group argued that the idea of an autonomy-based RNTK is incoherent because a person needs information (and knowledge that a decision needs to be made), in order to really exercise one's autonomy. RNTK skeptics also cited that choosing not to know information about oneself is almost never completely self-regarding because genetic information impacts relatives. This "harm to third parties" objection further undermines a claim that an individual should be allowed to keep themselves in the dark.

A second challenge is regarding the often-made claim that the legal right to refuse medical treatment includes a right to refuse learning about medical information. The right to refuse medical treatment jurisprudence is explicitly built on our history and tradition of protecting bodily integrity; relevant case law never mentions the distinct concept of psychological integrity raised by RNTK cases. Rather, in an RNTK case, the legal question is whether courts would expand established protection of bodily integrity to incorporate psychological integrity. Courts have been reluctant to expand constitutionally protected substantive due process liberty interests, particularly given how difficult it would be to establish the contours of protection for a concept as amorphous and potentially expansive as psychological integrity. In fact, courts have been willing to endorse the idea of imposing unwanted information on people in a number of realms (e.g., mandatory ultrasounds). Judicial acceptance of infringement on psychological integrity suggests that courts would find purchase in the distinction between physical and psychological integrity and would not find a clear history and tradition of protecting psychological integrity.

A third challenge is that it is necessary to conduct a *comprehensive* analysis of the harms and benefits that result from adhering to a strong RNTK position. Pro-RNTK commentators have been focused on autonomy, which has not allowed for a comprehensive analysis of the harms and benefits of honoring or ignoring the RNTK. The reality is that any policy will have potential negative consequences. Whichever option is chosen, we will necessarily be making a mistake in one of two directions: unwanted disclosure or lost opportunity for medical intervention. Arguably, the potential health benefits of abandoning a strong RNTK greatly outweigh the concomitant harms, thereby challenging the idea that psychosocial concerns should automatically get to trump the prospect of life-saving intervention.

In order to conduct this comprehensive analysis, there are three issues that need to be addressed in order to really understand the impact of a strong RNTK policy that requires solicitation of patient or participant preferences. First, how many people genuinely don't want to know genetic information about themselves, if it could have a profound impact on morbidity or mortality? Available data support the reasonable claim that the overwhelming majority of people would want to be given genetic risk information that will have a direct impact on their health. For example, in one study nearly all respondents wanted to learn about a range of genetic risk factors, with 90% wanting to learn about non-actionable health risks and 96% wanting to learn about actionable genetic risk factors (Kaufman 2008). Similarly, in the largest study to date of views toward the return of incidental findings resulting from sequencing research, nearly 5,000 members of the public were surveyed and nearly all of them (98%) wanted to learn about genetic risk for life-threatening conditions that can be prevented (Middleton et al. 2016).

Second, a comprehensive analysis also must include an examination of the magnitude and likelihood of harm that will occur if people are given genetic risk information that they would have preferred not to know. With respect to this, commentators often discuss psychological harms (e.g., depression, anxiety) that result from learning genetic risk information. However, the evidence about psychological harms suggests that we should be skeptical about claims that unfortunate genetic information is unduly debilitating. Generally, people are not as good as they think at affective forecasting or predicting the magnitude and duration of our future emotional reaction to negative events (Wilson and Gilbert 2005). When people receive such important information, they have an initial spike of emotion but gradually tend to return to their previous baseline level of happiness. Essentially, the body has a sort of psychological immune system, which helps people deal with negative information, often making the actual impact of negative information significantly smaller than the expected negative impact. However, when making a prediction about future emotional responses, we disregard our future ability to cope, thereby overestimating the negative impact of information. This is particularly true in the medical realm, where the literature suggests that an individual's predictions concerning the emotional consequence of learning about genetic disease risk do not square with people's actual ability to adapt to negative health information (Halpern and Arnold 2008). Therefore, the existing evidence suggests that negative reactions to unfortunate genetic information will be relatively mild and transient (Broadstock et al. 2000). More evidence about emotional reactions to genetic information would certainly be useful, but the existing literature at least raises important questions about whether we "systematically overestimate the durability and intensity of the affective impact of events on well-being," thereby creating a "culture of risk-aversion in which patients may be opting out of potentially beneficial diagnostic and treatment regimes" (Peters et al. 2014).

Pro-RNTK commentators also cite the possibility of economic harms (e.g., employment or insurance discrimination). The likelihood and magnitude of discrimination are somewhat more difficult to assess, but existing data suggest that perhaps there is less cause for concern than previously thought (Rothstein 2008). It appears that there are occasional instances of discrimination in these areas, but that they are primarily associated with untreatable single gene conditions like Huntington's disease, and it could be argued that they do little to determine whether there should be a broad RNTK for serious, actionable genetic information. Even with some scattered evidence of discrimination, a systematic review of existing data calls into question the need for a policy intervention (Joly et al. 2013), suggesting that there is a significant gap between the fears of genetic discrimination and reality.

The comprehensive analysis must also address a third issue: What is the cost of always soliciting preferences? It can be argued that a strong RNTK would necessarily result in some loss of opportunity to provide people with valuable information because there is good reason to doubt our ability to accurately and reliably assess people's true preferences. There are extensive data suggesting that people frequently do not carefully read consent forms and when they do, their understanding and appreciation of the content can often be lacking (Mandava et al. 2012). If subjects are signing consent forms with such incomplete understanding of the important details, it seems questionable to have confidence in the infallibility of any process designed to solicit preferences about knowing genetic incidental findings. This is particularly true, given the inherent complexity of genetic information and the associated difficulty patients will have in making a choice in that context. Many commentators have expressed a concern that the wide range of types of genomic findings will be overwhelming and could become a significant barrier to implementing truly *informed* consent (McGuire and Beskow 2010). Furthermore, it will even be difficult to adequately describe the variety of genomic information categories because of terminology confusion discussed above (Eckstein et al. 2014). There are also concerns about how preferences can shift over time and that there is the very real risk that a binding decision made at a single point in time could conflict with future preferences.

Taken together, this analysis suggests that we should be skeptical about a strong RNTK policy that always requires soliciting patient or participant preferences. As argued earlier, there is at least a small group of people who would not want to know and, arguably, those people are at a very low risk of experiencing significant, lasting psychological or economic harm. In contrast, there is a very real risk that a policy of actively soliciting preferences about knowing or not knowing genetic information could result in people making choices that do not reflect their true values and preferences, thus erroneously or accidentally not receiving potentially life-saving information. Arguably, the costs of a strong RNTK policy outweigh the benefits. Opinions differ, but it seems that this comprehensive set of questions is critical to rigorously analyzing the RNTK problem.

As a final argument, it is useful to consider genetic exceptionalism. Proponents of the RNTK are effectively arguing that the return of any genetic information requires explicitly soliciting patient consent. Since it is standard practice in many clinical situations to disclose certain kinds of non-genomic medical findings without asking for explicit permission, it seems fair to ask whether this instance of genetic exceptionalism is warranted.

Autonomy is obviously an important value in medical ethics; modern social norms have clearly and enthusiastically moved away from medicine's paternalistic history. However, it isn't true that patients are asked to make decisions about every single aspect of their health care. If a patient undergoes a specifically indicated scan, but that scan incidentally reveals a potentially cancerous tumor, a doctor isn't going to ask the patient if they want to learn about the unexpected but important result. Similarly, if a patient receives a routine blood panel to check for a specific indication, but the panel returns a panic value indicating a serious acute problem, the physician isn't going to ask before disclosing this urgent finding.

These examples aren't perfect; genomic findings generally aren't associated with conditions that require immediate attention, nor is genetic predisposition always equivalent to a diagnosis of manifested disease. But the question isn't whether genetic information is precisely analogous to the urgent cases presented above. Rather, the relevant question should be whether and why the kind of important genomic information being discussed here warrants special treatment.

To summarize, perhaps it is a mistake to actively solicit preferences for high-impact genetic information. We should inform patients that there is a default set of high-impact incidental findings that will be sought and returned. In the rare case that someone independently requests to not learn about this information, in-depth counseling should be provided to ensure that they fully understand the choice being made. But ultimately, their decision to remain uninformed should be honored if not knowing consistently remains their clearly stated preference. In short, for high-impact genetic information, any deviation from regular disclosure should be a clearly defined exception, rather than the basis for a broadly applied concept of the RNTK.

18.6 OTHER UNRESOLVED ETHICAL ISSUES RELATING TO RETURN OF GENETIC RESULTS

The increasing use of genomic sequencing creates or exacerbates a handful of additional ethical problems. First, as we continue to utilize sequencing more broadly, it will be increasingly more common to have situations where the proband has died, raising questions about how to handle subsequent results that might have relevance to the proband's relatives. On the one hand, it would be quite burdensome to ask researchers to return information to family members with whom they have no relationship and might not even know how to contact. On the other hand, if the results could be sufficiently medically important for relatives, there could be a strong beneficence justification for trying to return them. While any obligation to a family member has to be less than that owed to the proband herself, it seems like a compromise position might be warranted. When genetic results are of medical value (using a very high threshold) researchers should make their best effort to contact a single person (e.g., spouse, executor of estate, etc.) who can then disseminate the information to the rest of the family (Chan et al. 2012).

Second, the increase in the utilization of genomic sequencing to analyze trios (typically two parents and a child) will inevitably raise questions about how to approach findings of misattributed parentage. For example, take the following case:

A child with a mysterious condition is being seen by a team of specialists to see if they can use genetic tests to better understand her illness. When they analyze the girl's DNA, the team finds evidence that neither of the parents is biologically related to their daughter. The child had been conceived by *in vitro* fertilization, using the parents' own egg and sperm. The team assumes that a mistake had been made and that the parents don't know that their child is not biologically related to them. There is no medical reason to tell them this fact and members of the research team disagree about whether the parents would want to know. Should the research team tell the patient's parents what they found?

While arguments can be made on either side of this question, it can be argued that nondisclosure should be the default in the research context. There are a variety of possible harms and benefits associated with disclosing misattributed parentage and, in most cases, it will be very difficult to accurately assess whether disclosure would result in net benefit or harm. Since researchers have a strong obligation to minimize or mitigate harms to participants and, in the face of this uncertainty, non-disclosure should be the default policy. Although, there are cases (e.g., helping to bring a diagnostic odyssey to an end) where disclosure might be allowable. Any worries about creating a false belief or violation of a trust relationship can be mitigated by a rigorous and transparent consent process (Mandava et al. 2015).

Third, given that our knowledge of the links between genetic variation and human disease is constantly evolving, there are questions about when it is necessary to go back to reanalyze already-generated genomic data to reclassify already recognized variants or identify recently discovered variants. While clinical laboratories generally "do not have a duty to hunt" for variant reclassifications or identifications (Bombard et al. 2019), the ACMG encourages clinical laboratories to be proactive in reclassifying variants as needed and to provide those updates to patients and clinicians (Richards et al. 2015). While ASHG does not recognize an affirmative duty to reclassify or identify variants, it does affirm that laboratories "are responsible for the validity of variant classification[s]" (Bombard et al. 2019), which can trigger a corresponding obligation to recontact participants, especially if the variant is reclassified from pathogenic or likely pathogenic to a lower status.

Since researchers are constrained by finite resources and inadequate reanalysis infrastructure, their duty to reanalyze justifiably has to be limited to some degree. However, as health care increasingly incorporates genomics, the costs of genomic reanalysis will likely decrease and the related infrastructure will probably improve, decreasing the burden of reanalysis. This declining burden then becomes a less convincing justification for limiting the duty to reanalyze because the benefits to participants will outweigh the costs. In the near term, researchers must clearly convey their policies regarding reanalysis to research participants. In the medium to long term, as technology evolves and the burden of reanalysis lessens, these policies should evolve to reflect this shifting calculus of benefits and burdens.

Finally, there are concerns about analytic validation. The Clinical Laboratories Improvement Amendments (CLIA) require that labs comply with a series of technical requirements to ensure that clinical results returned to patients are analytically valid (i.e., the result being reported is actually the one that exists in this patient). Research labs are not generally in the business of returning clinical results, so most are typically exempted from complying with the CLIA requirements. However, CLIA still requires that any research results that could be used "for the diagnosis, prevention, or treatment of any disease or impairment of, or the assessment of the health of, human beings" need to be CLIA-validated before return to a subject (Clinical Laboratories Improvement Amendments 2012). Some have argued that CLIA confirmation isn't necessary as long as researchers make it clear that the clinically relevant results they are returning would need to be validated before being relied upon (Jarvik et al. 2014). But, the Centers for Medicare and Medicaid (CMS, the regulatory agency under which CLIA falls) has made it clear that this isn't their interpretation and that CLIA confirmation is still required. There is merit to the more permissive view, but this might be a case where the ethically defensible course of actions is inconsistent with what the law (as currently written) requires.

18.7 CONCLUSION

The genetics and bioethics communities have been debating the ethical issues raised by our steady move into a genomic era. While this debate has been vigorous and productive, it has not resolved all of the outstanding questions that this transformative new technology presents. In this chapter, many of the difficult ethical questions that will require more careful consideration as investigators continue to incorporate genomic sequencing into their research have been presented.

REFERENCES

Berkman, B.E. (2017) Refuting the right not to know. *Journal of Health Care Law and Policy*, 19(1):1–72.

Berkman, B.E.; Hull, S.C. (2014) The "right not to know" in the genomic era: Time to break from tradition? *American Journal of Bioethics*, 14(3):28–31.

Beskow, L.M.; Burke, W. (2010) Offering individual genetic research results: Context matters. *Science Translational Medicine*, 2:1–5.

Bombard, Y.; Brothers, K.B.; Fitzgerald-Butt, S.; Garrison, N.A.; Jamal, L.; James, C.A.; Jarvik, G.P.; McCormick, J.B.; Nelson, T.N.; Ormond, K.E.; Rehm, H.L.; Richer, J.; Souzeau, E.; Vassy, J.L.; Wagner, J.K.; Levy, H.P. (2019) The responsibility to recontact research participants after reinterpretation of genetic and genomic research results. *American Journal of Human Genetics*, 104(4):578–595.

Broadstock, M.; Michie, S.; Marteau, T. (2000) Psychological consequences of predictive genetics testing: A systematic review. *European Journal of Human Genetics*, 8(10):731–738.

Burke, W.; Antommaria, A.H.; Bennet, R.; Botkin, J.; Clayton, E.W.; Henderson, G.E.; Holm, I.A.; Jarvik, G.P.; Khoury, M.J.; Knoppers, B.M.; Press, N.A.; Ross, L.F.; Rothstein, M.A.; Saal, H.; Uhlmann, W.R.; Wilfond, B.; Wolf, S.M.; Zimmern, R. (2013) Recommendations for returning genomic incidental findings? We need to talk! *Genetics in Medicine*, 15(11):854–859.

Chan, B.; Facio, F.M.; Eidem, H.; Hull, S.C.; Biesecker, L.G.; Berkman, B.E. (2012) Genomic Inheritances: Disclosing individual research results from whole-exome sequencing to deceased participants' relatives. *American Journal of Bioethics*, 12(10):1–8.

Clinical Laboratories Improvement Amendments. 42 U.S.C. § 263a (2012).

Collins, F.S. (1999) Medical and societal consequences of the human genome project. *New England Journal of Medicine*, 341:28–37.

Collins, F.S.; Hamburg, M.A. (2013) First FDA authorization for next-generation sequencer. *New England Journal of Medicine*, 369:2369–2371.

Collins, F.S.; Morgan, M.; Patrinos, A. (2003) The human genome project: Lessons from large-scale biology. *Science*, 300(5617):286–2890.

Darnell, A.J.; Austin, H.; Bluemke, D.A.; Cannon, R.O.; Fischbeck, K.; Gahl, W.; Goldman, D.; Grady, C.; Greene, M.H.; Holland, S.M.; Hull, S.C.; Porter, F.D.; Resnik, D.; Rubinstein, W.W.; Biesecker, L.G. (2016) A clinical service to support the return of secondary genomic findings in human research. *American Journal of Human Genetics*, 98(3):435–441.

Eckstein, L.; Garrett, J.R.; Berkman, B.E. (2014) A framework for analyzing the ethics of disclosing genetic research findings. *Journal of Law, Medicine and Ethics*, 42(2):190–207.

Feero, W.G.; Guttmacher, A.E.; Collins, F.S. (2010) Genomic medicine: An updated primer. *New England Journal of Medicine*, 362:2001–2011.

Gliwa, C.; Berkman, B.E. (2013) Do researchers have an obligation to actively look for genetic incidental findings? *American Journal of Bioethics*, 13(2):32–42.

Gliwa, C.; Yurkiewicz, I.R.; Lehmann, L.S.; Hull, S.C.; Jones, N.; Berkman, B.E. (2016) IRB perspectives on obligations to disclose genetic incidental findings to research participants. Genetics in Medicine, 18(7):705–711.

Green, E.D.; Guyer, M.S. (2011) Charting a course for genomic medicine from base pairs to bedside. *Nature*, 470:204–213.

Green, R.C.; Berg, J.S.; Grody, W.W.; Kalia, S.S.; Korf, B.R.; Martin, C.L.; McGuire, A.; Nussbaum, R.L.; O'Daniel, J.M.; Ormond, K.E.; Rehm, H.L.; Watson, M.S.; Williams, M.S.; Biesecker, L.G. (2013) ACMG recommendations for reporting of incidental findings in clinical exome and genome sequencing. *Genetics in Medicine*, 15(7):565–574.

Halpern, J.; Arnold, R.M. (2008) Affective forecasting: An unrecognized challenge in making serious health decisions. *Journal of General Internal Medicine*, 23(10):1708–1712.

Jackson, L.; Goldsmith, L.; O'Connor, A.; Skirton, H. (2012) Incidental findings in genetic research and clinical diagnostic tests: A systematic review. *American Journal of Medical Genetics*, 158A:3159–3167.

Jarvik, G.P.; Amendola, L.; Berg, J.S.; Brothers, K.; Clayton, E.W.; Chung, W.; Evans, B.J.; Evans, J.P.; Fullerton, S.M.; Gallego, C.J.; Garrison, N.A.; Gray, S.W.; Holm, I.A.; Kullo, I.J.; Lehmann, L.S.; McCarty, C.; Prows, C.A.; Rehm, H.L.; Sharp, R.R.; Salama, J.; Sanderson, S.; Van Driest, S.L.; Williams, M.S.; Wolf, S.M.; Wolf, W.A.; eMERGE Act-ROR Committee; CERC Committee; CSER Act-ROR Working Group; Burke, W. (2014) Return of genomic results to research participants: The floor, the ceiling, and the choices in between. *American Journal of Human Genetics*, 94(6):818–826.

Joly, Y.; Feze, I.N.; Simard, J. (2013) Genetic discrimination and life insurance: A systematic review of the evidence. *BMC Medicine*, 11:25–39.

Kaufman, D.; Murphy, J.; Scott, J.; Hudson, K. (2008) Subjects Mmatter: A survey of public opinions about a large genetic cohort study. *Genetics in Medicine*, 10(11):831–839.

Kohane, I.S.; Masys, D.R.; Altman, R.B. (2006) The incidentalome: A threat to genomic medicine. *JAMA*, 296(2):212–215.

Laurie, G.T. (1999) In defence of ignorance: Genetic information and the right not to know. *European Journal of Health Law*, 6:119–132.

Laurie, G.T. (2000) Protecting and promoting privacy in an uncertain world: Further defences of ignorance and the right not to know. *European Journal of Health Law*, 7:185–191.

Mandava, A.; Millum, J.; Berkman, B.E. (2015) When should genome researchers disclose misattributed parentage? *Hastings Center Report*, 45(4):28–36.

Mandava, A.; Pace, C.; Campbell, B.; Emanuel, E.; Grady, C. (2012) The quality of informed consent: Mapping the landscape. A review of empirical data from developing and developed countries. *Journal of Medical Ethics*, 38(6):356–365.

Manolio, T.A.; Chisholm, R.L.; Ozenberger, B.; Roden, D.M.; Williams, M.S.; Wilson, R.; Bick, D.; Bottinger, E.P.; Brilliant, M.H.; Eng, C.; Frazer, K.A.; Korf, B.; Ledbetter, D.H.; Lupski, J.R.; Marsh, C.; Mrazek, D.; Murray, M.F.; O'Donnell, P.H.; Rader, D.J.; Relling, M.V.; Shuldiner, A.R.; Valle, D.; Weinshilboum, R.; Green, E.D.; Ginsburg, G.S. (2013) Implementing genomic medicine in the clinic: The future is here. *Genetics in Medicine*, 15:258–267.

Mardis, E.R. (2011) A decade's perspective on DNA sequencing technology. *Nature*, 470:198–203.

McGuire, A.L.; Beskow, L.M. (2010) Informed consent in genomics and genetic research. *Annual Review of Genomics and Human Genetics*, 11:361–381.

McGuire, A.L.; Caulfield, T.; Cho, M.K. (2008) Research ethics and the challenge of whole-genome sequencing. *Nature Reviews Genetics*, 9:152–156.

McGuire, A.L.; Joffe, S.; Koenig, B.A.; Biesecker, B.B.; McCullough, L.B.; Blumenthal-Barby, J.S.; Caulfield, T.; Terry, S.F.; Green, R.C. (2013) Ethics and genomic incidental findings. Science, 340(6136):1047–1048.

Middleton, A.; Morley, K.I.; Bragin, E.; Firth, H.V.; Hurles, M.E.; Wright, C.F.; Parker, M. (2016) Attitudes of nearly 7000 health professionals, genomic researchers and publics toward the return of incidental results from sequencing research. *European Journal of Human Genetics*, 24:21–29.

Ormond, K.E.; O'Daniel, J.M.; Kalia, S.S. (2019) Secondary findings: How did we get here, and where are we going? *Journal of Genetic Counseling*, 28(2):326–333.

Peters, S.A.; Laham, S.M.; Pachter, N.; Winship, I.M. (2014) The future in clinical genetics: Affective forecasting biases in patient and clinician decision making. *Clinical Genetics*, 85(4):312–317.

Pike, E.R.; Rothenberg, K.H.; Berkman, B.E. (2014) Finding fault? Exploring legal duties to return incidental findings in genomic research. *Georgetown Law Journal*, 102:795–843.

Presidential Commission for the Study of Bioethical Issues (2013) Anticipate and Communicate: Ethical Management of Incidental and Secondary Findings in the Clinical, Research, and Direct-to-Consumer Contexts.

Prince, A.E.R.; Berkman, B.E. (2018) Reconceptualizing harms and benefits in the genomic age. *Personalized Medicine*, 15(5):419–428.

Richards, S.; Aziz, N.; Bale, S.; Bick, D.; Das, S.; Gastier-Foster, J.; Grody, W.W.; Hedge, M.; Lyon, E.; Spector, E.; Voelkerding, K.; Rehm, H.L. (2015) Standards and guidelines for the interpretation of sequence variants: A joint consensus recommendation of the American College of Medical Genetics and Genomics and the Association for Molecular Pathology. *Genetics in Medicine*, 17:405–423.

Rothstein, M.A. (2008) GINA, the ADA, and genetic discrimination in employment. Journal of Law, Medicine & Ethics, 36(4):837–840.

Sullivan, H.K.; Berkman, B.E. (2018) Incidental findings in low-resource settings. *Hastings Center Report*, 48(3):20–28.

Taber, K.A.J.; Dickinson, B.D.; Wilson, M. (2014) The promise and challenges of next-generation genome sequencing for clinical care. *JAMA Internal Medicine*, 174(2):275–280.

Tabor, H.K.; Berkman, B.E.; Hull, S.C.; Bamshad, M.J. (2011) Genomics really gets personal: How exome and whole genome sequencing challenge the ethical framework of human genetics research. *American Journal of Medical Genetics*, 155A(12):2916–2924.

Takala, T. (1999) The right to genetic ignorance confirmed. *Bioethics*, 13(3–4):288–293.

Teer, J.K.; Mullikin, J.C. (2010) Exome sequencing: The sweet spot before whole genomes. *Human Molecular Genetics*, 19(R2):R145–R151.

Trinidad, S.B.; Fullerton, S.M.; Burke, W. (2015) Looking for trouble and finding it. *American Journal of Bioethics*, 15(7):15–17.

Wetterstrand, K.A. (2019) The cost of sequencing a human genome. https://www.genome.gov/about-genomics/fact-sheets/Sequencing-Human-Genome-cost

Wilson, T.D.; Gilbert, D.T. (2005) Affective forecasting knowing what to want. *Current Directions in Psychological Science*, 14(3):131–134.

Wolf, S.M.; Annas, G.J.; Elias, S. (2013) Patient autonomy and incidental findings in clinical genomics. *Science*, 340:1049–1050.

19 Genomics, Big Data, and Broad Consent

A New Ethics Frontier for Prevention Science

Celia B. Fisher and Deborah M. Layman
Fordham University

CONTENTS

19.1 INTRODUCTION

Emerging technologies for the collection and analysis of biospecimens have led to advances in understanding the interacting role of genetics and environment on the development of mental health and behavioral risk and resilience and individual responsivity to prevention and intervention programs (Dick et al. 2011, Fisher and McCarthy 2013, Musci and Schlomer 2018). The proliferation of genomic research

DOI: 10.1201/9780429263286-22

is fueled by the ease of collecting DNA through cheek swabs or saliva, the decreasing costs of genotyping and DNA sequencing (Dick et al. 2011, Lunshof et al. 2008), and technological advances in genome-wide association studies (GWAS) (Calvin et al. 2012, Davies et al. 2016, Greven et al. 2009, Krapohl et al. 2014, Mandelli and Serretti 2013, McCrory et al. 2010, Rimfeld et al. 2015), gene by environment studies (GxE) (Belsky and Pluess 2009, Kegel et al. 2011), and gene by intervention studies (GxI) (Dick et al. 2011, Musci and Schlomer 2018). As a result, the growing field of genomics research has enriched the contributions of prevention science for understanding the unique and interacting roles of genetic and environmental factors in areas including academic achievement, sexual risk behaviors, substance use, internalizing and externalizing disorders, and responsivity to educational and development promoting preventive interventions within the growing field of implementation science (Bakermans-Kranenburg et al. 2008, Beach et al. 2018, Brody et al. 2009, Dick et al. 2011, Fisher 2017b, Glenn et al. 2018, Haworth and Plomin 2012, Leadbeater et al. 2018, Musci and Schlomer 2018, Russell et al. 2017, Zheng et al. 2018).

The progress in utilizing biospecimens in prevention science parallels the rise in integrating large datasets across all scientific disciplines. This trend, sometimes referred to as "Big Data", is marked by increased access to and use of individual-level data across administrative data systems with the potential to link genomic data to health, public benefits, child welfare, criminal and juvenile justice, and educational records and other personal information (Caspi et al. 2002, 2017, Perlman and Fantuzzo 2013, Wertz et al. 2018). The accumulation of personal information into large centralized datasets increases opportunities for secondary widespread and ongoing use by diverse investigators (Gilmore 2016, Kaplan et al. 2014).

Along with the scientific benefits, advances in genomic and Big Data analytic tools are the increasing ability of investigators to re-identify previously de-identified participant information (Hansson et al. 2016, Malin and Sweeney 2001). To adapt to ongoing technological advances, research aims, and expanding contexts in which biospecimens are collected, stored, and available for secondary use, the Office of Human Research Protections (OHRP 2017) has issued revised federal regulations for the protection of human subjects (known as the Final Rule) that include expanded requirements for obtaining informed consent in general and a new category known as broad consent. Broad consent requires investigators to offer participants a range of choices regarding consent to the ongoing storage and future use of their personally identifiable data. The revised guidelines, scheduled to go into effect in 2019, have important implications for how prevention scientists will obtain initial consent for research involving collection of biospecimens as well as consent for future use.

This chapter begins with a discussion of changes to federal regulations on the format, content, and transparency of informed consent across all aspects of prevention science, followed by a description of the rationale, requirements, and implications for obtaining broad consent for the storage and future use of potentially identifiable information and biospecimens. We conclude with a discussion of future challenges that will be raised involving ongoing transparency and protections for participants and their communities.

19.2 CHANGES IN FEDERAL REGULATIONS GOVERNING KEY ELEMENTS OF INFORMED CONSENT

The Final Rule is intended to modernize federal regulations for human subject protections to be in step with the genomic revolution, the rapidly changing Big Data technology, and perceived inefficiencies and gaps in protecting the rights of prospective participants (Emanuel and Menikoff 2011, Sugarman 2017). In federal regulations, participant autonomy in deciding whether to participate in a research study is protected through the informed consent process with three key preconditions: information disclosure, participant comprehension, and voluntariness (Sreenivasan 2003, Strauss 2017). However, according to many of the comments elicited during consideration of the federal rule changes, the increasing length and complexity of modern-day consent forms threaten participant autonomy by sacrificing the clarity needed for comprehension in favor of protecting the liability of institutions (Klitzman 2013). A meta-analysis of informed consent in clinical trials found comprehension difficulties for important components including randomization, placebo, and participation risks and benefits (Tam et al. 2015). The revisions to federal regulations were designed to address these problems through new requirements for the format and content of informed consent.

19.2.1 FORMAT CHANGES: A CONCISE SUMMARY OF KEY INFORMATION

In response to lengthy consent forms that often hinder an informed participation decision, the revised regulations emphasize the need to improve the quality and transparency of informed consent. This effort is consistent with recommendations of the Society for Prevention Research (SPR) Ethics Task Force (Leadbeater et al. 2018) underscoring the need for prevention scientists to respect the rights of those whose lives they hope to improve and empower them to make decisions concerning issues that affect them. This refocus on comprehension requires informed consent documents that "as a whole must present information in sufficient detail relating to the research, and must be organized and presented in a way that does not merely provide lists of isolated facts but rather facilitates the prospective subject's or legally authorized representative's understanding of the reasons why one might or might not want to participate" (§__.116 (2)(ii); OHRP 2017, pp. 7265–7266). To fulfill this aim, the Final Rule requires, prior to the full consent form, an initial concise summary of key information necessary for a prospective participant to make a decision. Topics covered in this initial summary are similar to requirements for the full informed consent, e.g., purpose, duration of participation, procedures, risks/discomforts, benefits, and alternative procedures/treatment. It is not intended to replace any of the required information or detailed information about procedures and risks, but rather, to highlight the most critical information that may be buried in a lengthy, cumbersome document (Menikoff et al. 2017, OHRP 2017).

Guidance for developing this concise summary and a more comprehensible informed consent is left to what a "reasonable person would want to have in order to make an informed decision about whether to participate" (§__.116 (4); OHRP 2017, p. 7265). The use of "reasonable person" is intended to increase comprehension and transparency across participant populations and as described later in this chapter is also applied to requirements for broad consent. However, requirements for the length and specific content are explicitly left to the discretion of Institutional Review Boards (IRBs) with only minor direction regarding the underlying purpose and rationale. In attempting to address this requirement, investigators and IRBs should consider that different participant populations will have distinct levels of genetic literacy and informational needs and be wary of a scripted approach to the concise consent summary that may ultimately fail to adequately guide prospective participants through decision-making (Condit 2010, Fisher 2017a, Fisher and Wallace 2000).

19.2.2 Suggested Key Elements for Consent

A reasonable consent decision for research involving genetic testing may require understanding that the rapid rate at which new genetic technologies develop and the fact that many genes are related to more than one trait (pleiotropy) means that investigators may discover genetic risk that is unanticipated or incidental to the original aims of the research (Cooper et al. 2006). Relatedly, the multifactorial and probabilistic nature of data acquired through collection of genetic information for prevention studies and the lack of clinical utility can confuse participants attempting to understand the personal relevance of research results, leading to unrealistic expectations regarding the possibility of direct benefits (Fisher 2017b, Henderson 2008). Fisher and McCarthy (2013) have provided a detailed list of key elements for informed consent that can guide development of concise summaries for prevention research involving genetic testing. Some of the key elements they identify include: (1) how and for how long genetic material will be stored; (2) if, when, and how materials will be destroyed; (3) confidentiality protections including de-identification and risks of identity linkage; (4) the nature of personal genetic information that will or will not be disclosed to participants and the rationale for disclosure decisions; (5) opportunities for and limitations on the right to withdraw data once it has been collected, stored or analyzed, and for pediatric research; (6) parental permission and child assent procedures, and plans at the time child participants become legal adults; and (7) the possibility that data may contradict assumed attribution of paternity or other biological bases of family relationships.

19.3 TRANSPARENCY REQUIREMENTS FOR CONSENT FORMS RELATED TO CLINICAL TRIALS

Maintaining high standards of transparency in representing themselves to stakeholders is a key recommendation from the SPR Ethics Task Force (Leadbeater et al. 2018). A significant change to the Common Rule that will have implications for prevention science is the new, broader definition of a "clinical trial" and transparency requirements for online posting of the consent forms for such trials online. The current proposed change in regulations defines a clinical trial as "a research study in which one or more human subjects are prospectively assigned to one or more interventions (which may include placebo or other control) to evaluate the effects of the interventions on biomedical or behavioral health-related outcomes" (§__.102(b);

OHRP 2017, p. 7260). Many social–behavioral scientists expressed concern that the absence of a clear definition of "intervention" inappropriately places nonintervention social and behavioral research involving manipulation of variables under the "clinical trial" umbrella and subject to these transparency requirements. In response to these concerns, Congress passed an omnibus bill ("Consolidated Appropriations Act, H.R. 1625" 2018) delaying the implementation of the new clinical trials definition for projects that historically do not fall under the clinical trials definition until it can undergo more thorough review and consultation (Society for Research in Child Development (SRCD) 2018). However, the National Institute of Health interprets the new bill to refer only to prior approved studies and therefore are instructing primary investigators for all new submissions to submit their study as a clinical trial if it corresponds to the regulatory definition. As a result, investigators conducting prevention trials may be required to post one version of the informed consent form online at a specified federal website within 60 days from the close of participant enrollment. To date, no additional guidance was provided identifying the online options for investigators, although readers may refer to the Food and Drug Administration (FDA) ClinicalTrials.gov as a potential model for what may be required.

The advantages and disadvantages of applying the FDA model designed for pharmaceutical and medical research to prevention science will need to be determined as compliance with this regulation moves forward. Some authors have argued that increased transparency through an online posting of informed consent forms may facilitate the development of clear and comprehensive documents that reflect the spirit of the regulations' focus on comprehension and decision-making (Bierer et al. 2017). However, this assumes that once such documents begin to be posted online, investigators will refer to these documents as a resource when developing their own consent process. More likely, the posting of consent forms will lead to greater transparency of the scope of intervention research, engendering expectations by the public and scientific community to examine study findings. This, in turn, may lead to pressure on prevention scientists to report null results, public pressure previously applied to pharmaceutical clinical trials (Fisher 2006a).

19.4 BROAD CONSENT

The rapid increase in biospecimen repositories and the ability to link this data with integrated administrative datasets are continuing to influence how potentially identifiable participant information and biospecimens are collected and shared across research, healthcare, educational, and criminal justice systems. At the potential cost of individual privacy, aggregating data requires identifying individuals across datasets and has several benefits. Often undetected by smaller, lower powered studies, large aggregated datasets provide a cost-effective method to identify complex associations between biology and environmental risk factors for poor outcomes. However, these integrated datasets require additional confidentiality protections both because researchers may need to utilize legitimate means of identifying and linking an individual's information across datasets and the increasing sophistication of individuals within and outside the research community to re-identify assumed protected de-identified information (Fisher 2017c, Homer et al. 2008, Lunshof et al. 2008).

The introduction of broad consent in federal regulations arose in response to these concerns as well as recognition that additional participant protections were required for the long-term secondary use of potentially identifiable information by investigators who were not involved in the original collection of data and who might use the data for research purposes significantly different from the original study to which participants consented. Prevention scientists planning to store and maintain potentially identifiable information and biospecimens for future use by other researchers may substitute broad consent for the traditional consent procedures as long as the broad consent includes the components described in the next section and the reasonable person standard discussed above.

19.4.1 Background and Rationale: Balancing Privacy Concerns with Advancing Technologies

How to protect the autonomy of participants without hindering an important avenue of research and discovery has been vigorously debated in recent years (Berkman et al. 201, Grady 2017, Grady et al. 2015). Under previous regulations, investigators wishing to use secondary data could re-consent participants from the original study, or more commonly, petition the IRB to waive consent for secondary use (OHRP 2017). The Final Rule recognizes that re-consent is potentially a costly, burdensome, and prohibitive process which may not only derail promising scientific advances but may introduce unnecessary risk of privacy violations during re-identification procedures. However, the new regulations also attempt to address instances in which waiver of consent for secondary analysis may lead to similar privacy risks and potential violations of participant autonomy. Broad consent is a regulatory attempt to achieve an appropriate balance between participant rights to determine the future use of their research data and the scientific benefits that may accrue when such use involves unspecified investigators and research aims.

19.4.2 Definition and Overview of Broad Consent Requirements

According to the new regulations, as part of the initial consent procedures, investigators may seek broad consent for the storage, maintenance, and secondary research use of identifiable private information or identifiable biospecimens collected for studies other than the initially proposed research or for non-research purposes (§__.116(d); OHRP 2017, p. 7265). When compared to the practice of obtaining a waiver of re-consent for secondary analysis, broad consent increases transparency and provides greater opportunities for participants to decide if their identifiable private information or identifiable biospecimens may be used by future researchers for specified or unspecified research purposes (Menikoff et al. 2017). When broad consent is obtained, future research covered by the broad consent may be subject to limited IRB review designed only to determine if the proposed research is within the scope of the broad consent. IRB waiver of consent to use previously collected data for secondary use remains an option under the Final Rule. However, if broad consent has been offered but refused, an IRB cannot waive consent for secondary research use of that person's identifiable private information or identifiable biospecimens.

The regulatory vision for broad consent for future research hinges on the extent to which participants are provided with details of the nature, storage, maintenance, and future uses of their identifiable data needed for the reasonable person to make an informed decision. To be sufficiently robust, the regulations mandate a series of information disclosures related to the type of data stored, time period for storage and use, types of future use, and with whom data may be shared. Mandates also include additional disclosures related to whole-genome sequencings, clinically relevant data, and when data may be de-identified or glean commercial profit. A discussion of the required disclosures is provided below.

19.4.3　Definition and Description of Identifiable Information or Biospecimens

A significant change in the Final Rule is the inclusion of "identifiable information and biospecimens" under the definition "human subject" (§__.102 (e) 1 (ii); OHRP 2017). This expanded definition has been quite controversial since it means that identifiable information and biospecimens require the same protections as persons. Since the Final Rule requires investigators to describe the identifiable information and biospecimens that will be collected and stored for future use, it is noteworthy that the term identifiable is defined as "private information [or biospecimen] for which the identity of the subject is or may readily be ascertained by the investigator or associated with the information [or biospecimen]" (§__.102 (e) 5–7; OHRP 2017, p. 7260). The inclusion of "may readily be ascertained" is in recognition of the evolving ability to re-identify previously de-identified genetic information. At present, what qualifies as an identifiable biospecimen is left to the discretion of the IRB, although the Final Rule includes a provision for convening a committee for periodic review of the definition. As a result, prevention scientists will need to keep abreast of continuously changing definitions of identifiable information and biospecimens for broad consent procedures. To date, the definition of sociodemographic identifiable information attached to biospecimens or as part of administrative systems linkages draws from the Health Insurance Portability and Accountability Act (HIPAA) and includes but is not limited to: name; place of birth and mailing address more specific than state residence; hospital admission or discharge date more specific than year; email, telephone, and fax; Social Security or health plan number (US Department of Health and Human Services 2012). The original participant ID number is also considered an identifier and will need to be recoded if data is defined as de-identified.

19.4.4　Time Period for Storage and Use

A second required component is the time period of storage and use of the identifiable data, which can be limited or in perpetuity. Determining and communicating a time period for data use is particularly relevant when working with members of American Indian Alaskan Native (AIAN) nations. Some tribal communities, such as the Havasupai, prohibit body fragmentation and biospecimens living outside the body or after death (Bardill and Garrison 2015, Pearson et al. 2014, Sahota 2014). Broad consent for AIAN populations should, therefore, consult with AIAN leaders and carefully specify conditions for storage, destruction, and blessing before destruction of biospecimens (Arbour and Cook 2006). Extended time periods for storage also have implications for biospecimens collected on minors with guardian permission. Investigators must consider whether child participants, when they become legal adults, will be notified as to where their biological materials are stored and conditions in which they will or will not have a right to re-consent or withdraw permission for further use of their data (Fisher et al. 2013). When unlimited time periods for data storage and use conflict with cultural values or rights of minors, investigators may consider a model of "DNA on loan" where donations remain the property of the participant who gift their biospecimen to researchers who agree to act as faithful stewards for a specific period of time and for a specific research project (Arbour and Cook 2006).

19.4.5 DISCLOSURE OF FUTURE USERS

Broad consent must disclose who may have access to a participant's stored identifiable data or clearly indicate that the identity of those with access to secondary use will remain unspecified. Most commonly, access will be limited to investigators affiliated with accredited universities, research, or medical institutions that have the institutional oversight and infrastructure to adequately protect data security and abide by restrictions on use outlined in the broad consent. When considering whether to conduct secondary research or deposit data into biobanks or other data repositories, prevention scientists should investigate whether the repository conforms to applicable regulations and policies. The University of California (2012) has an informative guide to evaluating biorepositories that includes but is not limited to procedures for: (1) identifying and ensuring that the aims of secondary usage requests are consistent with consent obtained from participants; (2) evaluating the qualifications of researchers and entities requesting access to data; (3) updating data security in response to emerging technologies; (4) including a submittal agreement from the original investigator attesting to the IRB approval and written informed consent of participants from whom data was collected; (5) providing a standard usage agreement that details conditions for receipt and future use of data or human specimens; and (6) continuing committee review and oversight.

19.4.6 COMMERCIAL USE OF DATA

The movement toward open science, including the availability of data from prevention trials to other scientists and stakeholders (Caulfield et al. 2012, Leadbeater et al. 2018) and growing interest in genetic responsivity to psychopharmacological medications for behavioral and other mental health disorders is likely to be paralleled by increased interest in secondary use of biobank data by pharmaceutical companies and in funding prevention scientists to conduct such research. As recommended by the SPR Ethics Task Force (Leadbeater et al. 2018), investigators need to disclose financial and professional conflict of interests to all stakeholders, especially when presenting the scientific findings to stakeholders that affect program adoption, dissemination, and implementation strategies.

The new broad consent regulations require disclosure to participants if their bio-specimens may be used for commercial profit, and whether they will receive any portion of these profits. To be in compliance, at the outset of commercial sponsor funding relationships, investigators need to: (1) reach an agreement on where data will be stored; (2) ensure data repositories meet current standards of informational security if deposited at a company facility; (3) have a clear understanding of which entity owns the data for future use; (4) whether such use will be for commercial profit; and (5) whether participants will receive any portion of these profits.

19.4.7 DISCLOSURE OF FUTURE USE

A fourth requirement of broad consent is a mandate to disclose how participants' identifiable information may be used, whether whole-genome sequencing may be conducted by other investigators, whether participants will be informed of future use, and if they are being asked to agree to future research that may not be aligned with the purpose of the original study. Although investigators are not required to return individual genomic results to participants, survey research indicates that genetic testing serves as a strong incentive for participation and individuals often prefer to be provided with incidental results that go beyond the original aims of the study (Kaufman et al. 2016). Ethical obligations for disclosure of clinically relevant genetic information uncovered during secondary analysis will increase as genetic research advances to adequately identify and successfully intervene to reduce vulnerability or enhance development for critical outcomes such as academic achievement, health, and well-being (Appelbaum et al. 2014, Fisher 2006b, Grandjean and Sorsa 1996, Jarvik et al. 2014, Ravitsky and Wilfond 2006). Broad consent must thus include a statement regarding whether participants will be informed of clinically relevant findings that may emerge.

19.4.8 PARTICIPANT PERSPECTIVES

Emerging empirical evidence on public willingness to provide broad consent or donate genetic information to biobanks for future research suggests that a majority of people are willing to consent for altruistic reasons if adequate privacy protections are in place, they are informed about who will use the data, and have a say in how their information will be used (Burstein et al. 2014, Hens et al. 2011, Kaufman et al. 2008, 2016, Lemke et al. 2010, McGuire et al. 2008, 2011, Oliver et al. 2012). However, willingness to consent varies by the type of future research and the background of the prospective participant. According to one survey study, participants willing to donate biospecimens for future disease-related research were more hesitant on its use for socially sensitive topics such as abortion, genetic influences on violence, or vaccines related to biological weapons (De Vries et al. 2016). In a survey on adults' opinions about a nationwide precision medicine initiative involving collection of genomic and environmental information, fewer respondents were willing to agree to the use of their data with researchers outside of the United States or pharmaceutical or drug companies than with American academic researchers or NIH researchers (Kaufman et al. 2016).

The perceived vulnerability of participants has also been shown to influence willingness to share DNA samples for future research. In several studies, parents providing broad consent for their minor child expressed concern about unknown future risks and future decision-making for themselves and for their children when their children become adults (Burstein et al. 2014, Hens et al. 2011, Kaufman et al. 2008). In one of the few studies examining youth attitudes, adolescents who were receiving outpatient oncology, cardiology, and orthopedics services were more willing to donate their specimens to biobanks than their parents or their healthy peers (Kong et al. 2016). In a large nationally sponsored epidemiological study on mental health and substance use, although donation rates were high overall, African Americans and individuals with less education and a history of drug abuse were less likely to consent to sharing their sample with other investigators (Storr et al. 2014). Attitudes toward collection, storage, and use of biospecimens may also differ by culture and social risk factors. For example, community members in Africa, Asia and the America's involvement in HIV prevention trials, indicated that in some instances, sexual partners and spouses of participants wanted information on where biospecimens would be stored and to be included in decision-making (MacQueen and Alleman 2008).

The public response to the expansion of genetic explanations for substance use, behavioral disorders, racial/ethnic differences in mental health, and other socially stigmatized behaviors has the potential to perpetuate health disparities by attributing vulnerabilities intrinsically tied to social and structural inequities to genetic characteristics (Fisher et al. 2013, Fisher and McCarthy 2013). The extent to which unspecified secondary use of biospecimens can pose a social risk to already vulnerable populations is difficult to anticipate or describe in broad consent procedures. Because participants may be unwilling to provide a blanket broad consent for future use of their specimens, prevention scientists may consider allowing participants to opt out of use of their data for specific future research purposes. This approach may, however, place unrealistic demands on researchers to identify all possible future uses and if not adequately specified, place an unachievable burden on IRBs to interpret whether proposed secondary research aims meet the original broad consent specifications. One solution is to engage community advisory boards in creating explicit opt-out procedures tailored to the unique characteristics of participant populations to create a goodness-of-fit between broad consent procedures and participant values and concerns (Fisher 2015, Fisher and Ragsdale 2006).

19.5 CONCLUSIONS

Researchers seeking broad consent are tasked with specifying the terms of the consent and engendering trust that the investigators, their institutions, and future researchers will be faithful stewards of participants' identifiable information and biospecimens. Until the Final Rule is widely applied and tested, prevention scientists who utilize broad consent will face the challenging task of identifying potential future uses of data collected and determining the degree of specification necessary for the reasonable person to make an informed broad consent decision. Furthermore, investigators need to consider whether adopting an open-ended, broad consent for future use of identifiable data may discourage research participation or engender unreasonable expectations regarding future return of results. Investigators will also need to determine how to specify essential details without creating scripted templates for informed consent that do not adequately fit the participant's health and genetic literacy. An additional responsibility falling on prevention scientists during this preliminary period is the need to determine whether their data repositories have the infrastructure to honor obligations made during broad consent. Infrastructure obligations include the ability to identify which participants in the original study refused broad consent to ensure their data is withheld from secondary research efforts, to enforce the limits promised on data access and the purpose to which the data will be used, and the destruction of biospecimens on the specified schedule promised during broad consent.

IRBs and their institutions face additional challenges. Policies will need to be developed that adequately determine if secondary researchers have the training and expertise to be a proper steward of participant protections for the use of identifiable information and biospecimens and can honor the obligations in the original broad consent. To support ongoing stewardship of identifiable genetic material, the SRCD Committee on the Common Rule recommended that institutions should develop procedures to ensure that researchers who have access to data in the future will be bound by the best practices in confidentiality protections at the time data was collected and new protections as they emerge (Fisher et al. 2013). As prevention scientists' grapple with the current ambiguity and evolving interpretations of the Final Rule, an ethical awareness of the values and preferences with which participants approach the future use of their personal data will produce informed consent procedures that minimize informational risk, optimize participants' informed choice, and promote prevention science.

ACKNOWLEDGMENTS

The text for this chapter is reprinted with permission from the following publication: Fisher, C. & Layman, D. (2018). Genomics, big data, and broad consent: A new ethics frontier for prevention science. *Prevention Science*, 19. doi:10.1007/s11121-018-0944-z.

REFERENCES

Appelbaum, P. S., Parens, E., Waldman, C. R., Klitzman, R., Fyer, A., Martinez, J., ... Chung, W. K. (2014). Models of consent to return of incidental findings in genomic research. *The Hastings Center Report*, 44(4), 22–32. doi:10.1002/hast.328.

Arbour, L., & Cook, D. (2006). DNA on loan: Issues to consider when carrying out genetic research with aboriginal families and communities. *Community Genetics*, 9(3), 153. doi:10.1159/000092651.

Bakermans-Kranenburg, M. J., Van Ijzendoorn, M. H., Mesman, J., Alink, L. R., & Juffer, F. (2008). Effects of an attachment-based intervention on daily cortisol moderated by dopamine receptor D4: A randomized control trial on 1- to 3-year-olds screened for externalizing behavior. *Developmental Psychopathology*, 20(3), 805–820. doi:10.1017/S0954579408000382.

Bardill, J., & Garrison, N. A. (2015). Naming indigenous concerns, framing considerations for stored biospecimens. *American Journal of Bioethics, 15*(9), 73–75. doi:10.1080/152 65161.2015.1062164.

Beach, S. R. H., Lei, M. K., Brody, G. H., & Philibert, R. A. (2018). Prevention of early substance use mediates, and variation at SLC6A4 moderates, SAAF intervention effects on OXTR methylation. *Prevention Science, 19*(1), 90–100. doi:10.1007/s11121-016-0709-5.

Belsky, J., & Pluess, M. (2009). Beyond diathesis stress: Differential susceptibility to environmental influences. *Psychological Bulletin, 135*(6), 885. doi:10.1037/a0017376.

Berkman, B. E., Wendler, D., Sullivan, H. K., & Grady, C. (2017). A proposed process for reliably updating the common rule. *The American Journal of Bioethics, 17*(7), 8–14. doi:10.1080/15265161.2017.1329478.

Bierer, B. E., Barnes, M., & Lynch, H. F. (2017). Revised 'Common Rule' shapes protections for research participants. *Health Affairs, 36*(5), 784–788. doi:10.1377/hlthaff.2017.0307.

Brody, G. H., Beach, S. R., Philibert, R. A., Chen, Y. F., & Murry, V. M. (2009). Prevention effects moderate the association of 5-HTTLPR and youth risk behavior initiation: Gene× environment hypotheses tested via a randomized prevention design. *Child Development, 80*(3), 645–661. doi:10.1111/j.1467-8624.2009.01288.x.

Burstein, M. D., Robinson, J. O., Hilsenbeck, S. G., McGuire, A. L., & Lau, C. C. (2014). Pediatric data sharing in genomic research: Attitudes and preferences of parents. *Pediatrics, 133*(4), 690–697. doi:10.1542/peds.2013-1592.

Calvin, C. M., Deary, I. J., Webbink, D., Smith, P., Fernandes, C., Lee, S. H., ... Visscher, P. M. (2012). Multivariate genetic analyses of cognition and academic achievement from two population samples of 174,000 and 166,000 school children. *Behavior Genetics, 42*(5), 699–710. doi:10.1007/s10519-012-9549-7.

Caspi, A., Belsky, D. W., Moffitt, T. E., Houts, R. M., Harrington, H., Hogan, S., ... Poulton, R. (2017). Childhood forecasting of a small segment of the population with large economic burden. *Nature Human Behaviour, 1*(1). doi:10.1038/s41562-016-0005.

Caspi, A., McClay, J., Moffitt, T. E., Mill, J., Martin, J., Craig, I. W., ... Poulton, R. (2002). Role of genotype in the cycle of violence in maltreated children. *Science, 297*(5582), 851–854. doi:10.1126/science.1072290.

Caulfield, T., Harmon, S. H., & Joly, Y. (2012). Open science versus commercialization: A modern research conflict? *Genome Medicine, 4*(2), 17. doi:10.1186/gm316.

Condit, C. M. (2010). Public understandings of genetics and health. *Clinical Genetics, 77*(1), 1–9. doi:10.1111/j.1399-0004.2009.01316.x.

Consolidated Appropriations Act, H.R. 1625, Public Law No. 115–141 (2018).

Cooper, Z. N., Nelson, R. M., & Ross, L. F. (2006). Informed consent for genetic research involving pleiotropic genes: An empirical study of ApoE research. *IRB: Ethics and Human Research, 28*(5), 1–11. Retrieved https://www.jstor.org/stable/30033207.

Davies, G., Marioni, R. E., Liewald, D. C., Hill, W. D., Hagenaars, S. P., Harris, S. E., ... Deary, I. J. (2016). Genome-wide association study of cognitive functions and educational attainment in UK Biobank (N=112 151). *Molecular Psychiatry, 21*(6), 758–767. doi:10.1038/mp.2016.45.

De Vries, R. G., Tomlinson, T., Kim, H. M., Krenz, C., Haggerty, D., Ryan, K. A., & Kim, S. Y. (2016). Understanding the public's reservations about broad consent and study-by-study consent for donations to a biobank: Results of a national survey. *PLoS One, 11*(7), e0159113. doi:10.1371/journal.pone.0159113.

Dick, D., Latendresse, S., & Riley, B. (2011). Incorporating genetics into your studies: A guide for social scientists. *Frontiers in Psychiatry, 2*(17). doi:10.3389/fpsyt.2011.00017/full.

Emanuel, E. J., & Menikoff, J. (2011). Reforming the regulations governing research with human subjects. *The New England Journal of Medicine, 365*(12), 1145–1150. doi:10.1056/NEJMsb1106942.

Fisher, C. B. (2006a). Clinical trials results databases: Unanswered questions. *Science*, *311*(5758), 180–181.

Fisher, C. B. (2006b). Privacy and ethics in pediatric environmental health research: Part I: genetic and prenatal testing. *Environmental Health Perspectives*, *114*(10), 1617–1621. doi:10.1289%2Fehp.9003.

Fisher, C. B. (2015). Enhancing the responsible conduct of sexual health prevention research across global and local contexts: Training for evidence-based research ethics. *Ethics and Behavior*, *25*(2), 87–96. doi:10.1080/10508422.2014.948956.

Fisher, C. B. (2017a). *Decoding the Ethics Code: A Practical Guide for Psychologists* (4th edn). Thoasand Oaks, CA: Sage Publications.

Fisher, C. B. (2017b). Ethical risks and remedies in social behavioral research involving genetic testing. In E. L. G. S. Bourgy, S. R. Latham, & M. Tan (Eds.), *Current Perspectives in Psychology: Education, Ethics, and Genetics*, (pp. 263–283). New York: Cambridge University Press.

Fisher, C. B. (2017c). Rethinking individual and group harms in the age of genomics and big data. *Paper Presented at the Icahn School of Medicine at Mount Sinai IRB Retreat*, New York.

Fisher, C. B., & McCarthy, E. (2013). Ethics in prevention science involving genetic testing. *Prevention Science*, *14*(3), 310–318. doi:10.1007/s11121-012-0318-x.

Fisher, C. B., & Ragsdale, K. (2006). A goodness-of-fit ethic for multicultural research. In J. Trimble, & C. B. Fisher (Eds.), *The Handbook of Ethical Research with Ethnocultural Populations and Communities*, (pp. 3–26). Thousand Oaks, CA: Sage Publications.

Fisher, C. B., & Wallace, S. A. (2000). Through the community looking glass: Re-evaluating the ethical and policy implications of research on adolescent risk and psychopathology. *Ethics and Behavior*, *10*(2), 99–118. doi:10.1207/S15327019EB1002_01.

Fisher, C. B., Brunnquell, D. J., Hughes, D. L., Liben, L. S., Maholmes, V., Plattner, S., ... Susman, E. J. (2013). Preserving and enhancing the responsible conduct of research involving children and youth: A response to proposed changes in federal regulations. *Social Policy Report, Society for Research in Child Development*, *27*(1), 3–15.

Gilmore, R. O. (2016). From big data to deep insight in developmental science. *Wiley Interdisciplinary Reviews: Cognitive Science*, *7*(2), 112–126. doi:10.1002/wcs.1379.

Glenn, A. L., Lochman, J. E., Dishion, T., Powell, N. P., Boxmeyer, C., & Qu, L. (2018). Oxytocin receptor gene variant interacts with intervention delivery format in predicting intervention outcomes for youth with conduct problems. *Prevention Science*, *19*(1), 38–48. doi:10.1007/s11121-017-0777-1.

Grady, C. (2017). Informed consent. *The New England Journal of Medicine*, *376*(20), e43. doi:10.1056/NEJMc1704010.

Grady, C., Eckstein, L., Berkman, B., Brock, D., Cook-Deegan, R., Fullerton, S. M., ... Wendler, D. (2015). Broad consent for research with biological samples: Workshop conclusions. *The American Journal of Bioethics*, *15*(9), 34–42. doi:10.1080/15265161.2015.1062162.

Grandjean, P., & Sorsa, M. (1996). Ethical aspects of genetic predisposition to environmentally-related disease. *The Science of the Total Environment*, *184*(1–2), 37–43. doi:10.1016/0048-9697(95)04986-X.

Greven, C. U., Harlaar, N., Kovas, Y., Chamorro-Premuzic, T., & Plomin, R. (2009). More than just IQ: School achievement is predicted by self-perceived abilities—but for genetic rather than environmental reasons. *Psychological Science*, *20*(6), 753–762. doi:10.1111%2Fj.1467-9280.2009.02366.x.

Hansson, M. G., Lochmüller, H., Riess, O., Schaefer, F., Orth, M., Rubinstein, Y., ... Posada, M. (2016). The risk of re-identification versus the need to identify individuals in rare disease research. *European Journal of Human Genetics*, *24*(11), 1553–1558. doi:10.1038/ejhg.2016.52.

Haworth, C. M. A., & Plomin, R. (2012). Genetics and education: Toward a genetically sensitive classroom. In K. R. Harris, S. Graham, T. Urdan, C. B. McCormick, G. M. Sinatra, J. Sweller, K. R. Harris, S. Graham, T. Urdan, C. B. McCormick, G. M. Sinatra, & J. Sweller (Eds.), *APA Educational Psychology Handbook, Vol 1: Theories, Constructs, and Critical Issues*, (pp. 529–559). Washington, DC: American Psychological Association.

Henderson, G. E. (2008). Introducing social and ethical perspectives on gene: Environment research. *Sociological Methods and Research*, *37*(2), 251–276. doi:10.1177%2F0049124108323536.

Hens, K., Nys, H., Cassiman, J. J., & Dierickx, K. (2011). The storage and use of biological tissue samples from minors for research: A focus group study. *Public Health Genomics*, *14*(2), 68–76. doi:10.1159/000294185.

Homer, N., Szelinger, S., Redman, M., Duggan, D., Tembe, W., Muehling, J., ... Craig, D. W. (2008). Resolving individuals contributing trace amounts of DNA to highly complex mixtures using high-density SNP genotyping microarrays. *PLoS Genetics*, *4*(8), e1000167. doi:10.1371/journal.pgen.1000167.

Jarvik, G. P., Amendola, L. M., Berg, J., Brothers, K., Clayton, E., Chung, W., ... Wolf, W. (2014). Return of genomic results to research participants: The floor, the ceiling, and the choices in between. *American Journal of Human Genetics*, *94*(6), 818–826. doi:10.1016/j.ajhg.2014.04.009.

Kaplan, R. M., Riley, W. T., & Mabry, P. L. (2014). News from the NIH: Leveraging big data in the behavioral sciences. *Translational Behavioral Medicine*, *4*(3), 229–231. doi:10.1007/s13142-014-0267-y.

Kaufman, D. J., Baker, R., Milner, L. C., Devaney, S., & Hudson, K. L. (2016). A survey of U.S adults' opinions about conduct of a nationwide Precision Medicine Initiative® cohort study of genes and environment. *PLoS One*, *11*(8), e0160461. doi:10.1371/journal.pone.0160461.

Kaufman, D., Geller, G., Leroy, L., Murphy, J., Scott, J., & Hudson, K. (2008). Ethical implications of including children in a large biobank for genetic-epidemiologic research: A qualitative study of public opinion. *American Journal of Medical Genetics Part C: Seminars in Medical Genetics*, 148C(1), 31–39. Hoboken, NJ: Wiley Subscription Services, Inc., A Wiley Company. doi:10.1002/ajmg.c.30159.

Kegel, C. A., Bus, A. G., & van IJzendoorn, M. H. (2011). Differential susceptibility in early literacy instruction through computer games: The role of the dopamine D4 receptor gene (DRD4). *Mind, Brain, and Education*, *5*(2), 71–78. doi:10.1111/j.1751-228X.2011.01112.x.

Klitzman, R. L. (2013). How IRBs view and make decisions about consent forms. *Journal of Empirical Research on Human Research Ethics*, *8*(1), 8–19. doi:10.1525/jer.2013.8.1.8.

Kong, C. C., Tarling, T. E., Strahlendorf, C., Dittrick, M., & Vercauteren, S. M. (2016). Opinions of adolescents and parents about pediatric biobanking. *Journal of Adolescent Health*, *58*(4), 474–480. doi:10.1016/j.jadohealth.2015.12.015.

Krapohl, E., Rimfeld, K., Shakeshaft, N. G., Trzaskowski, M., McMillan, A., Pingault, J. B., ... Dale, P. S. (2014). The high heritability of educational achievement reflects many genetically influenced traits, not just intelligence. *Proceedings of the National Academy of Sciences*, *111*(42), 15273–15278. doi:10.1073/pnas.1408777111.

Leadbeater, B. J., Dishion, T., Sandler, I., Bradshaw, C. P., Dodge, K., Gottfredson, D., ... Smith, E. P. (2018). Ethical challenges in promoting the implementation of preventive interventions: Report of the SPR task force. *Prevention Science*. doi:10.1007/s11121-018-0912-7.

Lemke, A. A., Wolf, W. A., Hebert-Beirne, J., & Smith, M. E. (2010). Public and biobank participant attitudes toward genetic research participation and data sharing. *Public Health Genomics*, *13*(6), 368–377. doi:10.1159/000276767.

Lunshof, J. E., Chadwick, R., Vorhaus, D. B., & Church, G. M. (2008). From genetic privacy to open consent. *Nature Reviews Genetics*, *9*(5), 406–411. doi:10.1038/nrg2360.

MacQueen, K. M., & Alleman, P. (2008). International perspectives on the collection, storage, and testing of human biospecimens in HIV research. *IRB*, *30*(4), 9–14. Retrieved from https://www.ncbi.nlm.nih.gov/pmc/articles/PMC4413897/.

Malin, B., & Sweeney, L. (2001). Re-identification of DNA through an automated linkage process. *Proceedings, Journal of the American Medical Informatics Association*, 423–427. Retrieved from http://www.cs.cmu.edu/~malin/papers/reid_AMIA.pdf.

Mandelli, L., & Serretti, A. (2013). Gene environment interaction studies in depression and suicidal behavior: An update. *Neuroscience and Biobehavioral Reviews*, *37*(10), 2375–2397. doi:10.1016/j.neubiorev.2013.07.011.

McCrory, E., De Brito, S. A., & Viding, E. (2010). Research review: The neurobiology and genetics of maltreatment and adversity. *Journal of Child Psychology and Psychiatry*, *51*(10), 1079–1095. doi:10.1111/j.1469-7610.2010.02271.x.

McGuire, A. L., Hamilton, J. A., Lunstroth, R., McCullough, L. B., & Goldman, A. (2008). DNA data sharing: Research participants' perspectives. *Genetic Medicine*, *10*(1), 46–53. doi:10.1097/GIM.0b013e31815f1e00.

McGuire, A. L., Oliver, J. M., Slashinski, M. J., Graves, J. L., Wang, T., Kelly, P. A., … Hilsenbeck, S. G. (2011). To share or not to share: A randomized trial of consent for data sharing in genome research. *Genetic Medicine*, *13*(11), 948–955. doi:10.1097/GIM.0b013e3182227589.

Menikoff, J., Kaneshiro, J., & Pritchard, I. (2017). The common rule, updated. *New England Journal of Medicine*, *376*(7), 613–615.

Musci, R. J., & Schlomer, G. (2018). The Implications of genetics for prevention and intervention programming. *Prevention Science*, *19*(1), 1–5. doi:10.1007/s11121-017-0837-6, doi: 10.1056/NEJMp1700736.

Office for Human Research Protections (OHRP). (2017). Federal Register Federal Policy for the Protection of Human Subjects. Retrieved from https://www.gpo.gov/fdsys/pkg/FR-2017-01-19/html/2017-01058.htm.

Oliver, J. M., Slashinski, M. J., Wang, T., Kelly, P. A., Hilsenbeck, S. G., & McGuire, A. L. (2012). Balancing the risks and benefits of genomic data sharing: Genome research participants' perspectives. *Public Health Genomics*, *15*(2), 106–114. doi:10.1159/000334718.

Pearson, C. R., Parker, M., Fisher, C. B., & Moreno, C. (2014). Capacity building from the inside out: Development and evaluation of a CITI ethics certification training module for American Indian and Alaska Native community researchers. *Journal of Empirical Research on Human Research Ethics*, *9*(1), 46–57. doi:10.1525/jer.2014.9.1.4.

Perlman, S., & Fantuzzo, J. W. (2013). Predicting risk of placement: A population-based study of out-of-home placement, child maltreatment, and emergency housing. *Journal of the Society for Social Work and Research*, *4*(2), 99–113. doi:10.5243/jsswr.2013.7.

Ravitsky, V., & Wilfond, B. S. (2006). Disclosing individual genetic results to research participants. *IRB: Ethics and Human Research*, *29*(3), 10.

Rimfeld, K., Kovas, Y., Dale, P. S., & Plomin, R. (2015). Pleiotropy across academic subjects at the end of compulsory education. *Scientific Reports*, *5*(11713), 1–11. doi:10.1038/srep11713.

Russell, M. A., Schlomer, G. L., Cleveland, H. H., Feinberg, M. E., Greenberg, M. T., Vandenbergh, D. J., … Redmond, C. (2017). PROSPER intervention effects on adolescents' alcohol misuse vary by GABRA2 genotype and age. *Prevention Science*, *19*(1), 27–37. doi:10.1007/s11121-017-0751-y.

Sahota, P. C. (2014). Body fragmentation: Native American community members' views on specimen disposition in biomedical/genetics research. *American Journal of Bioethics: Empirical Bioethics*, *5*(3), 19–30. doi:10.1080/23294515.2014.896833.

Society for Research in Child Development (SRCD). (July 21, 2018). Member Resource on NIH Clinical Trials. Retrieved from https://www.srcd.org/membership/member-resource-nih-clinical-trials.

Sreenivasan, G. (2003). Does informed consent to research require comprehension? *Lancet*, *362*(9400), 2016–2018. doi:10.1016/S0140-6736(03)15025-8.

Storr, C. L., Or, F., Eaton, W. W., & Ialongo, N. (2014). Genetic research participation in a young adult community sample. *Journal of Community Genetics*, *5*(4), 363–375. doi:10.1007/s12687-014-0191-3.

Strauss, D. (2017). Changes to the Common Rule: Implications for Informed Consent. *Paper Presented at the Fordham University HIV and Drug Abuse Prevention Ethics Training Program*, Bronx, New York. Retrieved from https://www.fordham.edu/downloads/file/8959/changes_to_the_common_rule_implications_for_informed_consent.

Sugarman, J. (2017). Examining provisions related to consent in the revised common rule. *American Journal of Bioethics*, *17*(7), 22–26. doi:10.1080/15265161.2017.1329483.

Tam, N. T., Nguyen, T. H., Le Thi, B. T., Nguyen, P. L., Nguyen, T. H. T., Kenji, H., & Juntra, K. (2015). Participants' understanding of informed consent in clinical trials over three decades: Systematic review and meta-analysis. *Bulletin of the World Health Organization*, *93*(3), 186–198H. doi:10.2471/BLT.14.141390.

U.S. Department of Health and Human Services. (2012). Guidance Regarding Methods for De-identification of Protected Health Information in Accordance with the Health Insurance Portability and Accountability Act (HIPAA) Privacy Rule. Retrieved from https://www.hhs.gov/sites/default/files/ocr/privacy/hipaa/understanding/coveredentities/De-identification/hhs_deid_guidance.pdf.

University of Southern California. (August 17, 2012). University of Southern California (USC) Policy: Biorepositories. Retrieved from https://policy.usc.edu/biorepositories/.

Wertz, J., Caspi, A., Belsky, D., Beckley, A., Arseneault, L., Barnes, J., ... Morgan, N. (2018). Genetics and crime: Integrating new genomic discoveries into psychological research about antisocial behavior. *Psychological Science*, *29(5)*, 791–803. doi:10.1177/0956797617744542.

Zheng, Y., Albert, D., McMahon, R. J., Dodge, K., Dick, D., & Conduct Problems Prevention Research. (2018). Glucocorticoid Receptor (NR3C1) gene polymorphism moderate intervention effects on the developmental trajectory of African-American adolescent alcohol abuse. *Prevention Science*, *19*(1), 79–89. doi:10.1007/s11121-016-0726-4.

Index

Note: **Bold** page numbers refer to tables; *italic* page numbers refer to figures.

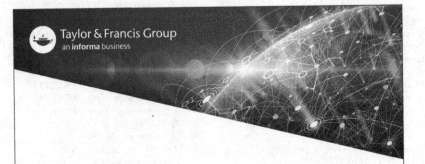

Printed in the United States
by Baker & Taylor Publisher Services